Communication in
Interprofessional Care:
Theory and Applications

NOTICE

The authors and publisher have made every effort to ensure the accuracy and completeness of the information presented in this book. However, the authors and publisher cannot be held responsible for the continued currency of the information, any inadvertent errors or omissions, or the application of this information. Therefore, the authors and publisher shall have no liability to any person or entity with regard to claims, loss, or damage caused or alleged to be caused, directly or indirectly, by the use of information contained herein.

Communication in Interprofessional Care:
Theory and Applications

Zubin Austin, PhD, FCAHS
Professor and Murray Koffler Chair in Management
Leslie Dan Faculty of Pharmacy and the Institute for Health Policy,
Management, and Evaluation–Faculty of Medicine
University of Toronto, Canada

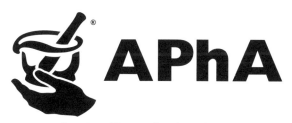

American Pharmacists Association
Washington, D.C.

Senior Director, Books and Digital Publishing: John Fedor
Director, Content Development: Janan Sarwar, PharmD
Acquisitions Editor: Janan Sarwar
Editorial Services: Absolute Service, Inc.
Cover Design: Scott Neitzke APhA Integrated Design and Production
Illustrations and Mind Maps: Diana Tabak

©2020 by the American Pharmacists Association
APhA was founded in 1852 as the American Pharmaceutical Association.

Published by the American Pharmacists Association
2215 Constitution Avenue, NW
Washington, DC 20037-2985
www.pharmacist.com
www.pharmacylibrary.com

Library of Congress Cataloging-in-Publication Data

Names: Austin, Zubin, author. | American Pharmacists Association,
    publisher.
Title: Communication in interprofessional care : theory and applications /
    Zubin Austin.
Description: Washington, D.C. : APhA, American Pharmacists Association,
    [2020] | Includes bibliographical references. | Summary: "Day-to-day
    clinical practice in the health and care professions is filled with
    challenging situations rooted in interpersonal psychology. Beyond their
    technical and profession-specific knowledge and skills, clinical
    practitioners must have extraordinary communication and observation
    skills to manage the complexities of their daily work. This can be
    particularly challenging for individuals educated within one profession
    when they are working within interprofessional teams where
    collaboration, consensus, and cooperative decision making are expected.
    Communication in Interprofessional Care: Theory and Applications
    approaches this important topic with a new perspective, supporting
    learners and teachers through practical application of psychological and
    communication theory. KEY FEATURES: Contains 14 real-world clinical
    cases and vignettes; Explains the role of motivation, trait, and
    social-psychological context in influencing behaviors; Uses theory to
    provide practical guidance around interpersonal communication; A model
    for understanding the psychology of empathy; Uses personal emotional
    intelligence as a tool for enhancing quality of interpersonal and
    interprofessional communication"-- Provided by publisher.
Identifiers: LCCN 2020025224 (print) | LCCN 2020025225 (ebook) | ISBN
    9781582123431 (paperback) | ISBN 9781582123448 (epub)
Subjects: MESH: Communication | Interpersonal Relations | Patient-Centered
    Care
Classification: LCC R727.3 (print) | LCC R727.3 (ebook) | NLM W 62 | DDC
    610.69/6--dc23
LC record available at https://lccn.loc.gov/2020025224
LC ebook record available at https://lccn.loc.gov/2020025225

How to Order This Book
Online: www.pharmacist.com/shop
By phone: 800-878-0729 (770-280-0085 from outside the United States)
VISA®, MasterCard®, and American Express® cards accepted.

Table of Contents

Preface

Taking care of patients is both a tremendous responsibility and an incredible privilege. Health care professionals have unique opportunities to work with, support, and help individuals at some of the most important times of their lives. The experience of being trusted, relied upon, and having others invest their confidence in your knowledge, skills, and expertise makes health care work meaningful and rewarding.

We owe it to those for whom we care to ensure we are practicing our professions to the best of our abilities. Not only do we need to fully engage and remain focused, we also need to find innovative ways of working better together. Interprofessional person-centered care has emerged as a central organizing paradigm for enhancing the quality of care and the impact of what we do. Central to interprofessional practice is the need to communicate effectively.

Communication is the common clinical skill shared by all health care professionals. We communicate through observation, listening, responding, speaking, hearing, gesturing, and simply being present. While each profession has its own unique and important technical and scientific knowledge base, this information is trapped without an effective vehicle for sharing it with patients and colleagues.

Communication in Interprofessional Care: Theory and Applications was written to provide health care professionals at all stages of their career with opportunities to enhance the quality and impact of their patient-focused practice and in the process amplify their own professional satisfaction. As the title suggests, the book is divided into two sections. The theory section is designed to help readers understand the science and art of communication. Learning and understanding theory provides a lifelong foundation for personal and professional development, as circumstances and requirements evolve with time. Rather than simply tell you how to communicate in specific situations, an understanding of communication theory can help you to better develop natural, authentic responses that are suited to your personality, temperament, and specific situation. Communication theory also provides you with a vocabulary to think about, analyze, and discuss complex interpersonal situations in a more systematic way. Theory for this section draws upon diverse literature in the social sciences, including personality psychology, social psychology, sociology, cognitive science, and anthropology.

The applications section is based around a series of real-world situations that I or my colleagues in practice have experienced. These situations range from touching to tragic to terrifying, and they are all in a day's work for any health care professional. It is tempting to hope that the case studies in the applications section can provide easy answers and perfect outcomes to complex human interactions; of course, this is not the case. Instead, this section provides you with opportunities to reflect on the Theory section, think about your own strengths and challenges as a communicator, then imagine "what-if" scenarios of alternative approaches to dealing with difficult situations.

I have been a researcher for 20 years, an educator for 25 years, a pharmacist for 30 years, and a human being for several more years than that. Regardless of the role we play or the job we hold, interacting with other human beings is one of the most difficult, important, rewarding, frustrating, and essential things we do in our day-to-day lives. Although communication is the focus of much of my teaching, research, and practice, I have learned so much writing this book and am so appreciative of the opportunity to share this with you. Interpersonal communication is a lifelong journey. I hope this book will be one small but helpful step on your pathway.

Acknowledgments

For the great communicators I have known and who have shaped me:

For Doris, my teacher who inspired my interest

For Emily, my preceptor who was my first role model

For Chris, my first boss who showed me how it was done

For Lesley, my colleague who shepherded my academic career

For Scott, my living laboratory for theory and application

For Diana, the most amazing communicator I will ever meet

1 | Interprofessional Person-Centered Care

Health care systems are transforming at an unprecedented rate. Heightened public expectations, increased scrutiny by government and payers, calls for accountability by patient advocacy groups, and the need for cost-containment or cost-justification all point to the necessity for health care workers—as professionals and as individuals—to leverage their knowledge and skills in new and more effective ways.

At the center of these changes are patients and their caregivers who are struggling as never before to cope with life-changing diagnoses, manage complex medication regimens, deal with difficult or unclear diagnoses, and optimize their health and quality of life. These patients and their families and communities need to know they can rely on a team of health care professionals who will work effectively together and have their best interests at heart. Those who provide care to patients—whether they prefer the label provider, practitioner, clinician, or professional—have both a tremendous responsibility, and opportunity, to help people live better and healthier lives.

How can health care professionals do better? How can we as individual practitioners help patients live better lives? The need for our health care systems as a whole to elevate the quality of patient care is clear: The pathway forward for each of us as individual practitioners will be different.

1.1 People and Their Care Providers

As scientifically educated and clinically trained individuals, health care professionals possess a wealth of knowledge and facts about health, wellness, illness, and treatment options. Knowing facts and accurately recalling details does not automatically translate into better patient care and a healthy and happy outcome. At the center of each care provider's practice is the unique and important relationship between the practitioner and the patient that allows knowledge to become mobilized, skill to be applied, and ultimately, effective care to be provided.

1.1.1   Communication: Our Core Clinical Skill

All health care professionals share the same common core clinical skill: We translate our professional and scientific knowledge into action and theory into patient care through good communication. We observe, we listen, we watch, we speak, and we respond. This is the way in which scientific and clinical knowledge is applied in order to help patients and their caregivers. We also document (or write), read, and communicate using social media and other Web-based methods.

Communication is more than simple literacy. Communication is a complex and nuanced dynamic between two people that relies on thinking, noticing, emotions, checking-in, and a variety of other dynamics.

1.1.2   What Is Communication?

There are many different ways of defining communication; in most cases it is described as **a reciprocal dynamic between receivers and senders involving verbal and nonverbal cues**. Let's examine what that means for you as a health care provider—and as a human being—in closer detail.

Reciprocal: Communication is a two-way interaction, with each person in a conversation giving and taking, or transmitting and receiving. Even when one person may appear quiet (i.e., not saying anything), they may still be communicating through their body language, their eye contact, or their facial expressions.

Dynamic: Communication is not a static event but a process that evolves moment to moment. Partners in a conversation are constantly changing roles (e.g., one person speaks, one person listens), the rules or tone governing a conversation can change almost instantly (e.g., when someone raises an eyebrow or grimaces), and it requires both partners to constantly be interpreting what the other is saying and not saying.

Receivers: At any time in a conversation, both partners are receiving information from one another, and having to interpret and understand its meaning. Sometimes this information can involve spoken words; at other times, it can involve behaviors (called *nonverbals* because no words are used) such as eye contact, body stance, hand gestures, or facial expressions.

Senders: At any time in a conversation, both partners are sending information to one another. Sometimes, a partner may be consciously aware of the information they are sending (e.g., when we carefully select our words or a gesture). Other times, a partner may not be aware of the unconscious verbal or nonverbal information that is being sent (e.g., when an inadvertent or accidental smile crops up, or when we do a double take in response to something startling).

Verbal Cues: The words and sentences we select when we speak are an important part of communication. They are, however, only one component of what we communicate. Words and word choice are of course significant—think of the difference when someone gives you a *reason* as opposed to an *excuse*. Selecting the correct word can make all the difference between a tense standoff and an amicable conversation, but communication is about much more than simply word choices.

Nonverbal Cues: When we communicate (as opposed to just talk), we are simultaneously sending and receiving both verbal and nonverbal cues. Nonverbal cues are all the forms of communication that do not involve words, everything from the way we carry ourselves, to the distance we leave between each other while speaking, to the facial gestures we use, to the eye contact we maintain, and the unconscious tics and movements we make in response to what we are seeing and hearing from the other person.

1.1.3   Communication Is Complicated

Communication can be challenging to manage and control, but it is only the first step in what a health care professional needs in order to truly elevate patient care. Communication is the primary vehicle by which we as professionals interact with patients and we as human beings interact with our friends, our family, and our social networks. It is the patient's first insight into who we are as professionals and as human beings. Our first impressions of others are generally made through verbal and nonverbal communication, and over time, our second, third, and fourth impressions are shaped by subsequent communication until we build a picture of one another that helps us guide future interactions.

Repeated, positive communication experiences between individuals can eventually build rapport. Rapport develops between individuals when they start to anticipate and look forward to future interactions with one another, and can reasonably expect such interactions to be positive and mutually beneficial. Rapport is an essential feature of human existence: It forms the foundation for the social interaction we all need in order to thrive as people. Rapport cannot be established instantly. It takes time, repeated exposure, and predictable positive experiences.

We all know the experience of rapport with others: There is an easiness to a conversation, a series of communication shortcuts that evolve that are unique to the pair as they get to know each other, and a genuine sense of comfort. A key feature of rapport is often a shared sense of humor or a common understanding of the rest of the world. Rapport is sometimes described as a connection between two people that allows them to move from formal to informal communication patterns that are more efficient, more effortless, and ultimately more rewarding for both.

1.1.4   Rapport: The Foundation of Trust

As rapport between individuals evolves and matures, a new and important subjective, emotional feeling will often occur between people: trust. Trust is one of the most important and essential attributes of human interaction. In most cases, trust is built over time and testing. As communication grows into rapport, trust may (or may not) emerge as the reliability of each partner in a dynamic is tested. Trust requires not only time to build but testing to confirm it. Difficult situations or conversations are among the most frequent ways in which trust is tested, confirmed, and amplified over time.

As health care professionals, it is sometimes tempting to assume that everyone immediately and automatically trusts what we say simply because we ARE health care professionals and therefore should deserve trust from others. Although a degree, a professional title, or a lab coat are considered external symbols of someone who is trustworthy, for many people, the reality is that the emotional feeling of "trusting" someone requires time and testing to truly occur. Trust is not earned by simply not telling lies: It involves a genuine belief by the patient that the health care professional truly has his or her best interests at heart.

Trust cannot be built overnight. It is not built when we are distracted by phone calls or other patients. Trust does not evolve when all we do is ask yes-or-no questions, or hand a patient a leaflet with how-to directions on it. Trust evolves when we prove to patients that we really are genuinely interested in them and their health, and that we are willing to take the time and provide the attention needed to prove it.

1.1.5   From Trust Comes Empathy

As relationships between patients and health care professionals evolve, the trust that is earned may further develop into empathy. Empathy is an invisible, almost chemical, connection between individuals who have proven themselves to one another in a way that no longer requires ongoing testing. Empathy is both a way of describing a highly evolved interaction between individuals and a concrete communication technique signaled by appropriate and well-timed verbal and nonverbal responses to what another person is saying. When empathy between individuals actually occurs, it provides both parties with a sense of comfort, confidence, and security.

Why does empathy matter so much in health care settings? It is sometimes said that patients will only care about what you say if they know you care about what they feel. If we are genuinely interested in helping patients with their health-related needs, then they will be genuinely interested in our suggestions, our advice, and what we say. Simply telling or lecturing a patient isn't helpful. They may smile and nod and politely agree, but in the absence of empathy, or trust, or rapport, or true communication, is it realistic to believe patients will take us seriously, actually listen to us, and follow our good advice? When patients feel empathy with their health care professional, they are in a primed emotional state. They are more attuned and more interested in what we say because they have an emotional investment in our professional relationship. With empathy, both patients and health care providers hear more, listen more attentively, can recall more details, and are more likely to understand what was said. Without empathy, it can be in one ear and out the other.

1.1.6   Communication to Rapport to Trust to Empathy and, Eventually, Care

It is sometimes tempting to believe that care can be reduced to a simple formula or a series of steps. This chapter has provided a model for how empathy develops through a series of stages beginning with effective communication leading to rapport resulting in trust. Although this model can be helpful in highlighting the time and effort required to actually build the high-quality relationships with practitioners and patients that result in the best health care outcomes, it is a mistake to believe it is a straightforward and linear sequence that only progresses in one direction.

As you will know from your personal experience, all human interactions and relationships are complex and sometimes rise and fall and advance and retreat in seemingly unpredictable and random ways. Sometimes, despite doing everything right, empathy may never truly develop between individuals for reasons that cannot be clearly identified.

If such unpredictability is an essential feature of all human relationships, including patient–practitioner interactions, why should we bother studying them and trying to learn how to improve them? Health care professionals study communication and applied psychology because, although it may not be the only thing that matters in good quality health care, it is clearly necessary and irreplaceable. The experience of caring for another person, or being cared for by another person, is emotionally complicated and does not proceed in a straight-line fashion. Instead, it is built gradually over time through literally thousands of small gestures, words, glances, smiles, laughs, and tears. Simply telling someone "I am your health care professional" does not translate into emotional acceptance by that person of your role.

Remember that when people require health care professionals, they may be very vulnerable, confused, sad, and anxious. The experience of receiving a surprising and negative diagnosis, hearing bad news about a loved one, being asked to change a pattern of behavior that has been a feature of daily life for decades, or discussing uncomfortable and intimate personal details with a relative stranger is difficult. For patients to feel truly comfortable, truly open, and truly safe to disclose their emotions and feelings, they need to experience the continuum of positive communication, rapport, trust, and ultimately, empathy and care. If any of this is missing, or if the foundation of the practitioner–patient relationship has not had sufficient time to ripen and blossom, patients will withhold, lie, or attempt to save face rather than tell you what's truly important, and ultimately, they may simply ignore, forget, or overlook the good advice you provide.

A caring relationship between practitioner and patient cannot develop instantaneously; it is not automatically conferred as soon as you point out your diploma or license on an office wall and say, "See, I'm really smart and graduated from a tough program, so you really should trust me and do as I say."

1.1.7 You Knew All of This Already Because You're a Person Too

In the education and clinical training of health care practitioners, a great deal of time is spent encouraging students to be professional and to check their personal feelings at the door before coming into the clinic. Of course, there is good reason for this: Personal bias must be carefully managed to ensure it does not interfere with the provision of care.

However, at times, it is particularly useful for professionals to remind themselves of the personal. As you reflect on the model presented in this chapter of effective communication leading to rapport which establishes trust necessary to support empathy and, ultimately, care, think about experiences in your own life with teachers, coaches, music instructors, friends, and relatives. Think about what has worked for you, and what hasn't worked for you, in helping to build strong, caring relationships with others in your personal life. Your personal reflections on these experiences can help you articulate some of your foundational strengths in establishing, building, maintaining, and growing the kinds of relationships that are necessary to provide the best possible patient care. Thinking about situations where a relationship has not succeeded, and what you and the other person may have done or avoided doing that resulted in the relationship not succeeding, can provide you with important personal clues as to where your strengths and areas for personal growth may be in communication. Such reflection may feel unnatural or forced to you, or it may provoke discomfort and a strong negative emotional response. However, as human beings, we must constantly reflect on our interactions with others to continuously nurture them, learn from our previous mistakes, and grow in a positive direction. As health care professionals, such reflection is even more crucial if we are to understand how we can be more effective, more satisfied, and ultimately, more impactful for our patients.

1.2   Interprofessional Care

There is general agreement that team-based models of care provide much better outcomes for patients and result in better, higher quality decision making. Interprofessional practice is now the standard and most widely used model of care delivery across all health care systems.

1.2.1   What Is Interprofessional Practice?

Within any health care system, there will be a large number of health care providers, each of whom will have different roles, responsibilities, strengths, limitations, educational preparation, knowledge, and skills. The reality of modern health care work is that no one person or professional actually has the intellectual capacity, time, or expertise to manage all aspects of a patient's health care needs effectively and efficiently.

Interprofessional practice is frequently described as a situation where providers from two or more different professions provide care to the same patient and collaborate with one another in a complementary way. There are many different models for interprofessional practice, but all of them require clear and efficient communication between and among health care team members and the patient in order to ensure safe and effective health care delivery and optimal outcomes.

Interprofessional practice requires trust. Each individual care provider must trust the work, the skills, and the professionalism of the other members of the team. Importantly, the same mechanisms that underlie the development of trust between patients and health care providers are necessary when building trusting relationships between team members. Effective communication builds rapport, which in turn generates trust, and which ultimately can build to empathy.

1.2.2   Who Are These Interprofessionals?

Traditionally, health care practitioners are educated in profession-specific silos: Future pharmacists go to pharmacy schools, those wishing to become nurses attend nursing college, and students wanting to become physicians go to medical programs. This is of course important: Each profession has its own unique and important foundation of scientific and clinical knowledge and skills that must be acquired by students before they can actually practice that profession safely and effectively. Profession-specific education is also important developmentally. It helps to socialize younger members of a profession into the culture of the field, to learn some of the secrets of the trade, and to learn the ways of performing and successfully navigating a complex, profession-specific world.

Despite the necessity of profession-specific education, there may be unintended consequences to this model of clinical teaching and learning. Profession-specific education can sometimes result in the formation of tribes, a psychological sense of us versus them with respect to our future colleagues. We may not adequately understand or respect the knowledge, skills, and talents of other professionals simply because we haven't been sufficiently exposed to all they have learned and experienced in their programs. We may instead fall prey to easy stereotypes about certain professions based on nothing more than what we see on our screens or what we have heard over the years from uninformed chatter by others.

Perhaps most importantly, a significant limitation of profession-specific education is that it does not adequately equip us for the reality of day-to-day work out in the field. Virtually every health care system today functions interprofessionally specifically because health care is too complicated for one person alone to manage all aspects of it safely and effectively. Health care teams are the central organizing principle of most systems today; however, the word *team* may be broadly applied. In some cases, interprofessional teams work together side by side on a daily basis, seeing each other's faces, handing each other documents, and taking coffee breaks at the same time. In other systems, interprofessional teams may only virtually meet using video or phone conversations. In yet other systems, teams never connect all together at any one time; instead, one person communicates with another who passes on information to a third professional to communicate to a fourth person. Recognizing that interprofessional teams can have very different styles, structures, and workflows can sometimes make it challenging to actually recognize when one is working in a team environment or not. Across any kind of health care team—regardless of structure or style—will be a group of caring and committed professionals with diverse backgrounds, education, and skills.

1.2.2.1   *The Professionals on a Team*

Every team will be different, but every health care team is composed of two or more practitioners committed to providing care to patients. The term *health care professional* or *practitioner* may mean different things in different geographical jurisdictions. In most cases, these individuals will be regulated or licensed by an administrative or governmental body. A key feature of health care work today is the need for objective oversight and control of the work of professionals to ensure it conforms to standards and expectations of society. Health care teams most typically will be composed of such regulated health care professionals.

Regulation of health professionals' work is a process for establishing standards and ensuring quality, safety, and effectiveness of the care provided by these individuals. Depending on the geographical jurisdiction, regulators may have different titles or labels. In the United States, most regulators of health professionals are referred to as *boards*; for example, the Federation of State Medical Boards (FSMB) is a group representing all the individual state medical boards in the United States that govern and oversee the practice of medicine across the country. Although each state may have its own state-specific board with state-specific practices, the FSMB provides continuity across the country and standardization to help ensure that the quality and safety of medical practice is more or less similar regardless of where within the United States a patient happens to be. In Canada, most regulators of health professionals are called *colleges*; for example, the College of Physiotherapists of Ontario is not an educational institution but instead a regulatory body that governs the practice of physiotherapists in Canada's largest province. This terminology can be confusing because, in some cases, individuals may receive their education from a college as well. In the United Kingdom, regulators of health professionals are called *councils*; for example, the General Pharmaceutical Council (GPhC) regulates the practice and profession of pharmacists and does so by not only requiring pharmacists to undertake annual continuous professional development activities to maintain their competency but also by inspecting individual pharmacies to ensure they are clean, have the appropriate and required equipment, and do not store or sell expired or substandard medications to the public.

Regardless of naming, boards (or colleges or councils) have an important role to play in determining what educational and training requirements exist before people are licensed (or registered) to practice their profession and what continuous professional development expectations exist to ensure each and every practitioner maintains their competence in their field in the decades after graduation. This highly developed and rigorous system of professional oversight is meant to ensure public protection and provide reassurance to all stakeholders that those who practice a profession are indeed safe and qualified to do so.

Importantly, this structure of professional regulation may mean that in some states, provinces, or countries, some individuals are regulated and some are not; for example, in many parts of Canada, homeopathy is a regulated health profession, whereas in some parts of the United States, it is not regulated and therefore perhaps not recognized within a health system as a member of the health care team. In the United Kingdom, the profession of midwifery is highly regulated, independent, and highly esteemed and has been an established part of the British birthing system for generations. In some parts of the United States, midwifery is not recognized or regulated, or it may be considered subordinate to obstetricians.

For historical, safety, and liability reasons, health care teams have traditionally been composed of regulated health care professionals. Increasingly, and because of a lack of consistency and uniformity across different geographical jurisdictions, health care teams may be composed of both regulated and unregulated health care providers who have different skills and knowledge to contribute to the care of a patient. In your own geographical jurisdiction and health system, it will be important to familiarize yourself with the specific and unique nuances of health care personnel regulation.

Reflect on the following list of health care providers. In your geographical jurisdiction and health system, which of the following would be considered regulated? What might be the implications for patient care for unregulated health care providers?

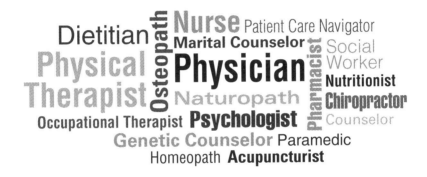

1.2.3 How Does Interprofessional Practice Work?

At its best, interprofessional practice works by focusing on the unique and specific needs of each individual patient. For example, a patient who is recovering from a sports-related knee reconstructive surgery may have a team consisting of a surgeon (to monitor and manage postoperative surgical complications), a nurse (to provide self-care education to the patient and to manage and monitor the healing of surgical incisions), a physical therapist (to provide support for muscle and joint mobilization that will enhance recovery and postoperative functioning), an occupational therapist (to help prepare a patient for discharge home following the procedure, to prepare the patient to navigate the home environment, and to take care of activities of daily living outside of a hospital or institution). If the patient is also receiving medications (e.g., pain-control drugs to manage postoperative pain), a pharmacist may or may not be required for the team. If the patient is not taking medications but instead is managing pain through use of acupuncture, massage, or complementary/alternative medicines, other kinds of professionals (regulated or not) may be important members of that patient's care team. Alternatively, in some cases, the pharmacist may be a central member of a patient's care team. Conditions such as diabetes or post–cardiac arrest care can be incredibly medication intensive, in which case the team may involve a family physician, the pharmacist, and a nutritionist. Not every interprofessional team necessarily requires every single possible health professional to be involved; the specific needs, preferences, and requirements of the patient should determine who is involved in the team and the level of care provided.

1.2.3.1 Scope of Practice

An important concept in interprofessional practice to help better understand the structure and functioning of teams is *scope of practice*. Scope of practice refers to the specific jobs, tasks, and responsibilities that each interprofessional team member is expected to safely perform. Scope is usually based on the nature and level of education and clinical training received prior to becoming licensed or registered and working, and it is also connected to legal expectations about what some professionals are allowed to do in a specific geographic jurisdiction. For example, in most jurisdictions around the world, the scope of practice for physicians will typically involve prescribing medications. In many parts of the United States, pharmacists (as well as some types of nurses) may be legally allowed to independently (i.e., without authorization of or supervision by a physician) prescribe certain medications. In Canada and the United Kingdom, pharmacists are legally allowed to independently extend (i.e., renew) and adapt (i.e., change or modify) prescriptions written by physicians in order to better achieve health outcomes for patients. In most health systems at the current time, scopes of practice are evolving and changing rapidly, and it is essential that all members of a health care team are constantly keeping up to date as to what each profession is authorized and expected to do within a specific system and jurisdiction. This can be particularly complicated because health care professionals may move frequently in their career. They may go to school in one place, undertake postgraduate training in another place, get a first job in a third city, and ultimately settle down in a fourth jurisdiction. Each of these jurisdictions will have different scopes of practice for different practitioners, and this can cause confusion unless each member of the health care team takes the time to truly learn and understand everyone else's scope of practice rather than assuming it is the same everywhere you go.

1.2.3.2 Scope of Practice and Delegation

Scope of practice can be further complicated by the use of delegation protocols and authorizations. In many health care systems, many professionals working in teams come to trust and rely on one another in unique ways. In busy and complex practices, where practitioners have worked closely with one another for many years, there is a strong incentive and need to try to enhance the efficiency of care delivery to benefit both patients and the professionals themselves. For example, certain medications (such as lithium [most often used for mental health conditions], or warfarin [most often used as an anticoagulant to control the thickness of blood], or phenytoin [most often used to manage or control seizure disorders]) have known but manageable side effects and toxicities that are best managed through careful monitoring of the blood concentration of the drug. This means patients on such medications must have routine blood tests that measure the concentration of the medication in the blood stream; once this is known, the dose can be titrated (i.e., adjusted upward or downward) to try to achieve the most appropriate target concentration for safety and efficacy. This process can be time consuming and laborious but is essential for optimizing use of these medications and preventing toxicities. In many jurisdictions, this is legally the job (i.e., scope of practice) of physicians. The time required to do such monitoring and titration can be significant; in jurisdictions where pharmacists are not legally allowed to independently modify or adapt prescription drug doses, a physician can authorize—through a delegation protocol—the pharmacist to perform this important task on his or her behalf without direct supervision or sign-off each time a dose is adjusted based on a blood concentration level. This type of delegation protocol recognizes the education and expertise of pharmacists in general, and the particular experience and judgment of the individual pharmacist to whom the delegation protocol has been issued. It is a legal document in which liability and responsibility are carefully spelled out, but one that allows a pharmacist to transcend a traditional scope of practice limitation in the name of providing better and more efficient, cost-effective patient care.

Beyond a legal document, of course, effective communication between practitioners and within a health care team is essential to ensure success of a delegation protocol. Patients may not understand why one practitioner is now doing something another practitioner used to do, and this misunderstanding can become upsetting or alarming without effective communication and clarification. Similarly, other health care professionals who are not aware of a specific delegation protocol may not understand new and evolving roles and responsibilities. Clear and effective communication is necessary to prevent these misunderstandings that could compromise patient care.

When used appropriately and accompanied by effective communication to prevent misunderstanding, delegation protocols can be an important tool to improve the efficiency and effectiveness of health care. Simply relying on legal documentation without paying attention to communication with others can undermine this objective and create additional, unanticipated problems that could be prevented.

1.2.4 Interprofessional Person-Centered Care

At its best, interprofessional person-centered care allows multiple practitioners with complementary skills to focus their strengths and attention on each person's unique needs and concerns. At its worst, interprofessional care can be confusing, inefficient, and ineffective. In most cases, the difference between the best and the worst delivery of interprofessional person-centered care is the quality of communication among team members and with the patient. Communication—whether it is face-to-face, in writing, in person, or virtually mediated—is integral to success.

Communication in interprofessional teams can be complex and further complicated by the need to involve multiple individuals at different times, sometimes spread across different geographic spaces. Understanding the unique complexities of each individual team is important to allow for planning and to implement communication systems that are comprehensive, timely, appropriate, and meaningful for all those involved.

It may be tempting to wonder if all this complexity is actually worth the additional effort required in order to communicate effectively. Perhaps the following quotation from a family physician may help explain why the time and effort required to ensure effective communication in interprofessional teams will help you to better understand its importance.

> *I'm a family doctor and for many years worked on my own, with a secretary and nurse to support me. Recently, I started working in a large interprofessional health clinic and honestly, it was challenging. There were a lot of different professionals, it wasn't clear to me all the time who did what, and there was a lot of time spent in meetings, talking to other people and explaining my decisions. Sometimes, frankly, I wondered if it was actually worth it or a waste of time. All the time I spent talking to others and in meetings, I could spend actually meeting with patients instead. Well, I learned my lesson a few years later. You see, in this team, I was the only person who could speak French. One day, a new patient who only spoke French came to see us, and I was the only person in the team who could actually communicate with her. Suddenly I realized for the first time in years, I had to do EVERYTHING. Instead of having the pharmacist there to explain how to use medications and how to deal with side effects, instead of having the nurse there to take the history and check blood pressure, instead of having the nutritionist there to help her manage her diet and lifestyle, and instead of having the psychologist there to provide counseling support—everyone in the team—for the first time in years, I had to do it all. And immediately I realized, I couldn't do any of this as well as these other team members. Worse, in the past, when I used to do this all on my own, I realized, I never did these jobs as well as the professionals who are trained in these specific jobs. Now because I was the only person who could actually speak French with the patient, I had to do it all, and it really made me realize I can't. No one can. I was so grateful for my team after that.*

1.3 Summary

Interprofessional patient-centered care is at the heart of the health care system. Without effective communication within and across a team, with the patient, and with the patient's caregivers, the quality of health care will be suboptimal. Recognizing that effective communication is as important to patient care and health outcomes as the technical, scientific, and clinical knowledge and skills of a profession is essential in helping to unleash the potential of all practitioners to elevate the care of patients.

1.4 Mind Map Chapter 1

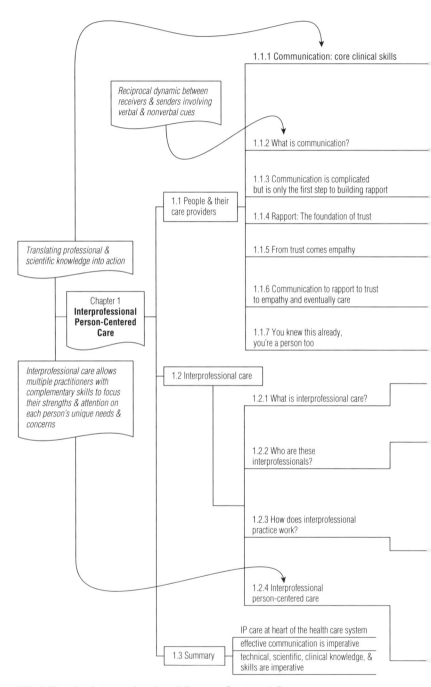

Mind Map for Interprofessional Person-Centered Care

listen
watch
speak
respond
write/document
read
social media
Internet

dynamic
receivers
senders
verbal cues
nonverbal cues

common understanding developed over time
efficient, effortless connection

essential attribute
earned & evolves through genuine interest

acknowledges what a person is saying & experiencing
requires genuine interest
provides comfort, confidence, & security

nonlinear
nonformulaic

communication
positive continuum
rapport
trust
self-reflection
empathy

2 or more different professions caring for the same patient
collaborate & complement each other

group of caring & committed professionals with diverse backgrounds, education, & skills
profession-specific education to navigate
complex profession-specific world

unintended consequences
different styles, structures, workflows

working together side by side or virtually or in a team chain

1.2.2.2 The professionals on a team

regulated or licensed
professional regulation requirements are not uniform

focused on the unique & specific patient needs

1.2.3.2 Scope of practice

specific jobs, tasks, & responsibilities
evolving
not the same for each team member
requires learning & understanding each team member's scope of practice

1.2.3.3 Scope of practice and delegation

important tool to improve efficiency & effectiveness
legal document codifying liability & responsibility
recognizes education & expertise
effective communication is essential to ensure its success

At its best: allows multiple practitioners with complementary skills to
focus their strengths on each person's unique needs & concerns
At its worst: confusing, inefficient, & ineffective
Key - effective communication!

For Further Reading:

Bendaly L, Bendaly N. *Improving Healthcare Team Performance: The 7 Requirements for Excellence in Patient Care.* Ontario, Canada: John Wiley & Sons Canada, Ltd.; 2012.

Kurtz S, Silverman J, Draper J. *Teaching and Learning Communication Skills in Medicine.* 2nd ed. Oxon, UK: CRC Press; 2006.

Lake D, Baerg K, Paslawski T. *Teamwork, Leadership, and Communication: Collaboration Basics for Health Professionals.* Canada: Brush Education; 2015.

McCorry L, Mason J. *Communication Skills for the Healthcare Professional.* Baltimore, MD: Lippincott Williams & Wilkins; 2011.

Moss B. *Communication Skills in Health and Social Care.* 4th ed. London: Sage Press; 2017.

2 | Personality Psychology: Learning About Ourselves

Throughout your education as a health care professional, there are abundant opportunities to learn more about the scientific, clinical, and technical aspects of your work. Rarely, however, do learners in such programs have opportunities to learn more about themselves and about their own psychological strengths, limitations, and areas for development. Personality psychology is a branch of psychology that focuses specifically on the concept of "self" and how it varies among individuals. Simply because we are all health care professionals, we share the same educational background or preparation, or do the same work, does not mean that we are all the same as human beings. Personality psychology is valuable because it helps us to remember that each of us, regardless of degree, job title, or professional designation, are first and foremost individuals. Throughout our education and training, we are frequently told it is important for us to act professional or check your personal feelings at the door. Increasingly, there is recognition that health care professionals cannot simply divorce who they are from what they do. Our personalities are central to the way we practice our profession and the way we interact with and communicate with patients, colleagues, and other health care professionals. Learning more about personality psychology and applying it to our day-to-day work as health care professionals can be an important tool for professional development and can help us to become more effective communicators and care providers.

2.1. What Is Personality?

The word *personality* originally comes from the Latin word *persona,* meaning mask. From this perspective, a personality is a mask or costume we wear when we are interacting with others. Today, most psychologists describe personality as a set of characteristics possessed by each of us as individuals that influences our thinking, feeling, motivations, and behaviors.

Your personality is unique and reflects many complex processes in your past and in your present that will ultimately influence your future. Human beings rely on assessments of one another's personalities in order to predict reactions. For example, as a child you may have known that a certain teacher's personality would allow you to get away with certain things in a classroom, whereas another teacher—a person with the same educational qualifications, background, and job as the first teacher—would respond entirely differently.

Personality is an important but rarely discussed variable in understanding patient care, interprofessional collaboration, and health care outcomes. Part of the reason that personality is rarely discussed within professional education is that even among psychologists, there is no clear understanding of what personality is, how it evolves, and how it influences our interactions with each other.

2.1.2   Personality Psychology 101

One of the central challenges in studying personality and attempting to apply personality theories to professional practice is the fact that there are a significant number of unanswered or unanswerable philosophical assumptions at the heart of what it means to be a human being. There are at least five major categories of questions—and disagreements—about personality that must first be considered before we can think further about the role of personality in interprofessional person-centered care.

- Is personality formed by nature or nurture?

  There is no clear consensus as to whether one's personality is born or made (i.e., is personality determined by genetics and biology, or is it shaped by childhood environment, parental influence, and early life experiences). Today, the emerging consensus is "all of the above." Most psychologists today believe that human beings are born hardwired with a foundational series of personality traits and that early childhood experiences refine and shape these traits into adult personalities. The interaction of genetics and environment, of biology and experiences, most likely results in the formation of the personality you possess today. It is a complex and reciprocal process in which individual preferences may or may not be rewarded by the specific parent, teacher, or environment, and consequently, individuals adapt their genetic preferences accordingly.

- Is personality fixed or is it situational?

  All of us can relate to the experience of behaving in one manner around certain people (e.g., parents) and in another, sometimes completely opposite, manner around other people (e.g., friends). For those who have the experience of being children of recent immigrants to a new country, there is a well-documented phenomenon known as *code shifting*, which describes how one's accent will actually shift when speaking to parents and older family members as opposed to conversations with friends or even nonimmigrant parents of friends. There is much speculation as to whether personality is fixed and predictable or whether we are literally different people in different situations. Of course, there may be great individual differences that make this a difficult question to answer. Some people behave exactly the same regardless of situation or context, whereas others seem to morph even fundamental characteristics and traits to different circumstances. Similar to the nature-versus-nurture argument, there is no single or clear answer to the question of whether personality is fixed or situational; however, in this case, the extent to which one willingly or eagerly changes one's personality depending on the audience in front of them is likely a core personality trait in and of itself.

• Can personality be changed with training, circumstance, or sheer force of will?

Are personalities stable and unmovable, or can we find ways to actually change aspects of ourselves that we (or others) may not necessarily like? Perhaps you are change-averse and much prefer routine and predictability rather than novelty and constant uncertainty, yet you find yourself in a job or with a group of friends where the dominant preference is for change rather than stability. Can you make a choice, or take a course that will help you to change a fundamental preference? Most psychologists believe the answer to this question is "probably not." Certainly today there is broad acceptance that some aspects of our personality (e.g., sexual orientation) cannot be changed; although it may be possible to fake a certain sexual orientation for a period of time in order to achieve some objective, it is clearly faked, consumes psychological energy, and in the long run can neither be sustained nor ever actually result in a true shift in orientation. On the other hand, many students find that when they are in school they are night owls, preferring to go to sleep at 2, 3, or 4 in the morning and wake up after noon, yet when they actually start working for a living, such a pattern is not possible and they eventually become morning people. Most psychologists today believe some elements of certain personality characteristics can, to a limited degree, actually be changed, but the more foundational aspects of who we are as people are notoriously resistant to significant change despite our best efforts and thousands of dollars spent on self-help books or courses.

• Are there better and worse personality types?

As human beings, we all know there are some people we get along with and others we don't. We have our own preferences for interacting with other individuals with specific clusters of personality traits and characteristics, and of course a preference to avoid others. We tend to filter our worlds—and make our decisions about who we like and who we don't—based on a hierarchy of personality traits and dimensions. For example, some of us prefer to interact with nice people who are kind, thoughtful, altruistic, and generous. Others of us prefer to interact with fun people who are edgy, unpredictable, spontaneous, and who in some cases may not be particularly nice (e.g., kind, thoughtful, altruistic, and generous). As we mature, we begin to realize that everyone has personality strengths and simultaneously characteristics that are irritating or off-putting, and that no one is perfect. Every individual has their own preferences and weightings for different personality types and attributes, and engages in a series of trade-offs in negotiating friendships and relationships. Your best friend may be selfish (insofar as she talks about herself and her problems all the time) and, weirdly, also very generous (insofar as she spends lots of money on your birthday present every year). Human beings, including you, can be contradictory, illogical, and simultaneously demonstrate seemingly opposite personality traits and behaviors. It is sometimes said that the more you get to know anyone, the weirder everyone appears to become. Personality psychologists believe there are not necessarily good or bad personality types, but instead there are characteristics that in specific situations may be more or less advantageous in achieving a specific goal or objective.

- Do personalities produce culture or does culture produce personality?

Culture is a complex idea; it refers to the unspoken and unwritten rules that govern our day-to-day interactions with others and form the common substrate upon which we understand social relationships. Culture is sometimes described as the air we breathe. It is around us all the time and essential to day-to-day functioning, yet few of us actually bother thinking about it unless it's not there. Culture helps us to understand how we are supposed to address certain people (by their first name? by their professional designation?), how long to maintain eye contact with them when speaking, or whether we should shake hands with them when we meet them or give them one (or two or three) kisses on the cheek. Failure to adhere to a cultural norm can result in swift judgment from others, and ultimately being labeled as someone who "doesn't fit in here."

In our increasingly multicultural communities, the issue of culture's influence on personality has produced significant interest and discussion. Do cultures shape who we are, or do we contribute to the norms of a culture because of our personalities? For example, East Asian cultures have traditionally been associated with a high degree of respect for authority figures, such as parents, grandparents, and teachers. A culture that rewards respect for authority will produce individuals who tend to be very compliant—they will sit quietly in class, listen attentively, do their homework, and do what they are told. In contrast, North American culture has traditionally been associated with a high degree of individuality and competitiveness. Compliance is less of a cultural norm than beating other people in competitions. A culture that rewards competition and individuality will produce very different kinds of students. Individuals who may be ethnically or culturally East Asian but who are fully immersed from birth in North American culture may, at best, have access to a much broader repertoire of personality and behaviors than those who are locked in monocultural environments. Conversely, at worst, these individuals may feel confused, pressured, or uncertain about what the right way to behave actually is.

The broader society or culture in which we find ourselves can sometimes be at odds with our foundational personalities. In this context, culture is not necessarily a country or society; it can also refer to a much smaller group of people, like a health care team. Some of the tensions experienced in interprofessional teams may be a result of cultural differences among the health care professionals themselves and the challenges associated with navigating these differences (more about this in Chapter 3). For now, most psychologists believe that culture, whether broad or narrow, has an important role in shaping both behavior and, to a lesser extent, personality, and that it is quite unusual or rare (but not unheard of) for an individual's personality to have the ability to actually shape or change a culture.

2.2 The Big Five

One of the best-known and most enduring theories in all of psychology is the Big Five personality traits. The Big Five refers to a cluster of dimensions upon which our personalities, and our selves, are based. The Big Five theory suggests that human beings can be understood as the intersection of five distinct but interdependent functions. When these functions are combined, they give rise to the uniqueness that characterizes each human being (i.e., our personalities).

2.2.1 What Are the Big Five?

The Big Five personality traits are openness, conscientiousness, extroversion, agreeableness, and neuroticism. Let's look at each of these dimensions in greater detail.

Openness is the personality dimension that describes one's psychological comfort and preference for innovation, change, and spontaneity. Those who are more open typically grow bored of routine, stability, and predictability and instead crave newness and surprise. Those who are more open typically prefer thinking on their feet to rigorous rehearsal and preparation. Those who are less open find greater psychological comfort in consistency and constancy, and are at their best in situations that are familiar to them.

Conscientiousness is the personality dimension that describes one's psychological need for rules and guidance and the comfort derived from actually adhering to them. Those who are more conscientious typically crave the organization and certainty associated with clear structure, policies, and procedures. Those who are less conscientious are *not* irresponsible or lazy; instead, they have a psychological preference for flexibility and situational thinking and tend to feel constrained in environments where rules are rigid and behavior is prescribed.

Extroversion, in common use, usually refers to a pattern of behavior associated with those who like the company of others, enjoying parties and social interaction, or who have no difficulty meeting new people. Psychologists use the term *extroversion* somewhat differently to describe a kind of psychological energy that flows within social situations. Extroverted individuals gain psychological energy from the presence of others, whereas introverts spend or lose psychological energy in the same situation. Curiously, many people who make a living from public speaking (e.g., professors or actors) are actually introverts. They have no difficulty speaking in front of large groups of individuals and are not shy, but the act of doing so drains them of energy and they must consequently recharge after performing. In contrast, a true extrovert is actually energized by such a situation and will not need to recharge. In fact, an extrovert may feel psychologically depleted being on their own and not having others around them with whom to interact.

Agreeableness refers to the extent to which you as an individual feel psychological comfort from being liked or being right when it is not possible in a particular situation to experience both simultaneously. In many situations in life, we must choose between being liked and being right. We cannot be both at the same time. Those who are more agreeable may find themselves going along with a majority opinion or belief even if personally they are opposed to it simply to avoid conflict and to be liked by the crowd. Those who are less agreeable may experience only minimal psychological distress in asserting their beliefs and are fine to live with the social consequences that may follow.

Neuroticism refers to the extent to which individuals are psychologically comfortable in their own skin. It describes the sense of accurate self-appraisal and self-acceptance an individual possesses about their own strengths and weaknesses, and describes the behavior associated with changing yourself to please the person you happen to be with at any given time. Those who are more neurotic may not truly know or accept who they are and consequently may find themselves morphing their opinions, behaviors, and attitudes to those who are around them, or presenting a social face to others that they believe these others actually want or expect from them. Less neurotic individuals are more stable in their presentation to different individuals and groups and have a greater degree of and more grounded self-awareness and self-acceptance.

According to the Big Five personality theory, the intersection of these five interdependent processes produces the individual person each of us is today. Because we all possess different aliquots of each of these five dimensions, the admixture of all of these produces the unique, interesting, and highly variable personalities we encounter in our day-to-day lives.

The Big Five is a foundational theory in psychology and has many practical applications for both understanding oneself and better understanding others. It is the basis for a diverse array of pop psychology interventions as well as more scientifically oriented personality tests and profiles, including the Myers-Briggs Typology Inventory (MBTI), which have been used for career planning and other purposes.

2.3 Emotional Intelligence

An important application of the Big Five personality theory is *emotional intelligence*. You may have heard the term *emotional intelligence* before; it is used frequently to describe individuals who have certain strengths or people skills. It is frequently used as a shorthand way of describing a constellation of behaviors related to social interactions and is most often thought of as a positive attribute. In contrast with intelligence, emotional intelligence describes so-called soft skills that are essential for personal and professional success.

Many different models and theories of emotional intelligence have been proposed, each of which have different features and strengths. Emotional Intelligence has emerged as a method used by organizations and employers in an attempt to diagnose individual employee's emotional intelligence for the purpose of team building or sorting individuals into appropriate roles. In some cases, emotional intelligence testing and training can take months and cost thousands of dollars. Although there may be great value in such in-depth examinations of personal emotional intelligence, few individuals have dedicated time and resources to focus on this, so alternative methods for assessing and interpreting emotional intelligence have evolved that provide a shortcut to better understanding one of the Big Five personality dimensions and one's emotional intelligence.

2.3.1 The Health Professionals' Inventory of Learning Styles

One such shortcut that has been used for many years is the Health Profession-als' Inventory of Learning Styles (or H-PILS) tool. This instrument—initially devel-oped within and for pharmacy education but now more broadly used and applicable across the health professions—can help individuals assess and reflect on their own emotional intelligence and Big Five profiles and offers opportunities to consider alter-native approaches in difficult professional and personal circumstances.

The H-PILS is derived from the pioneering work of David Kolb, who developed the concept of Learning Styles Theory. Because health professionals' work is intimately connected to learning—and health professionals are constantly learning, whether they are in a formal degree program or in the workplace—Learning Styles Theory is an appropriate framework for helping better understand personal psychology and emotional intelligence.

2.3.1.1 *Learning Styles Theory*

Learning Styles Theory (LST; sometimes referred to as Learning Preferences Theory) is a model to explain how human beings interact with their environment when they are learning new things. As you will know for yourself (and will have observed in others), people have very different ways of learning. Some of us like to cram for an exam the night before, whereas others prefer to do all the homework and problem sets on a regular basis. Some of us will actually read the instructions for how to assemble a barbecue grill before we attempt to do so, whereas others simply start fiddling with the parts and go along with trial and error. When learning new software, some of us want someone beside us explaining step by step how to use it, whereas others prefer to be left alone and just figure it out.

These observed differences in learning behaviors reflect broader underlying differences in Big Five dimensions and in emotional intelligence. To Kolb, learning is best understood as the interaction between one's external environment (e.g., a classroom, a lab, a clinic) and one's internal psychology. From this perspective, learning consists of two interdependent processes: When we learn something, we first have to take in information from the outside world, then secondly, we need to actually find of a way of internalizing it.

How do people take in information from the outside world? We all fall some-where along a continuum in terms of our preference (or style). On one extreme of this continuum are the kind of people who like to take in information by watching, reading instructions, and observing. These people do not want to get involved or participate directly with something new but instead need time to actually see others doing something so they can learn from observation. In contrast, others will take in information in a more direct or active manner; they need to actively be engaged in a task, learning with their hands, or learning by trial and error. These individuals may have difficulty learning by reading or get bored watching others do something and instead want to jump in with both feet and just try it.

Once we've taken in information from the outside world, we need to internally (cognitively and psychologically) process it. How do people process information?

Again, we all fall somewhere along a continuum. Some people, once they've taken in information, immediately need to apply or use it. They need to actively experiment and use new knowledge or skills. If not, it will be quickly forgotten or deteriorate. In contrast, others of us, once we've taken in information, need time to think further about it, reflect, or rehearse. These people do not like being put on the spot or being put on their feet. Instead, they need time and space to internally reflect rather than actively participate in something.

Importantly, there is no right or wrong way of learning, but it is clear that as human beings we demonstrate a wide difference in our learning styles and preferences. Consider the following example. A student on a clinical rotation is asked to educate a patient on how to use a new device such as an inhaler. The student is not familiar with that device. Some students will feel perfectly comfortable saying to a patient, "I don't know how this thing works, but let's get the instructions out and we can learn this together" or "This device is new to me but I'm pretty confident I can figure this out without help. And worse comes to worst, we can just look up directions for use on the Internet." In contrast, another student may say, "I have no idea how to use this device. Let me do some research, read about this, then before I actually talk to a patient, I will practice on my mother so I am confident I am saying the right things in the right way."

There is nothing inherently right or wrong or good or bad about any of these different approaches, as long as the information is correct and the patient is well-served. Your individual learning style and preference in a situation like this does not make you better or worse than anyone else. However, in some situations, workplaces, or contexts, certain learning styles or emotional intelligences may be better suited to solving day-to-day issues or are more highly rewarded by the workplace culture. Learning more about your personal learning style and emotional intelligence can therefore provide you with important clues for how to best fit in to your workplace environment and how to best leverage your strengths to meet the needs of your patients.

2.3.1.2 Using the H-PILS

At the end of this chapter, you will find the H-PILS inventory. Prior to reading the remainder of this chapter, experiment with the inventory for yourself so you can then compare your results to the learning styles and emotional intelligence theories that follow.

The H-PILS inventory provides an assessment of your emotional intelligence and learning style using the Big Five dimensions. It does this by integrating your responses to a series of 17 questions focused on self-assessed behaviors in different situations involving learning. The strength of your responses (e.g., hardly versus frequently) helps provide an indication of the strength of your preferences. When you tally up the frequency with which you circled answer options A, B, C, or D, you will identify a dominant and secondary emotional intelligence style.

In many cases, individuals completing this inventory will have a tie or very close numerical scores for A, B, C, and D. This simply means that such individuals are relatively even in their emotional intelligence strengths. For the purposes of the commentary below, if you have a tie in your dominant emotional intelligence identified by the H-PILS, or if the numbers were very close, simply read the paragraph descriptions associated with each emotional intelligence factor and pick the style that most closely resembles who you believe you are.

The H-PILS provides a diagnosis of four different emotional intelligence styles or types: divergers, assimilators, convergers, and accommodators. Let's look at each of these in more detail. Of course, it may be natural to gravitate to the description of your dominant emotional intelligence style; however, you are strongly encouraged to review all four of these styles or types because you will be working with people with different emotional intelligences during your career and it is useful to know more about each of them.

2.3.1.3   *The Four Emotional Intelligences and You*

Divergers: If there were a single sentence that would best summarize divergers, it may be "Let's just all get along, okay?" Divergers have an emotional intelligence that is oriented toward interpersonal interactions and, in particular, harmonious, nonconfrontational, positive relationships with others. In terms of Big Five dimensions, divergers typically trend toward being very open, moderately conscientious, very agreeable, and somewhat neurotic. They may be introverts or extroverts. The first impression made by most divergers is one of friendliness. They tend to rely strongly on the strength of their personality, like to use humor, and are generally regarded as warm people by others. On the other hand, divergers can be somewhat overly sensitive to criticism or questioning, or any kind of direct communication that threatens their belief that they are liked by others. In difficult situations, divergers typically rely on their personal charm rather than logic, forceful argumentation, or any other technique to defuse tension. To be at their best, divergers need to feel secure and comfortable and believe that everyone around them is positive and cooperative. Divergers generally do not perform well in highly political, gossip-intensive situations that are highly competitive or where individuals routinely jockey for position or power.

Assimilators: The strongest assimilators firmly believe that "a lack of organization on *YOUR* part should be no reason for an emergency on *MY* part." A dominant characteristic of these individuals is the value they place on clarity and the faith they have in organization and processes. Most assimilators tend to be only moderately to weakly open, and instead prefer routine, predictability, and stability over surprise or spontaneity. They are highly conscientious and most frequently are introverted rather than extroverted. They are moderately agreeable. Whereas they might prefer to be liked (rather than disliked), they are more comfortable being right than divergers may be. They tend to be somewhat neurotic and concerned about the image they project to others. The first impression assimilators make is one of being methodical, earnest, organized, and rule-following. They are somewhat open to criticism and feedback provided it is based on structured and clear criteria and is fair. Assimilators sincerely want to improve and believe perfection (or at least excellence) is possible, but it frustrates them when teachers (or parents or supervisors) provide vague feedback that doesn't really help them to learn or develop. A key attribute of assimilators is their strong need to learn *without* being watched by others. Assimilators typically dislike learning on their feet or learning as they go along, and instead require time to rehearse or practice in private before going public with what they know. Assimilators may be most vulnerable to confusing confidence with competence. Whereas the words sound the same, they are of course completely different concepts. Assimilators are somewhat easily blinded by other, more confident individuals and may erroneously assume that simply because they display confidence (e.g., they volunteer to go first, they answer a teacher's question), they are actually smarter or better. Of course, this is not necessarily the case!

Convergers: Of all the emotional intelligence types, convergers are likely the ones most stimulated by competition and the prospect of winning. They tend to rise to the occasion when pitted against others and enjoy the idea of competitions, debates, or other opportunities to demonstrate their mastery. They tend to be moderate to strongly open. Convergers may get bored easily by routine or repetition and enjoy thinking on their feet. They are moderately to slightly conscientious. Although they understand the reason for rules, they also have sufficient self-confidence to believe that rules are not absolute and that their judgment and wisdom are equally important tools for decision making. Most convergers are extroverts and enjoy activities that involve interactions with others (particularly competition). They are not particularly concerned about the image they present to others and are only weakly neurotic. If there were one sentence to summarize convergers, it may be: "Relax everyone. I'm here to help!" Convergers are typically natural leaders, although they may be somewhat short on patience with others. The first impression they make may be built on appearing larger than life, dynamic, and inspiring. Rather than rely on logic, facts, or charm to deal with difficult situations, convergers may rely heavily on the force of their own personality and the loudness of their voice instead. They are direct in communication and can sometimes be overly directive with others. The opposite of assimilators, convergers may sometimes confuse their own self-confidence with competence.

Accommodators: If there were a single sentence to sum up the strongest accommodators, it might be: "Are we there yet?" Accommodators tend toward action rather than reflection and prefer decision making to deliberation. They tend to be moderately open but only weakly conscientious. At their worst, accommodators may value efficiency (getting things done) at the expense of effectiveness (getting things done well or properly). Strong accommodators may argue back, "Most times, good enough IS actually good enough. You don't need perfection in everything." As can be seen, accommodators are typically only weakly agreeable, and prefer to be right rather than liked, and are not particularly concerned about how others' appraise them so they are not particularly neurotic. The first impression they make may be one of valuing getting things done rather than valuing interpersonal connections or people. In some cases, accommodators may actually resent the interpersonal overhead time and social chitchat associated with most modern workplaces; instead, they value being left alone and simply trusted to get things done.

There are of course many more nuances and dimensions to each of these different emotional intelligence styles, but for now it may be useful to reflect on the dominant and secondary styles you have self-identified. Such reflection can help you to better understand the face you present to others and how you interact in difficult situations, and can provide you with a vocabulary to describe the real interpersonal differences you encounter in your personal and professional life.

You may wonder whether emotional intelligence is stable in all circumstances or whether people shift depending on the specific situation or context in which they find themselves. The answer to that will likely depend on your individual score on the H-PILS. Those who are relatively evenly distributed across two, three, or all four styles will likely find it easier and more natural to adopt different kinds of emotional intelligences based on situation-specific circumstances. Those who have very high scores in a dominant area and very low scores across all others may find it more difficult to consciously or unconsciously adapt responses and personal emotional intelligence to different situations and contexts. Although there is undoubtedly fluidity in the way our emotional intelligence may express itself in a particular social situation, our personal degree of flexibility is a reflection of our unique emotional intelligence makeup.

Importantly for this book, understanding your personal emotional intelligence and personal psychology will help you to better interpret and integrate the communication strategies we will be discussing. In the past, many communication skills references and books tended to present solutions to difficult problems in a one-size-fits-all manner. Your understanding of emotional intelligence should help you better understand that in communication skills, as in interpersonal interactions and day-to-day life in general, there is rarely a one-size-fits-all solution. What works for a diverger may be toxic for an accommodator; the strategies that can be helpful for assimilators may backfire spectacularly for convergers. Customizing communication skills to your emotional intelligence—and to the emotional intelligence of those you interact with—is time consuming and requires thinking and planning, but in the long run it is more likely to yield a more beneficial outcome than simply using a canned phrase in a one-size-fits-all manner.

2.4 **Summary**

Understanding your personal psychology and your own emotional intelligence is a crucial first step in enhancing the quality of your communication with different audiences. Although you cannot control or manage anyone else's psychology, you can understand yourself better to help you predict and maintain greater control over your responses. Understanding emotional intelligence and reflecting on your own emotional intelligence can help you to adjust your communication and presentation style to different audiences. It may also help you to better understand the communication and behaviors of others as you use this knowledge to think about others' emotional intelligence styles. The emotional intelligence model presented in this chapter is built on the work of Learning Styles Theory; it is simply one model for understanding emotional intelligence and has the benefit of being fairly straightforward and simple. This theory, however is neither perfect nor exhaustive, and other models and theories may provide additional lenses through which human personality can be understood. Other more nuanced or in-depth models and tools are available for those who seek further study in the area.

THE HEALTH PROFESSIONALS' INVENTORY OF LEARNING STYLES (H-PILS)

Think about a few recent situations where you had to learn something new to solve a problem. This could be any kind of situation: while you were taking a course at school, learning to use new software, or figuring out how to assemble a barbecue grill.

Now, circle the letter in the column that best characterizes what works best for you in situations like the ones you've thought about.

When I'm trying to learn something new	Usually	Sometimes	Rarely	Hardly
1. I like to watch others before trying it for myself.	B	D	C	A
2. I like to consult a manual, textbook, or instruction guide first.	B	C	D	A
3. I like to work by myself rather than with other people.	A	C	B	D
4. I like to take notes or write things down as I'm going along.	B	C	D	A
5. I'm critical of myself if things don't work out as I hoped.	B	C	D	A
6. I usually compare myself to other people just so I know I'm keeping up.	B	D	C	A
7. I like to examine things closely instead of jumping right in.	B	D	C	A
8. I rise to the occasion if I'm under pressure.	C	A	B	D
9. I like to have plenty of time to think about something new before trying it.	D	B	C	A
10. I pay a lot of attention to the details.	B	C	A	D
11. I concentrate on improving on the things I did wrong in the past.	C	A	D	B
12. I focus on reinforcing the things I got right in the past.	B	D	A	C
13. I like to please the person teaching me.	D	B	A	C
14. I trust my hunches.	D	C	A	B
15. I'm usually the first one in a group to finish whatever we're doing.	A	C	D	B
16. I like to take charge of a situation.	C	A	B	D
17. I'm well-organized.	B	A	C	D

Now, add up the number of times you circled each letter.

A = _____   B = _____   C = _____   D = _____

Your **DOMINANT** learning style is the letter you circled most frequently.
Your **SECONDARY** learning style is the next most-frequently circled letter.

A = Accommodator

You enjoy dealing directly with people and have little time or patience for indirect or soft-sell jobs. You enjoy looking for, and exploiting, opportunities as they arrive, and you have an entrepreneurial spirit. You learn best in a hands-on, unencumbered manner, not in a traditional lecture-style format. Though you don't take any particular pleasure in leading others, you do so because you sense you are best-suited for the job. You are confident, have strong opinions, and value efficiency. You are concerned about time and like to see a job get done. Sometimes, however, your concern with efficiency means that the quality of your work may suffer and you may not be paying as much attention to others' feelings and desires as you ought to.

B = Assimilator

You generally prefer working by yourself, at your own pace, in your own time, or with a very small group of like-minded people. You tend to avoid situations where you are the center of attention, or you are constantly being watched—you prefer to be the one observing (and learning) from others. You have an ability to learn from your own, and others', mistakes. You place a high priority on getting things done properly, according to the rules but, at times, you can be your own worst critic. You value organization and attentiveness to detail.

C = Converger

You are focused, practical, and to the point. You usually find yourself in a leadership role and enjoy this challenge. You have little time or patience for those who dither or are indecisive or who spend too much time on impractical, theoretical matters. You are good at coming to quick, decisive conclusions, but you recognize that at times your speed may result in less than perfect results. You would rather get a good job done on time than get an excellent job delivered late. You like being in a high-performance, high-energy, fast-paced environment.

D = Diverger

You enjoy out-of-the-box environments where time and resources are not particularly constrained. You have a flair for keeping others entertained and engaged, and sincerely believe this is the way to motivate others and get the best out of everyone. You are most concerned—sometimes too concerned—about how others perceive you, and you place a high priority on harmony. You find little difficulty dealing with complex, ambiguous, theoretical situations (provided there is not a lot of pressure to perform), but sometimes you have a hard time dealing with the practical, day-to-day issues.

Now, as a group of individuals with the same dominant learning style, think about the following questions and share your opinions.

> 1) What professional, social, or personal characteristics do you have in common?
> 2) What teaching and learning methods work best for you?
> 3) What teaching and learning methods do not work well for you?
> 4) What are some examples of the type of feedback that motivates you?
> 5) What are some examples of the type of feedback that discourages you?

Now, share your group's discussion with members of the other learning-styles' groups.

2.5   Mind Map 1 Chapter 2

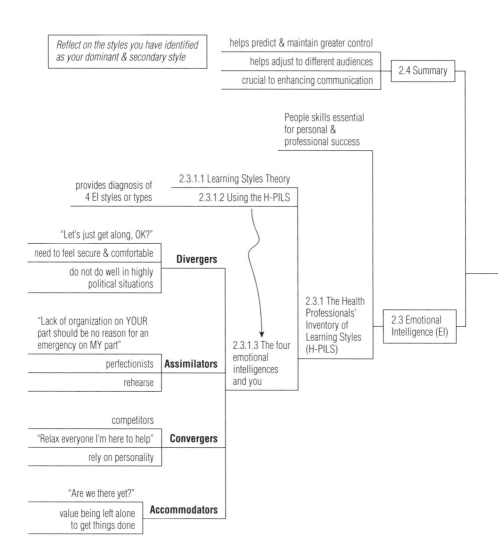

Mind Map for Personality Psychology - Learning About Ourselves

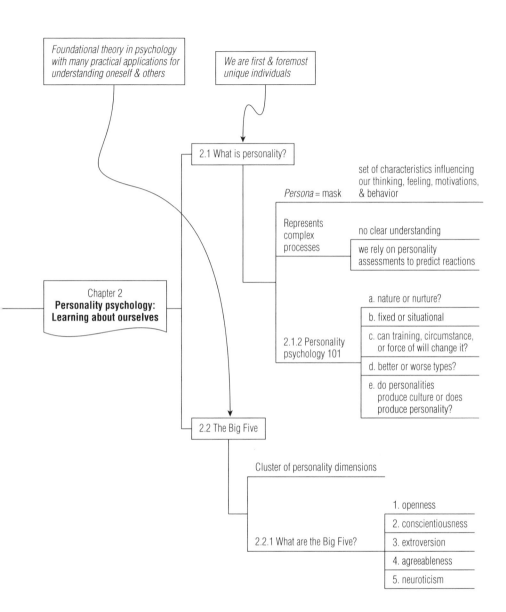

2.6 Mind Map 2 Chapter 2

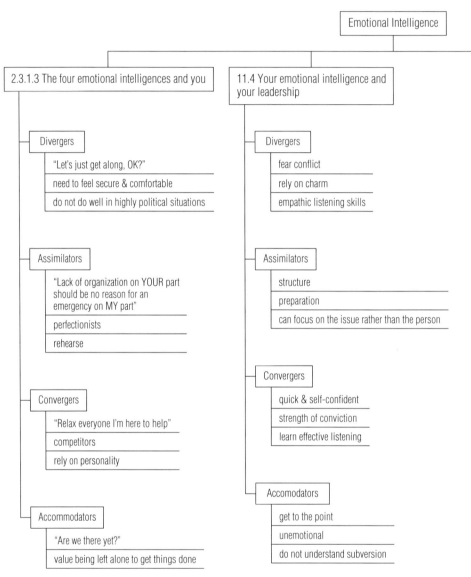

Mind Map for Emotional Intelligence

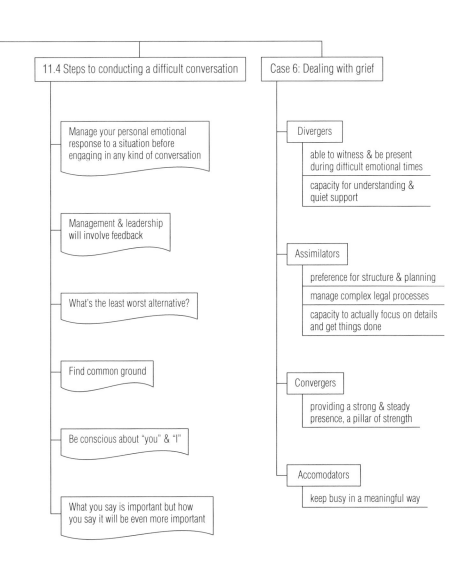

11.4 Steps to conducting a difficult conversation

Manage your personal emotional response to a situation before engaging in any kind of conversation

Management & leadership will involve feedback

What's the least worst alternative?

Find common ground

Be conscious about "you" & "I"

What you say is important but how you say it will be even more important

Case 6: Dealing with grief

Divergers
able to witness & be present during difficult emotional times
capacity for understanding & quiet support

Assimilators
preference for structure & planning
manage complex legal processes
capacity to actually focus on details and get things done

Convergers
providing a strong & steady presence, a pillar of strength

Accomodators
keep busy in a meaningful way

For Further Reading:

Akerjordet K, Severinsson E. Emotionally intelligence nurse leadership: a literature review study. *J Nurs Manag.* 2008;16:565–577.

Austin Z. Learning styles of pharmacists: impact on career decisions, practice patterns, and teaching method preferences. *Pharm Educ.* 2004;4(1):13–22.

Birks YF, Watt IS. Emotional intelligence and patient centered care. *J R Soc Med.* 2007;100: 368–374.

Fergusson E. Personality is of central concern to understand health: toward a theoretical model for health psychology. *Health Psychol Rev.* 2013;7(Suppl 1):S32–S70.

Goleman D. *Emotional Intelligence: Why It Can Matter More Than IQ.* New York: Bantam Dell; 2016.

Kolb AY, Kolb DA. Learning styles and learning spaces: enhancing experiential learning in higher education. *Acad Manag Learn Ed.* 2005;4(2):193–212.

Luca J, Tarricone P. Does emotional intelligence affect successful teamwork? Paper presented at: Meeting at the Crossroads. Proceedings of the 18th Annual Conference of the Australasian Society for Computers in Learning in Tertiary Education. December 9–12, 2001; Melbourne, Australia. Available at: http://ro.ecu.edu.au/cgi/viewcontent.cgi?article =5833&context=ecuworks.

McAdams D, Pals J. A new Big Five: fundamental principles for an integrative science of personality. *Am Psychol.* 2005;61(3):204–217.

McCallin A, Bamford A. Interdisciplinary teamwork: is the influence of emotional intelligence fully appreciated? *J Nurs Manag.* 2007;15(4):386–391.

Raggatt P. Putting the five-factor model into context: evidence linking Big Five traits to narrative identity. *J Pers.* 2006;74(5):1321–1348.

Shatalebi B, Sharifi S, Saeedian N, Javadi H. Examining the relationship between emotional intelligence and learning styles. *Procedia Soc Behav Sci.* 2012;31:95–99.

Suliman WA. The relationship between learning styles, emotional social intelligence, and academic success of undergraduate nursing students. *J Nurs Res.* 2010;18(2):136–143.

3 | Team Psychology: Learning About Those with Whom We Work

It is sometimes said that "there is no I in TEAM," meaning individual egos and interests should have no place in teamwork. Although it is true the word team has no I in it, it has an E and an M, which spells *me*, suggesting individual egos and interests must always be considered in team functioning despite best intentions and hopeful wishes.

In Chapter 2, we reviewed principles of individual psychology to help you to better understand yourself in diverse interpersonal and social settings (including in health care work). In this chapter we will be examining an important element of your day-to-day life as a health care professional—the other health care professionals with whom you work, also known as the *health care team*.

3.1 What's a Team?

There are many different definitions of what constitutes a team, both in health care and in other industries or settings. Mosser and Begun (2014) suggest that a team is "a group of people with a full set of complementary skills required to complete a task, job, or project"; other definitions state that teams are "collections of people with a strong sense of mutual commitment, creating synergy and thus generating performance greater than the sum of its individual members." More technical definitions of teams suggest that they are "groups operating with a high degree of interdependence, sharing authority and responsibility for self-management, accountability for collective performance, while working toward a common goal."

Regardless of the definition of team one selects, there are common characteristics of teams and teamwork that are central to their functioning. For teams to work they must have agreed-upon goals and objectives. Although they may disagree in the details or quibble about methods, all teams require some common understanding of their purpose in order to function effectively. Teams generally are built of people who complement—rather than reinforce—one another. If everyone in a team had the same beliefs, skills, talents, and strengths, there would be little need for them all to work together. We need teams precisely because no single individual can possibly do everything well, and as a result, they need to combine forces (and skills) as efficiently as possible. Finally, teams need to develop sophisticated mechanisms for communicating within and across the team itself and with outsiders who are involved and interested in their work.

3.2 Team Models in Health Care

Although it is tempting to believe health care work is highly unique and specialized—and therefore health care teams are unlike any other teams anywhere else—the reality is that health care teams are composed of diverse individuals struggling to work together just like any other team in any other industry, sport, or group activity such as an orchestra or band.

Much of what we know about health care teams is actually based on research in other sectors and applied to health care work. Among the most important issues with any team is the model that governs its organization and functioning. Bringing a diverse group of individuals together to do something important and collaborative requires these individuals actually know and accept their roles and responsibilities and understand what is expected of them.

Within health care teams, there are at least three standard models for how teams can form: division of labor, sharing of labor, and undifferentiated labor. Let's look at each of these in turn.

Division of labor: A team that is structured around division of labor is one where each individual's role is clearly known and understood, accepted by all team members, and has a clear perimeter or boundary around it to protect that person's role from other individuals encroaching upon it. In a division of labor team model, there is no or only minimal overlap in jobs, responsibilities, and tasks. Each individual knows specifically what to do: who hands them work and who they hand work off to once they have completed it. One of the best known examples of division of labor outside of health care would be an assembly line. Each worker on an assembly line has a specific job or task to do, and rarely does this individual know any other jobs or tasks so they cannot step in. The assembly line is carefully controlled to allow each person sufficient time to do the assigned job, and there is a clear process in which one person hands off to another who completes work and then in turn hands off to the next person on the line. Within health care settings, division of labor models of teamwork are most likely to be seen in highly technical or proceduralized environments that follow strict processes and protocols—for example, operating rooms where surgical staff each have a job to do and everyone's work is important, but it is very rare for one person to "step in" for another.

Sharing of labor: A sharing of labor team model occurs when there is some overlap with boundaries and some flexibility in who does what based on circumstances and context. Sharing of labor typically begins as division of labor, but with time and positive experience working with one another, team members start to become more flexible in their roles, more willing to share responsibilities, and more ready to trust one another. Sharing of labor has several important advantages over division of labor. First, when labor is shared, redundancy is possible, which means there is backup available for crucial roles in case of illness or vacation. Second, sharing of labor allows individuals with different backgrounds opportunities to do the same job; this can result in different perspectives and talents being brought to a job, which can result in improvements in the longer run. On the downside, sharing of labor can take time to evolve and may be highly dependent on a positive interpersonal chemistry evolving between team members. At its worst, sharing of labor may produce role confusion and operational inefficiency where people simply assume others are doing certain jobs when in fact they are not, or having multiple people repeat the same job in a way that is wasteful and unnecessary. In primary school, teachers may share labor with one another; the assigned music teacher may suddenly have to step in to be a gym teacher for a day if there is illness or absence. In high school, the degree of specialization required to teach students is greater; such "stepping in" becomes problematic. By the time you reach university, it is extremely unlikely that a chemistry professor can step in for a sociology professor.

Within health care teams, there is increasing use of sharing of labor in primary health care teams. In some cases, this sharing occurs through the use of delegation protocols (see Chapter 1) where, for example, a family doctor may delegate certain rights and responsibilities for prescribing and medication management to a pharmacist or other health care professional to improve the overall efficiency and effectiveness of care delivered by the entire team.

Undifferentiated labor: At the other end of the spectrum from division of labor is a team model described as undifferentiated labor. In this model, there is significant role overlap and role fluidity; each member of a team is ready and capable to assume some, many, or all the responsibilities of any other team member. Day-to-day tasks are generally negotiated based on specific needs and requirements of the moment (e.g., who happens to be on vacation, who happens to be busy doing other things). The great advantage of undifferentiated labor is that it offers maximum flexibility in terms of scheduling and work allocation because everyone is capable of filling in for everyone else. A significant disadvantage of undifferentiated labor is the overlap and redundancy it produces, which may lead to operational inefficiencies. The communication requirements for team members operating with undifferentiated labor are extraordinarily high; they must be in constant communication and clearly communicating what they are doing to ensure nothing gets overlooked or things are not done twice. In many families, the traditional roles once played by mothers and fathers have now been replaced by undifferentiated labor, where each parent can do most things the other parent stereotypically may have done in the past. Today, in many families, fathers cook dinner and do the laundry, and mothers may be the primary breadwinner until the time comes for these roles to be reversed. In a health care team, truly undifferentiated labor is rare due to legal requirements related to scope of practice (see Chapter 1). Where it is most frequently seen is in contexts that have a high psychosocial or emotional element associated with care provided, for example, in psychiatric or rehabilitation settings, or in palliative care.

Understanding the structure of teams is essential to understanding how they work and how they can be improved. Unfortunately, in most health care settings, little time or attention is paid to formally deciding how to structure a team, and even less time is spent explaining team structure to individual team members or the patients they serve. As a result, confusion may arise, particularly if one team member believes the team is structured one way and another assumes it is structured differently. Clarity in describing and defining team structure is essential to optimize the team's ability to provide care.

3.3. How Do Teams Make Decisions and Get Things Done?

Some people dread the idea of teamwork as they fear it becomes an excuse for indecision and unnecessary bureaucracy and chitchat. At the end of the day, teams—like the individuals who make up these teams—have a job they need to accomplish, one that inevitably involves making decisions. Although the structure of the team (Section 3.2) can be helpful in predicting certain features of team functioning, it is useful to also establish clarity around the issue of how teams make decisions and take action and whose voices matter most in difficult situations. There are at least six different models that can be used to describe team-based decision making: hierarchical, majoritarian, alliance based, consensual, isolative, and facilitative.

Hierarchical: Hierarchical decision making, sometimes described as top-down or militaristic decision making, is a model of team functioning most often associated with division of labor (although not always). In hierarchical decision making, the most important determinant of decisional power is authority: Who is the most senior, important, or skilled person on the team? Authority is central to hierarchical decision making; although the most responsible individual may consult, ask for opinions, or seek advice from others, ultimately in this decision-making model, the final decision rests solely with this person. The advantage of hierarchical decision making is that it can be undertaken rapidly, with a minimal amount of discussion, which of course is also its most significant disadvantage. There are circumstances—for example, in an emergency department or an intensive care unit—where authority-driven hierarchical decision making makes most sense. These are frequently time-pressured and chaotic settings where there is no time for the luxury of collaborative discussion and where impactful decisions must be made quickly and confidently. On the downside, where hierarchical decision making is used in other settings that are more nuanced or linked to psychosocial or emotional needs (e.g., a psychiatric unit), it may be less successful. Some health care professionals have a difficult time functioning in a hierarchical team environment and may bristle at the militaristic style, whereas others may appreciate the clarity it brings to decision making.

Majoritarian: In a majoritarian decision-making model, teams make decisions collectively rather than rely solely on the most responsible or senior members. In such settings, typically each team member gets a single vote, regardless of their position, expertise, or role. When making decisions, the majority rules and dictates actions in a one-person one-vote system. In team-based majoritarian decision making, there is great emphasis on persuasive expertise. Opinions are formed, minds are changed, and decisions ultimately get made through the process of discussion and debate, and those who are most persuasive frequently win. Importantly, majoritarian decision making is NOT democratic decision making, although there may be some superficial similarities. Democratic decision making has important safeguards in place to ensure that 51% of people do not take undue advantage of the remaining 49% by simply claiming majority rules. In a majoritarian system, 51% indeed does rule, and this can lead to suboptimal decisions being made in some instances. At its best, this system is effective at ensuring team members with different perspectives have their voices heard, even if they are eventually unhappy with the outcome. In practice, certain individuals and certain professions may occupy unique power advantages that can be amplified in this model. The veneer of a more inclusive decision-making style may mask the reality that one person or a few people are still really running things. Worse, majoritarian decision making can alienate some team members over time. In health care settings, this model of decision making is becoming more prevalent across diverse settings.

Alliance based: Alliance-based decision making is focused on the principle of reciprocity and involves the principle of trade-offs. In such a model, individuals do not focus on a single immediate decision but instead on a wide array of decisions and behaviors and horse trade with one another to accomplish specific outcomes at the expense of other ones. In this model, temporary alliances (or agreements or partnerships) may form between different individuals so that together (collectively) they can accomplish a mutually desired outcome. Although this can sometimes give the impression of some team members "ganging up" on another team member in order to get their way, alliance-based decision making involves a complex negotiation among members of the alliance as to what each is willing to trade or give up in order to get something else of importance. This model of teamwork is complex and can sometimes lead to political infighting and hurt feelings due to the issue of feeling ganged up on. At its best, alliance-based decision making allows those who are traditionally less powerful or disadvantaged to surface their opinions and voices by first proving their value to a smaller group prior to establishing a team-wide platform. In this way, alliance-based decision making not only allows for a broader array of perspectives and voices to be brought forward and discussed but it actually helps these perspectives to be translated into decisions and behaviors.

Consensual: Consensual decision making is focused on establishing and maintaining team cohesion at all costs. Unlike majoritarian or alliance-based decision making, which risks alienating individuals within a team, consensual decision making prioritizes maintenance of positive working relationships among team members by ensuring no decision gets made unless everyone agrees to it. At its purest, this implies that a single dissenting view means a decision will not be made. The cost of consensual decision making is frequently a high degree of conversation, listening, and communication, which may be exhausting, irritating, or simply unrealistic in some settings. For example, consensual decision making in an emergency department is likely not practical; by definition, many things in an emergency department are in fact emergencies, which require quick decisions and where there is simply not enough time to build consensus. In contrast, some health care settings, particularly unionized workplaces, prioritize consensus building in making decisions (such as a shift scheduling for staff) knowing that failure to build consensus now will only lead to bad feelings, which will undermine team functioning in the future.

Isolative: Particularly within division of labor settings, isolative decision making may predominate. In this model, decisions are not made in a group-based manner, but each individual has a high degree of control regarding decisions based on his or her expertise and specific tasks and responsibilities. Isolative decision making has the advantage of being efficient, but sometimes at the cost of sacrificing the big picture perspective. Where one person's decision has material impacts on the work of another person on the team, this model of isolative decision making, although efficient, may ultimately be ineffective as teams may splinter apart. Isolative decision making is rare in health care settings due to this concern regarding team cohesion and dynamics. Where it is most frequently seen is in highly skilled trades where individual tradespeople have a unique skill set and can be trusted with the responsibility to exercise decision making within the remit of their specific area.

Facilitative: Facilitative decision making attempts to bring together some of the best elements of the previous decision-making models and in the process address some of the deficiencies noted previously. Facilitative processes are most frequently the ideal in primary care settings where patients' complex needs require multiple perspectives and multiple skill sets to coordinate effectively. In this model, there are strong elements of the majoritarian model (in that each team member is given a vote), but there may be deference given to the hierarchical model insofar as the most responsible or senior person's vote may simply carry more weight. The ultimate goal of facilitative decision making is the attempt to balance outcomes with processes to ensure both are respected and valued but that one does not overrule the other.

It is important to remember that these six decision-making styles used by teams are simply descriptive; there is not one style that is inherently superior to another in all cases. Depending on the workplace situation or health care context, one style may be preferred and be more effective. For example, in a time-pressured, crisis-driven health care environment such as emergency medicine, it will be more appropriate to rely on more hierarchical decision making in some (but not all) circumstances because of course not every health care decision and situation in emergency medicine actually IS a crisis. Conversely, although a facilitative or consensual decision-making model might be generally more appropriate in adolescent psychiatry, sometimes hierarchical or majoritarian decision making might be necessary.

The key is for the health care team themselves to possess a broad repertoire of decision-making behaviors and styles that allows them to adapt to an immediate situational need rather than be stuck in a predetermined pattern that may or may not be fit for a specific purpose.

3.4 Clinical Decision Making

Thus far, much of the discussion of teams has focused on the structure and organization of teams and has not addressed any potential differences among individual team members. Although Chapter 2 helped us to reflect on the importance of individual emotional intelligences in shaping interpersonal interactions, there is a unique and important additional layer of individual difference that must be considered in health care teams: clinical reasoning.

Clinical reasoning refers to the methods used by individual practitioners to identify, prioritize, and solve health-related problems faced by patients. Although clinical reasoning will be influenced by individual temperament and emotional intelligence, and may be affected by how teams are structured and how decisions are made, there is strong evidence to suggest the way that individual health care professionals approach clinical problems is very much influenced by the way they were educated and socialized in their profession-specific curricula.

The influence of professional education and socialization on clinical reasoning is significant and, unfortunately, in some cases can be a barrier to effective collaboration among health care professionals who have different ways of approaching and solving clinical problems. Although this is a broad, complex, interesting, and very important area of research in the health professions, for the purposes of this discussion, a simplified model of clinical reasoning will be presented to help support you in better understanding how differences in thinking about patient problems influences team functioning and effectiveness.

3.4.1 Story-Oriented and Problem-Oriented Practitioners

There are important differences in the way health care professionals with different designations and backgrounds approach similar patient-care problems. Two broad categories of clinical reasoning have been identified: *story oriented* and *problem oriented*. Traditionally and historically, physicians (psychiatrists and other medically trained individuals) were thought to approach patient care issues with a problem orientation; in contrast, most other nonmedically oriented health care professionals (nurses, psychologists, rehabilitation professionals, social workers, etc.) were thought to approach the same issues with a story orientation. Today, across all health professions, there has been significant change in the way students are recruited, admitted, and taught, and as a result, these categories and distinctions between different professional designations are far less rigid than in the past.

Problem-oriented professionals see patient care as a series of problems surrounded by a great deal of extraneous information that potentially clouds speedy and accurate access to a solution. For problem-oriented individuals, the goal of clinical reasoning is to reduce the noise—to remove extraneous information, narrow the focus, and use laserlike precision to accurately and specifically focus and target problems in order to identify best possible solutions. This is usually done through a process of rapid questioning, hypothesis generation, hypothesis testing, and elimination of hypotheses that fail such tests in order to narrow one's focus as much as possible.

In contrast, *story-oriented professionals* see problems as embedded within abundant context that is essential to understand in order to truly comprehend the dimensions, depth, and significance of the problem itself. Rather than work to reduce complexity and narrow the focus, story-oriented individuals demonstrate a form of clinical reasoning characterized by actually expanding the definition and scope of the problem broadly, to take in as much information as possible to make as fully informed a decision as possible. Story-oriented professionals generally recognize that their model of practice appears, superficially, to take more time; however, in the long run, considerable time is saved simply because a deeper understanding of a patient's true needs occurs more quickly.

In practice, these differences produce a series of very different clinical behaviors and interactions with patients. Problem-oriented practitioners typically ask patients many questions that have yes or no answers; if the patient starts to tangent toward other issues deemed nonrelevant to the problem at hand, the practitioner will redirect the patient back to a narrower focus to ensure attention is not lost and specificity is not diluted by talking about too many different things. In contrast, the story-oriented practitioner tends to ask fewer questions but those that require patients to speak more and provide more personal information and context; these questions typically do not yield yes or no answers and instead produce subjective impressions and opinions. Story-oriented individuals use this additional information as a vehicle to gain greater insight into problems and understand the patient's perspective in more detail.

There is nothing inherently right or wrong about either approach, although in any specific situation, one approach is likely to be superior to the other. For example, when treating an unconscious patient who is bleeding profusely and trying to understand what happened by speaking to his friend, asking yes or no questions in a focused, problem-oriented manner is probably more appropriate. In contrast, when speaking with a family discussing medical aid in dying (also known as medically assisted death), a story-oriented perspective is likely to be more effective and desired. And of course, few individuals are pure versions of either story- or problem-oriented professionals; each of us is a complex amalgam of both styles.

Generally, health professional education does not necessarily equip students with the skills to effortlessly switch between these different modes of clinical reasoning smoothly and effectively as the context requires. Historically, medical students (and the physicians they eventually became) were rooted in a problem orientation, whereas most other health professional students (and the practitioners they eventually became) were in a story orientation. It was very difficult for anyone educated and socialized in one orientation to simply switch to the other. This reality, of course, helps us to understand why team-based care is so important—we need both problem- and story-oriented individuals to provide care to people based on the specific context of the situation and needs of the patient, and it is difficult for any one individual to do both. Fortunately, today, there is greater understanding of the value of both approaches, and there are concerted attempts by educators to ensure both problem and story orientations are presented to students in all professions to help better prepare them for future clinical practice. Increasingly, curriculum, professional education, or professional designation may matter less than the individual's personal emotional intelligence style; for example, strong convergers and accomodators will be more inclined toward problem orientation, whereas strong divergers are likely more comfortable with a story orientation.

3.4.2 Thinking About Clinical Problems

Cognitive psychologists have identified three dominant modes of clinical reasoning common across health care professionals: reasoning from first principles, application of rules, and pattern recognition. Let's look at each of these in more detail.

Reasoning from first principles: Sometimes referred to as scientific thinking, reasoning from first principles is a form of clinical reasoning that is most frequently seen among novices or early learners in any profession or field. It involves a form of problem solving that values a methodical, systematic approach utilizing current data and foundational scientific principles. To use a non–health care-related example, imagine a novice or inexperienced driver changing lanes while driving on a highway. A more experienced driver may simply do a quick blind spot check, then change lanes. Our novice, inexperienced driver approaches this "problem" as a scientific problem to be solved. They focus all their attention and emotional strength on solving this risky new challenge; they firmly grasp the steering wheel at the 10-and-2 position. Our novice notes the speedometer in the car indicates a velocity of 60 mph. Our driver notes the adjacent car appears to be going somewhat faster, say at 65 mph, and estimates that the adjacent car is approximately 200 feet behind. The driver estimates a minimum of 120 feet of safe distance between his car and the adjacent car is needed to safely execute the lane change. All of this data is plugged into the formula $d = v/t$ and a calculation is made as to whether it is safe, or not, to change lanes.

Wow. Think about how long that previous paragraph took to read, and think of how long it would take if this is what you did every time you changed lanes on a highway. Experienced drivers simply could not function by reasoning from first principles all the time; however, if you reflect back on your own experience as a novice driver, you likely undertook a systematic approach to problem solving similar to this each time you did something new, scary, complicated, and potentially dangerous. The great advantage of clinical reasoning from first principles is that it is methodical, exhaustive, and affords the opportunity for the individual to independently verify a decision prior to implementing it. The great disadvantage of this approach is that it is exceptionally time consuming and inefficient, and gives the impression to others that one is hesitant, indecisive, and lacks confidence.

Application of rules: As novice and inexperienced drivers (and health care practitioners) start to do things over and over again, certain cognitive shortcuts start to emerge that allow for more rapid decision making. The next tier of decision making is referred to as application of rules, and as the label suggests it is a form of clinical reasoning that involves use of an established principle, guideline, algorithm, or rule to solve problems, thereby avoiding the need to do the calculation oneself. Consider another driving example: parallel parking. Many drivers intensely dislike parallel parking, and for some, being a good parallel parker is a badge of honor and a mark of distinction as a driver. Most confident parallel parkers are not actually thinking when they parallel park but instead are simply applying a predigested rule for how to get a car into a tight spot: Pull you car up about 10 feet away from the car you'd like to park behind, line up your rearview mirror with the back tires of that other car, then turn the steering wheel hard, and—presto!—you'll be a great parallel parker. Application of rules has the advantage of being fast and generally resulting in the outcome desired, without the cognitive overload required to constantly think about angles, speeds, and directions. It sometimes gives the illusion of mastery but, because it is a behavior that is rooted in application rather than actual thinking, it can sometimes lead to inappropriate overconfidence. For those readers who consider themselves great drivers and parallel parkers, how confident would you be parallel parking on the other side of the road? Or parallel parking in a congested city like Mumbai or Shanghai? A challenge with reliance on application of rules as a tool for clinical reasoning is that once the context for problem solving has been radically changed, the rule may no longer be applicable and you may have then lost the ability to actually reason it through from first principles.

Pattern recognition: How does an experienced, confident driver—someone who has done this every day for years and years—change lanes on a busy highway? They don't reason from first principles (takes too long and is too exhausting) and they don't apply rules (too many variables on a busy highway to actually have a hard-and-fast rule to apply). Instead, experienced drivers rely on pattern recognition, a system of matching previously encountered experiences to a current problem to arrive at a solution. An experienced and confident driver simply looks at the rearview mirror, does a cursory blind-spot check, and in an instant knows whether it is safe to change lanes. They are not reasoning in the way we traditionally conceptualize that word. Instead, they are instantaneously matching the pattern of cars around them to patterns buffered in their memory from the past, and if it was safe to change lanes then, it is probably safe to change lanes now. So—presto!—lanes are changed with a minimum of fuss, bother, or stress. To the novice or inexperienced driver, pattern recognition such as this looks like magic. The pattern recognizer is confident, speedy, and right 90% of the time (Groopman 2007). Of course, the great downside to pattern recognition as a form of clinical problem solving is that it can sometimes breed overconfidence, can be too speedy, and is only right 90% of the time (Groopman 2007).

In general, most experienced physicians, clinicians, and other professionals will rely heavily on pattern recognition as their dominant mode of clinical reasoning, whereas less experienced practitioners will rely on application of rules or reasoning from first principles. Interestingly, as scopes of practice of practitioners are evolving, particularly in primary care, a curious situation is arising. Take, for example, the experience of pharmacists who in many jurisdictions are now legally able to prescribe medications (rather than simply dispense them). Experienced pharmacists who have dispensed for many years will suddenly become novices when they are initially called on to prescribe. This can produce significant difficulties in practice. Experienced physicians may look at these "experienced" pharmacists who are relying on application of rules or reasoning from first principles in their prescribing work and erroneously think they are slow, lack confidence, and are behaving a bit like third-year medical students rather than coequal practitioners. In turn, these pharmacists may observe the confident pattern recognition demonstrated by physician colleagues and think, "Wow, they must be SO much smarter than me that they can do this so quickly. I can never catch up."

Within a health care team, clinical reasoning is the face we present to our fellow team members of not only our personal competencies but also the capacity of our profession to meaningfully contribute to the care of patients. Differences in modes of clinical reasoning are real and important, but this can sometimes mask a broader issue in collaborative care and teamwork.

It is easy to assume that pattern recognition is the right or best way for health care providers to make clinical decisions because it is confident, it is fast, and it is the way most experienced physicians operate. Unfortunately, this glosses over an important issue. If health care teams only rely on pattern recognition, they are more likely to make mistakes due to overconfidence and lack of reflection. Teams composed of health care providers who use different modes of clinical reasoning—reasoning from first principles, application of rules, as well as pattern recognition—have a broader repertoire of thinking strategies to rely on and can therefore potentially make better and safer decisions, even if on the surface they may appear to be slower and less confident.

Few if any health care professionals can truly and comfortably toggle between these three different types of decision making; instead, as a function of our professional education and socialization, each health care provider is likely to be somewhat stuck as a problem-oriented or story-oriented individual, and as someone who solves problems through pattern recognition OR through application of rules. In some cases, this can be seen as a negative. There are many pharmacists and pharmacy educators who despair at the slowness and seeming indecisiveness of pharmacists as prescribers and want to say, "Don't just stand there. Do something! Make a decision, stop just deliberating and weighing options!" This approach disproportionately and inappropriately values physician-oriented and problem-oriented pattern recognition, and diminishes the value of reasoning from first principles and application of rules with respect to making more thoughtful and safer evidence-based decisions. Perhaps instead of saying, "Don't just stand there. Do something!" to story-oriented individuals, we should be equally saying, "Don't just do something. Stand there!" to problem-oriented individuals who could benefit from some of the more deliberative modes of clinical reasoning other practitioners are more likely to utilize.

3.5 What Does This Mean for Health Care Team Functioning?

Health care professionals are generally smart, nice, well-intentioned people. They selected this line of work because they have a genuine desire to help others, not because they hoped for great power or influence. We naturally assume that when a group of individuals—each of whom is smart, nice, and well intentioned—assemble into something called a team that this means they should all get along well and be productive and happy together. As we've seen, however, there are some significant differences between individuals and among professions that can make teamwork challenging, particularly if structures and decision-making processes are unclear or not aligned with individuals' expectations. The psychological implications of these differences are important to understand because they directly influence communication, collaboration, and job satisfaction in health care teams.

Trust is defined as a firm belief in the reliability, truth, ability, or strength of someone or something. Trust is essential to the functioning of society. You trust that your teachers, your parents, your managers, and your textbook authors are telling you the truth, so you rely on this trust in order to undertake your daily activities. We trust road engineers who have designed highways, and as a result, we drive on these roads designed by complete strangers. Citizens must trust their governments; otherwise, there will be a breakdown of law, order, civility, and ultimately society as a whole. Similarly, individuals who work together on a health care team must trust one another to ensure day-to-day work can proceed. This means a physician must trust that the medication history completed by a pharmacist and the blood pressure taken by a nurse are accurate; otherwise, the physician would have to redo all this work. The pharmacist must trust that the physician has thoroughly assessed a patient and prescribed an appropriate medication. The physical therapist must trust the work of the medical laboratory technologist who is reporting laboratory findings. Without trust in one another, each health professional would need to constantly redo everyone else's work, and this would be inefficient and, frankly, impossible. As we have seen, however, this optimistic view of professionals simply automatically trusting one another when they are put together in a team may not always be the case. Research suggests the cognitive model of trust for physicians, some advanced practice nurse practitioners, and clinical specialists in other professions may be different than for other professionals. Story-oriented practitioners appear to have a cognitive model of trust that is shaped by externalities. If they are introduced to a person who is a doctor, who has won an award, who has written a book, or who has an impressive job title, these story-oriented practitioners are likely to automatically (or implicitly) trust them. In contrast, problem-oriented professionals—like physicians—are more influenced by personal history and relationships. They will trust other practitioners who have a track record of success and have already proven themselves personally. Rather than be impressed by a degree or title, they may ask, "What have you done to prove yourself to me that I can trust you?"

Although there is nothing inherently superior with either mental model of trust, it raises a problem in teams. If one practitioner (e.g., a pharmacist) gives trust freely based on title and degree, and another practitioner (e.g., a physician) can only trust after the pharmacist has proven himself to her, this introduces a major asymmetry in the relationship. One person gives trust; the other person needs to earn trust. To the pharmacist in this example, this feels unfair; this feels like the physician thinks she is better than everyone else, this feels like she doesn't respect me the way I respect her. As a result, it can lead to hurt or hard feelings among colleagues before they have even really started working together. At the base of this problem is the simple reality that different people have different mental models for what constitutes trust, but is it interpreted through an emotional filter that can produce barriers to collaboration among colleagues.

Communication is described as the exchanging of information. Interestingly, the psychological differences among health care professionals can influence the way they speak with and to one another. In a well-intentioned (but perhaps misdirected) attempt to be polite, respectful, and deferential to authority, story-oriented individuals frequently communicate indirectly. Rather than simply get to the point and say, "I think you made a mistake," they may say, "I was reviewing this chart note and saw something new, and as I wasn't sure, I thought I should do a little bit of further research on this. This intervention that was documented in the chart was quite unusual and I'm wondering if we might be able to discuss it further, just so I can understand it?" This long-winded way of saying, "I think you made a mistake" actually sends important subconscious signals relating to power, prestige, and hierarchy in a profession. If a nurse colleague feels he cannot say to a physician colleague "I think you made a mistake," it suggests the nurse may feel subconsciously or psychologically subordinate to the physician. If that is the case, the physician may subconsciously or psychologically think "If you are so circuitous in your speaking, maybe you aren't as confident or certain in what you're saying as I am, so why should I bother listening to you?" Of course, there is a world of difference between saying, "I think you made a mistake" and "Hey, dufus, you screwed up." Some may prefer to say, "I'm wondering if a mistake was made" rather than "You made a mistake." There are more polite and less polite ways of making a direct statement, but the important point here is that when we use too many words to say something relatively simple, it may suggest to other health care team members that we are lacking confidence in our own opinion. And if we lack confidence, why should they believe what we are saying?

Responsibility is defined as the state or fact of having a duty to deal with something, of being accountable, or to blame. All health care professionals think they are responsible people. Owing to differences among health care team members we have discussed here and in Chapter 2, it appears that there are substantial differences in the mental model of the word *responsibility* between problem-oriented and story-oriented professionals. For story-oriented health professionals, responsibility is about doing everything possible within the rules and being respectful of processes, but to break the rules or consciously disregard the processes is not only irresponsible, it is dangerous. In contrast, problem-oriented individuals may believe that responsibility means putting one's own neck on the line to break a rule when it is absolutely necessary to solve a problem. A good example of this different vision of responsibility may occur in the context of so-called off-label prescribing. Off-label prescribing occurs when a prescriber (usually a physician) prescribes a medication in a way that is not officially recognized. It is sometimes necessary to do because traditional prescribing guidelines simply have not worked for a patient and there is a need to go beyond these guidelines. Appropriate off-label prescribing is not uncommon and must always be based on some kind of evidence; prescribers do not simply make stuff up and invent new protocols or doses, but they will base off-label prescribing decisions on small trials, N-of-1 case studies, or other evidence that is not as strong or robust as a clinical trial but nonetheless provides some insight into a difficult problem. Off-label prescribing can be enormously stressful for pharmacists and nurses who are clinically trained and have a strong need to follow guidelines and algorithms. Exceeding guideline doses of medications puts these story-oriented individuals in a gray zone where they may feel very uncomfortable implementing a physician's prescription. To them, responsibility may mean "We follow the rules, we follow the guidelines," but to the physician, responsibility may mean "But we tried following the guidelines and it didn't work, so we have to try something new." Trying something new does not always succeed or work out as hoped, and this is exactly the sticking point for disagreement within a health care team. It is rooted in having different mental models for what it means to be responsible in a specific situation.

Self-confidence is defined as assurance or belief in oneself and one's abilities. For story-oriented individuals, clinical confidence means certainty in having the RIGHT answer: I will speak, I will suggest, and I will recommend only if I'm certain I know the best thing to do; otherwise, I'll keep my mouth shut. How can this be wrong? In contrast, problem-oriented individuals do not necessarily believe they are always right or always know everything, but they have a psychological bias toward action rather than deliberation. Consequently, they have a kind of serenity in believing that if (or when) what they think is best goes wrong, they will find a way of coping and dealing with it at the time. In a team context, this means that sometimes problem-oriented individuals may give the appearance of always wanting to try new things and pressuring others to "Don't just stand there. Do something!" In contrast, story-oriented individuals may give the appearance of being overly cautious and excessively careful to the point of never wanting to take any kind of risk (i.e., "Don't just do something. Stand there!"). Of course, depending on the specific circumstance, both perspectives can be right and both perspectives can be wrong. The issue in collaborative teams is that problem-oriented and story-oriented individuals get locked into one pattern and cannot demonstrate sufficient flexibility to acknowledge that sometimes, another team member's perspective is the best one in a particular case.

As highlighted, team functioning and team dynamics are complicated. Simply putting a group of smart, nice, well-intentioned people together and calling them a health care tem does not automatically mean they will get along and work well together. There are significant individual and profession-specific differences and these can influence team functioning in foundational ways involving trust, communication, responsibility, and self-confidence. There are no easy or immediate fixes for these differences. A first important step, however, is awareness that these differences exist, that they are real, and for each team member to not take it personally when this difference causes disagreement. If story-oriented individuals can anticipate that they will need to earn the trust of their problem-oriented colleagues, perhaps they will not experience hurt feelings when trust is not given freely. Problem-oriented individuals should anticipate that their story-oriented colleagues are going to be less than enthusiastic, uncomfortable, and question their judgment when they engage in activities like off-label prescribing. Perhaps then they will not feel as frustrated and annoyed by the risk-averse colleagues on their team, and instead recognize the value they bring by carefully questioning decisions to help prevent errors from occurring. Understanding and anticipating how these differences will play out in an interprofessional setting is crucial to help prevent small issues from becoming big problems.

3.6   The Development of a Collaborative Health Care Team

It is not necessarily easy or natural for health care teams to form and function. In many cases, different people are simply thrown together as a team because of workplace circumstances, not because of any particular desire to work with one another as individuals. Large employers such as hospitals or health systems may rarely consider issues of individual temperament or compatibility when assembling teams, and instead expect that everyone is a professional and can therefore just figure out how to make it work.

The literature on team development has pointed to a process by which individuals learn how to work with one another in a collaborative manner within a team structure. These stages of team development include the following.

Forming: When people first are assigned to teams, they may have a variety of different baseline thoughts and expectations. Some people may look forward to it, some people may resent it, others may think everyone thinks like they do, others may expect conflict and disagreement all the time. During this first phase of team development, individual team members must negotiate roles and responsibilities and jointly figure out what the culture of the team will become, such as what unwritten rules will govern their day-to-day interactions. The forming stage of team development is usually helped by social interactions and more informal and less work-related discussions so individuals can get to know each other as people first, to establish a foundation for future professional friendships and relationships. Learning about each other within a low-stakes, low-stress environment first facilitates formation of social relationships and communication patterns that will ultimately be tested in future stages of the process.

Storming: Eventually, the low-stakes, low-stress environment of team formation must give way to real-world performance, and this can lead to some initial disagreements and distress within a team. Storming is the process of testing the boundaries and limits of the team structures established during the forming stage when things were safe and less stressful. Storming is an essential part of team formation because it is the point at which real-world environmental constraints help each team member observe how everyone performs. Storming will often lead to conflict and disagreement, but ultimately it is necessary to help renegotiate team culture, hierarchies, and dynamics in light of real-world experiences.

Norming: After storming and renegotiation, there will likely follow a period of time when team members start to become comfortable in their revised roles and responsibilities. During this norming phase, ongoing adaptations will of course be necessary, but there is a growing comfort in working collaboratively based on a firmer foundation of relationships among team members. During this phase, individuals may experience less conflict and disagreement and feel more enjoyment and satisfaction in working collaboratively with others.

Performing: Through the norming phase, the team is solidifying its collaborative culture, leading the way to peak performance and success. In the performing stage, the team is functioning at optimal effectiveness and efficiency as they have managed to deal with the cultural, communication, and collaborative issues that potentially held them back in the past. High-performing teams not only like working with one another, but they also achieve outcomes that surpass the sum of any individual accomplishments.

Adjourning: Of course, in any group, there will be times when individual group members must leave (e.g., they retire, get new jobs, take parental leaves) or when the entire team must disband because the job they were to complete is now finished. When teams are performing, individuals have made both professional and personal commitments to one another, and the relationships that form in such teams are powerful and important. You may have heard the term *work wife* or *work husband* used to describe people on a team who work so closely with one another that they spend more time together as a team than they do with their own families. When such teams disband, there is a powerful, personal, and emotional loss that may be experienced. In adjourning, it is necessary to find ways of managing this personal relationship loss, which for some people can be similar to the feeling of watching their own child grow up and move out of the house, or grieving the loss of a loved one. Failure to effectively manage the adjourning process may make it difficult for team members to trust themselves to form strong work bonds again in the future for fear of the emotional loss associated with the inevitable end of a work-based team.

This five-stage model for team development is not perfect or universally applicable, but it helps to provide a framework for understanding how health care teams develop and what to expect. There is no strict timeline associated with each stage, nor do all teams successfully navigate all five stages. In some cases, teams never make it past storming, whereas in others, it may take months or years to achieve performing. Each team is as different as the individuals who constitute that team, but for all teams, attention must be paid to the process of team development in order to help them reach their best potential.

3.7 **Summary**

Teams are complex, ever-changing entities and understanding the complex psychological dynamics of team functioning is essential to unleash their true potential. The structure of a team will directly influence its functioning and, in particular, the style of decision making that is utilized. Building on our understanding of individual emotional intelligence and its influence in shaping our social and interpersonal interactions, insights into profession-specific clinical reasoning can help us to understand and better appreciate the differences among team members in the way they approach patient-care problems. Rather than seek a team where everyone thinks the same, there is great value in having not only a diversity of professional backgrounds but a range of different thinking strategies that can be applied to clinical problems to ensure that the optimal and safest alternatives are selected that will best help patients manage their health-related needs.

3.8   Mind Map Chapter 3

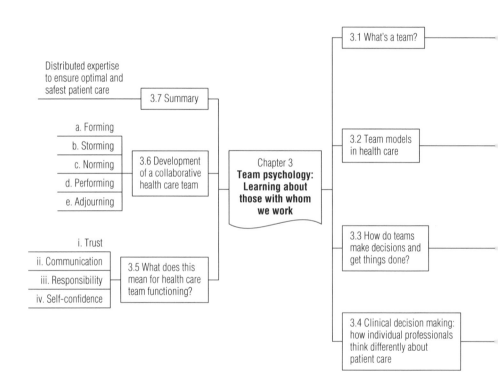

Mind Map for Team Psychology

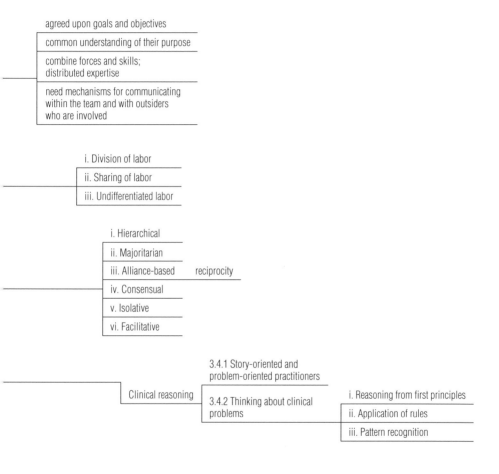

agreed upon goals and objectives

common understanding of their purpose

combine forces and skills;
distributed expertise

need mechanisms for communicating
within the team and with outsiders
who are involved

i. Division of labor

ii. Sharing of labor

iii. Undifferentiated labor

i. Hierarchical

ii. Majoritarian

iii. Alliance-based   reciprocity

iv. Consensual

v. Isolative

vi. Facilitative

Clinical reasoning

3.4.1 Story-oriented and
problem-oriented practitioners

3.4.2 Thinking about clinical
problems

i. Reasoning from first principles

ii. Application of rules

iii. Pattern recognition

For Further Reading:

Bendaly L, Bendaly N. *Improving Healthcare Team Performance: The 7 Requirements for Excellence in Patient Care*. Ontario, Canada: John Wiley & Sons; 2012.

Clarke P, Drinka T. *Health Care Teamwork: Interdisciplinary Practice and Teaching*. Westport, CT: Praeger; 2000.

Gordon S, Mendenhall P, O'Toole B, Sullenberg C. *Beyond the Checklist: What Else Health Care Can Learn From Aviation Teamwork and Safety*. Ithaca, NY: Cornell University Press; 2013.

Groopman J. *How Doctors Think*. Boston, MA: Houghton Mifflin; 2007.

Lake D, Baerg K, Paslawski T. *Teamwork, Leadership, and Communication: Collaboration Basics for Health Professionals*. Canada: Brush Education, Inc.; 2015.

Mosser G, Begun J. *Understanding Teamwork in Health Care*. New York: McGraw-Hill Education; 2014.

Reeves S, Lewin S, Espin S, Zwarenstein M. *Interprofessional Teamwork for Health and Social Care*. Oxford: Wiley-Blackwell; 2010.

Those We Serve: Patients, Clients, Customers, and Consumers

"What do these people want from me?"

At some point, every health professional will ask this question. There will be situations where the advice you provide will be disregarded or challenged, where the well-intentioned support you provide will be rebuffed, or the day-to-day pressures of your job will go unrecognized by those you serve. In such situations, it is quite natural to feel exasperated, frustrated, and perhaps even wonder whether health care work is the right job for you.

Regardless of your professional designation, degree, or background, the primary responsibility of any health professional is to serve and care for individuals, their families, and communities. The specific tasks each health professional undertakes is a function of their legal scope of practice, the knowledge and skills acquired during education and training, and workplace expectations. Beyond these tasks, however, each professional must consistently demonstrate the ability to care for others and care about the quality of the work being performed.

Health care work is, at its most basic, interpersonal in nature. Although some health professionals may spend much of their professional life working with electronic data or diagnostic equipment (e.g., radiologists, medical laboratory technicians), all health care professionals are required to communicate effectively and interact appropriately with different individuals. Success as a health care professional is, therefore, closely associated with success in managing interpersonal interactions. This can be particularly challenging and complicated, of course, because when people seek out health care professionals, they are frequently "not at their best." They may be ill, worried about being ill, or dealing with a variety of physical and psychological consequences associated with their health that may make it difficult for them to be understanding, lucid, or cooperative. As health care professionals, therefore, it is important to have an awareness of the complexities associated with human emotional responses as a way of better understanding and accepting the strong and sometimes negative reactions we encounter in day-to-day practice.

4.1   The Complexity of Human Beings

Each of us as human beings is aware of how complicated our thinking and emotions can become, particularly in times of difficulty or stress. We sometimes express astonishment—and sometimes outright disdain—at the seemingly contradictory behaviors demonstrated by some people. Why do those who are at highest risk for illness continue to smoke? (Shouldn't they know better?) Why do those who are the most financially impoverished continue to gamble at casinos or play the lottery? (Don't they know the odds, and shouldn't they save their money instead of wasting it this way?) Despite years of education and public health advertisements, why do people still engage in reckless and dangerous sexual behaviors such as unprotected intercourse? (What's wrong with them?)

The reality, of course, is that human beings are complicated, messy, and sometimes contradictory in their behaviors. Knowing what is the right thing to do does not necessarily translate into the best and most sensible actions. Increasingly, psychologists are explaining these seemingly self-destructive behaviors in terms of emotional rather than logical responses to the environment.

Since the earliest days, philosophers have been struck by the choices, behaviors, and motivations of human beings. Early philosophers recognized an important duality in all human beings—the constant, internal tug-of-war we experience between emotions and logic, between thinking and feeling. These early philosophers believed that our cognitive selves—the part of us that is focused on rational thinking and logic—was in an unending battle with our emotional selves, that part of us focused on immediate gratification and instantaneous emotional fulfillment. For centuries, the solution to this internal battle that plagues each of us was to simply ensure that the logical side won. Philosophers, psychologists, and other health care professionals worked very hard to encourage human beings to ensure they controlled their feelings, managed their emotions, and suppressed the impulses that lead to self-destructive or indulgent behaviors. The main tool for this control and management of emotion was through logic, reason, and thinking. To this day, the legacy of this approach continues in health professions' education. Every health care student, from their earliest days in school, will be told to be professional or to check your emotions at the door rather than allow your personal feelings to influence thinking or behavior.

In more recent times, psychologists' understanding of the human condition has evolved considerably. Rather than believing that thinking and feeling are two separate and distinct aspects of human psychology, there is growing awareness that our cognitive and emotional selves are much more closely interconnected than many of us would like to believe. Instead, emotions are actually the primary filter through which humans experience the world, and it is only through this emotional filter that logic, thinking, and reason can function.

4.1.2   How We Interpret Our World

In the past, it was believed that human beings made conscious and subconscious choices and decisions every moment of every day. Do I respond to what I see or hear in a logical, rational way, or do I respond to it in an emotional, feeling (and therefore illogical or irrational) way? The reality of human experience is, however, very different.

Humans experience the world through our senses—sight, sound, smell, taste, and touch. These five senses are the gateway through which we interact with our world and in turn interpret everything around us. A rudimentary understanding of the central nervous system helps us to understand an important reality. All of the sensory inputs we receive are processed through a central nervous system that is hardwired to first run through the emotional centers of our brain. It is only later in the sensory transmission process that higher order, cognitive centers of the brain are engaged. Human beings, it appears, are literally hardwired to feel before they think, to emote before they reason.

Emotions and our emotional selves, therefore, form the primary filter through which we experience everything. If we are happy and relaxed, we will literally see and hear things differently than if we are anxious and fearful. Our central nervous systems from a kind of protective barrier to the outside world, and our emotions forcefully filter out certain sensory inputs and similarly forcefully emphasize others. Thus, it is not actually possible for logic to control feelings or for thinking to manage emotions. Increasingly, there is an understanding that the process works the other way around, that our emotional state governs our thinking and our feelings dictate how logical we can be in any given circumstance.

4.1.3 Our Emotional Selves

Given the central role of emotions in governing human cognition, it behooves us not to ignore or suppress emotional responses, but rather to try to better understand them and their influence on our behavior. The field of personality psychology has made tremendous advances in helping to describe this complex interplay between feeling and thinking, but much more work is required before any definitive models can be confidently described.

As best as we currently understand, psychologists have named six core emotions that appear to be universal and hardwired into all human beings from birth. Before we can even lift our own heads or roll over on our own, human infants have already experienced powerful emotions that will be central to their experiences for the rest of their lives. These six core emotions are joy, sadness, fear, anger, disgust, and surprise. There is no need to further explain or define these emotions. Every reader of this book will have already experienced these emotions over and over again in day-to-day life.

It is intriguing to speculate on why four (perhaps five) of these six core emotions are feelings we traditionally think of as negative. If we are only hardwired with six core emotions, why are there a disproportionate number of them such as sadness, fear, anger, and disgust? Evolutionary psychologists have hypothesized that these strong, seemingly negative emotions are crucial for survival—they actually help protect us from a world where dangers (ranging from toxic plants that trigger disgust to monsters under the bed that stimulate fear) abound. From this perspective, these emotions are not negative; they are actually helpful and have allowed us to survive as a species.

Although environmental threats to our survival as infants are more or less managed by caring and doting parents who protect and nurture us, why do these negative emotions still persist? In today's more sheltered world, these negative emotions serve another very important function. They help infants (who cannot speak and who cannot yet think) to signal to parents when something is wrong, giving those parents the opportunity to sort out the situation.

Psychologists generally believe that thinking, logic, and reason (as we understand those terms) only occur as language starts to be acquired. Without language, human cognition does not really exist. As we all know, children do not begin to verbally articulate language until several years after they are born, and even then it can take many years before a vocabulary necessary to support complex thinking and reasoning can be developed. During this time, it is our core emotions that keep us safe, help us communicate, and allow us to interpret and interact with our world.

Emotions, therefore, are the primary filter through which we experience human interactions. Reflect on your own experiences. There may be certain teachers you have had who you liked, who you found funny or charming, and with whom you felt connected. You may have had no particular interest in the subject they teach, but the subjective, emotional experience of liking a teacher makes it easier for you to learn the subject (i.e., engage your rational, logical, thinking self). Conversely, there may be a politician whom you strenuously dislike. The simple sight of his or her face and the tone of voice completely disgusts you. This primary emotional filter of disgust (or anger) literally makes it impossible for you to hear what is being said let alone cognitively or logically manage that politician's arguments. In this case, the emotional filter serves as a wall or barrier, preventing calm, logical, reasoned thinking.

Of course, the story of our emotional selves becomes further complicated with time. From the six foundational core emotions, other emotions and the full array of different feelings human beings experience are derived, including emotions such as regret, loss, and gratitude. Learning to accurately identify and name emotions is an essential skill for self-management, and each person's capacity to do this increases as vocabulary and language skills evolve with time and with age. Many parents of young children intuitively understand this important concept. You will frequently hear parents encourage their child to "use your words" to describe the emotion the child is feeling, instead of simply acting on it. Importantly, the ability to name an emotion and use language to convey a feeling signifies an important developmental hallmark. Rather than simply feel anger and deal with it by punching something (or someone), engaging one's cognitive self by articulating "I feel angry" is the first step in helping to productively and appropriately manage it. With time, this interplay between thinking, use of language, and emotional experience is one of the most valuable life skills any human being can develop, and it allows that person to interact effectively with other human beings rather than simply act on emotional impulses. Although it may appear that this reflects the triumph of logic over feeling (or thinking over emotion), this is not entirely correct. Instead, by using words to express emotions (rather than violent actions), it opens up the possibility of other people similarly using words to express their emotions, which in turn can lead to a resolution rather than a fight. The emotions are still there and are strong, but with language and vocabulary, other options are now available to manage difficult situations in a more socially appropriate manner.

If this discussion of emotions strikes you as tiring and overly complicated, with time, it gets even more complicated! As our cognitive selves evolve—and in particular our language skills and vocabulary—so too do our emotional selves. Human beings begin to experience not simply a single predictable emotional response to a given situation, but we start to develop strangely and sometimes paradoxically contrary multiple emotional responses, and in particular, emotions that seem to contradict one another. Consider a parent attending the wedding of a much beloved child. In most cases, this event would trigger the emotion of happy-sadness. On the one hand, there may be great joy that the child has found immense love (particularly if the parent agrees with the child's choice of spouse); on the other hand, no matter how wonderful this spouse may be, most parents will feel sadness (or regret or melancholy) knowing their child has grown up and is launching on to his or her own life now. Similarly, despite the clichéd tropes found in most Hollywood movies, most long-married couples experience an emotional state best described as regretful-grateful after many years together. On the one hand, they are very grateful (or happy) about what a long and successful marriage represents; still, no matter how happy most couples are, most will also harbor some regret about missed opportunities or seemingly long-forgotten grievances.

At this point, where contradictory emotions simultaneously coexist, it is challenging for the English language and our vocabulary to manage such complexity. There is no word in English that means "happy-sad" or "regretful-grateful," and without a word to capture this emotional concept, it becomes cognitively very challenging to actually interpret, analyze, process, and manage such complex emotional responses. This is not a limitation of the English language; most languages (French, Spanish, Mandarin, Urdu, etc.) have similar limitations. Certain languages (including German and Scandinavian languages such as Norwegian) do have the ability to describe complex hybridized emotions through concatenation; for example, the German word *schadenfreude* describes the strange pleasure you may feel at witnessing a friend's misfortune. The inherent contradiction in experiencing joy at another person's sadness has a specific word in the German language, but no such equivalent exists in English. By having a word to describe such complex feelings, opportunities emerge to better manage and deal with such contradictory emotions—for German speakers or for those who can find a way to express it similarly in the language they speak.

Importantly, our emotions appear to engage before our logic; despite what you may believe (or want to believe), or what Ancient Greek philosophers have said, logic cannot be used to control emotion. Instead, emotion is the gatekeeper to thinking, and recognizing this reality is essential for health care professionals working with patients.

4.2   Applying the Psychology of Emotions to Your Professional Practice

As outlined in Section 4.1, human beings are complex and must be understood in terms of both emotions and logic. Perhaps then it should not be a surprise to us when we tell a patient to stop smoking because of the life-reducing risk factors associated with nicotine and that patient nods and agrees with us, but just keeps on smoking. In this particular example, you could argue this behavior occurs because of the powerful addictive properties of nicotine; however, there are abundant other examples of how well-intentioned, highly logical reasons to change behaviors appear to go unheeded. Why, after decades of public health advertising, do more and more young people engage in risky unprotected sex despite the known risks of sexually transmitted diseases? Put plainly and bluntly, because for many young people, the emotional satisfaction of sexual intimacy co-opts any logical, reasonable, or sensible thoughts about protection. Why, after decades of education, do so many middle-aged people (many of them well-educated and who should know better) still make poor dietary choices and carry excessive weight? Again, put plainly and bluntly, because for many middle-aged people the emotional satisfaction associated with a tub of ice cream or a perfectly grilled steak or a stack of bacon for breakfast inhibits thinking.

4.2.1   The Truth About the Truth

Regardless of your field, degree, or specialization, you as a health care professional will spend a considerable amount of your professional lifetime telling people to change their behavior. You will ask them to quit smoking, or lose weight, or use condoms. You will instruct them to take a certain medication three times a day, without food but with a full glass of water, for 10 days in a row without missing a dose, regardless of how disruptive this is to their day-to-day lives and routines. You will provide them with a routine of exercise designed to strengthen failing muscles and connective tissue, knowing that this routine will, over time, help to build strength and mobility and ultimately result in a higher quality of life, only to see these patients lose interest and stop.

For many young practitioners in every profession, the first few years of practice can be extremely frustrating and disheartening. Despite the optimistic (perhaps unrealistic?) rhetoric we've heard in school about the positive difference we will make in the world and in our communities, many young professionals experience disenchantment and disappointment early in their careers because no one seems to listen to what they have to say. Despite having years of university or college education and knowing what is the right thing to do, why do people still disregard our advice and do things that are actually harmful?

Most practitioners have unquestioned faith in the scientific underpinnings of their profession. We believe microbes cause disease; antibiotics can help but vaccines can actually prevent many diseases, yet a large and growing proportion of the population doesn't believe in them and therefore deprives their children of these potentially lifesaving medical interventions. When patients reject the truths we believe, we may respond by rejecting the patients themselves and thinking less of them, rather than trying to look for different ways of conveying these truths to patients that are more successful than simply telling them what to do.

It is sometimes easy for scientifically trained health professionals to forget that truth is a logical construct based on reason, thinking, and cognition. Truth is not rooted in emotion, and consequently, what we may perceive to be truth can easily be filtered out through the emotional sieve that influences our behaviors. Trying to fight the battle between cognition and emotion using data, facts, and logic may often be frustrating and pointless. Worse, health professionals sometimes grow fatigued or cynical, and start to experience their own emotional responses to patients who don't listen to them, sometimes labeling them in a highly uncharitable or insulting manner and then simply giving up trying to convince them to change.

In Chapters 5 and 6, we will discuss how this understanding of human psychology, and in particular the complex interplay between cognition and emotion, can be applied to use effective communication techniques and strategies with the aim of improving health care outcomes for patients and job satisfaction for health care professionals.

4.3   Different People at Different Times Need Different Things From You

Who are these people for whom we care? Traditionally, health professionals have referred to them as patients, but increasingly, other terms are being used, such as *clients*, *customers*, or in some cases *consumers*. These different terms are not simply a matter of labeling convenience; they are important distinctions about the different kinds of individuals who seek out the service of health professionals. Equally important, they reflect the reality that the same individual will have different levels of need and different expectations for care and service depending on the specific condition and context.

It is essential that health professionals recognize that not all individuals who seek service or care need, expect, or want the same things; that individuals, over the course of their lifetime, will require different levels of service and care; and the importance of accurately assessing and identifying what levels of care and service are needed and desired, and responding in an appropriate way.

There are many different models that have been proposed to help health professionals more accurately assess and identify what levels of care are wanted and needed by specific individuals. Such models are sometimes referred to as *taxonomies*. Taxonomies are intended as practical guides and can help match a health professional's responses more appropriately to a person's needs. A convenient and widely used taxonomy in the pharmacy profession suggests that there are four different levels of need in health care that point to varying responses that are expected from professionals:

Patients: Traditionally and historically, the term *patient* has been widely used in health professions' education to denote a very specific kind of relationship between professionals and those they serve. The term *patient* has been the foundation of much sociological research examining, for example, the patient role or the patient voice, and has been the basis of a model of care delivery referred to as patient-centered care. What exactly is a patient, and what do patients want, need, and expect, and what can health professionals do to most appropriately address these wants, needs, and expectations?

Traditionally, the term *patient* has been used in a way that implies an important asymmetry between individuals. Patients seek the expertise and care of health professionals because they are needful, less qualified, and as a result, vulnerable. The word *patient* has multiple meanings in the English language: It is used in health care to refer to a person who has needs (as in "Mohammed is a cardiac patient"), but it is also an adjective that describes someone who has little choice but to wait, who is uncomplaining, and who demonstrates a degree of long-suffering behavior (as in "Mohammed is a patient person but will eventually get the rewards he deserves"). The sociologist Talcott Parsons famously described the sick role: It is a socially accepted position in which someone who is ill (as defined medically) is exempted from certain activities (work, socializing, other responsibilities of day-to-day life), and in turn, must accept certain new tasks (e.g., doing what he is told by medical professionals, trying to get better) in order to maintain the title of patient.

When people feel as though they are patients, it is most frequently linked to the belief they have an illness or a sickness that cannot be managed on their own. The sense of dependency on others to provide instruction, support, interventions, and care to help the person move from illness to wellness is a crucial feature of the patient role. As a result, those who are patients may feel a unique and, in many cases, somewhat unpleasant sense of vulnerability to others—such as health professionals—who have more knowledge, greater skill, and more power than they do.

Not everyone who seeks out a health professional is a patient of course, but when someone is in the patient role, it is essential and an ethical imperative that these professionals discharge their responsibilities carefully. For example, a person who is undergoing surgery is very likely to feel like a patient. He is vulnerable, other people are doing things to his body, he will be unconscious for much of the procedure, and the technical and scientific basis of these things being done to him are likely beyond his knowledge base and skill set. He may feel he has no choice but to comply with everything these professionals are telling him for fear they may stop trying to help him or, worse, take advantage or punish him when he is unconscious. The vulnerability associated with the patient role introduces extraordinarily important ethical obligations on health professionals that are usually described in depth in each profession's code of ethics.

The experience of being a patient is strongly rooted in the emotional, rather than in the cognitive. Most frequently, patients feel they are ill, and this emotional experience can provoke a variety of simultaneous responses ranging from fear to anger to despair, or all three simultaneously. When these emotional filters are in place, patients will literally see what you do and hear what you say in different ways than you may intend. With such strong emotional filters in place, there may be a very limited role for facts, truths, or other cognitively oriented techniques to get people to change their behavior. Instead, it may become more important to actively engage with the emotional filters themselves. Rather than tell patients to be brave or to pull themselves up by their bootstraps, alternative forms of communication that allow for the expression and discussion of emotions as a first step may be required.

Who is a patient? Of course it can be anybody, but in most cases, the psychological experience of being a patient is usually linked to a subjective sense of uncertainty, lack of confidence, and fear. For example, a healthy 21-year-old college student receiving a prescription for an oral contraceptive may not see herself as a patient at all. She is healthy, many of her friends have been using contraceptives for several years with no problems, and for her, it is simply the reasonable, responsible, and totally typical thing to do at her age and stage of life. She has no emotional response to this decision; there is no fear, anger, or uncertainty she is experiencing. Treating this person as a patient would be inappropriate. However, if that same 21-year-old college student was receiving an oral contraceptive to treat an ovarian cyst of unknown origin, one that may or may not be cancerous, the same person receiving the same medication but in a different situation may feel very afraid and uncertain about her future. She may (or may not) want and expect to be treated as a patient and be assured both her medical and emotional and psychosocial needs are attended to adequately.

Clients: In some professions, all those who are served are routinely referred to as clients rather than patients, regardless of the complexity or intensity of their emotional and psychosocial needs. Traditionally, in the professions, clients have been those served by lawyers, accountants, or real estate agents rather than health practitioners. Today, and in particular with the easy availability of all information through the Internet, the client role in health care is emerging as a more important one.

The term *client* suggests a greater level of equality and a smaller power differential with the practitioner. Patients need or rely on practitioners, whereas clients select or choose. Of course, although clients may have complex psychosocial needs, the emotional component of these needs may not be as intense or overwhelming as for patients. Those with a client orientation gain comfort and strength from perceiving they have choices and control, which represents a source of power and self-confidence. Although a patient may feel they have no choice but to meekly comply with whatever a practitioner says for fear the practitioner may be disappointed in or fire him if he asks too many questions, a client will feel a level of self-confidence where they will freely ask questions and, if they don't get the answers they want or expect, they will be disappointed in the practitioner and may in fact fire him! Patients may perceive they have limited choices, whereas clients may perceive they have abundant options.

In some professions (e.g., social work, nursing), there is an ongoing debate as to whether practitioners have a duty to not only treat patients as clients, but also to support those in a patient role or with a patient orientation to shift toward a more empowered and confident client role. Some argue that the potential for abuse of authority and position with patient's demands that professionals relinquish their power and instead facilitate enhancement of client self-awareness and self-confidence.

The client–practitioner relationship may demonstrate different dynamics than the patient–practitioner relationship. For example, patients may refer to physicians as Dr. Jones, whereas clients may use the first name and refer to her as Sally instead, emphasizing their equality rather than a power difference. Clients typically ask more questions, seek alternative opinions and options, and have a level of health literacy and Internet savvy that allows them to double check claims made by practitioners. For example, a healthy and vigorous 21-year-old sexually active college student seeking oral contraceptives may not perceive her need as being medical in any way. She is not ill and, therefore, is not a patient. She is, however, a client of health services and will actively seek out practitioners she likes and who she connects with and will, without any hesitation, walk away from those she dislikes. So, if a well-meaning but paternalistic physician makes a comment such as, "But you're not married, are you sure you should be sexually active so young?" this client may rightly become offended and take her business elsewhere. To be clear, this individual still needs to secure contraceptives—prescribed by a physician, nurse, or pharmacist—and she cannot (in most jurisdictions) simply stop at a convenience store on her way home and pick up a package or two. However, she is not a patient requiring emotional support; she is a client expecting service, and it is incumbent upon health practitioners to recognize and acknowledge this important distinction.

Customers: Increasingly, with the widespread availability of virtually all medical information on the Internet, and with increasing accessibility to products such as laboratory tests and medications without need for a prescription from a physician, many people seeking health care think, feel, and behave like customers rather than clients or patients. For both clients and patients, there is still an emphasis on care of some sort being provided; for the empowered client, there will be expectations as to the nature and extent of that care that need to be satisfied, but still there is a recognition that clients need something from their health practitioner that they cannot get on their own. For customers, there may actually be an inversion of the traditional power differential with the practitioner, in which the customer now has greater power or responsibility and is willing to use it to get what she wants. Consider a situation where a person is experiencing gastrointestinal symptoms consistent with severe heartburn. A generation ago, this person would experience distress, become concerned, make appointment with a physician, have an assessment, and then get a prescription filled at a pharmacy. More recently, the person may go directly to the pharmacy and be assessed by the pharmacists, who would recommend a medication along with sensible lifestyle modifications around diet and exercise. In most jurisdictions, that person could simply look up their symptoms on a reputable website (because they are actually smart enough to figure out for themselves what is reputable and what is not), follow the algorithm provided, determine the best possible product for themselves, then simply go to the store and buy it. Of course, this person still could theoretically go to a physician and get a prescription, or speak to a pharmacist and have an assessment done, but now they really don't need to take these additional steps. If the physician or pharmacist added some significant value to the process, or if the additional time and effort required somehow improved the outcome for the person, they would certainly be open to it. However, as a customer, this person knows what they want and need and is looking for the most efficient way of getting it. Customers will sacrifice some efficiency if they perceive there is benefit. For example, if this particular person is taking other medications, it may simply be too much effort to look up all possible drug interactions, and this customer may then actually speak with a pharmacist to determine what the best medication is for heartburn that minimizes potentially harmful interactions. When in the customer role, individuals emphasize personalized, high-quality service rather than psychosocial care. They have high expectations and will quickly and happily walk away if the practitioner does not satisfy them. As the educational and information gap between practitioners and patients shrinks, more recipients of health services feel, think of themselves as, and will behave as customers, and expect a level of customer service—as opposed to patient care—that may be challenging for some practitioners to deliver. Customers want and expect choices, options, respect, and deference to their needs. For example, a physical therapist offering wellness and "stay healthy" education to seniors must contend with a variety of other competitors, including other physical therapists, the Internet, television programs, and simple inertia. This physical therapist will need to sell the service he offers with a smile rather than simply say, "Do it, it's good for you." Similarly, many customers of health services will no longer put up with long waiting times, delayed appointments, and other similar indignities; as customers (rather than clients or patients), they want what they want now and if they don't get it they will find other ways of accessing it.

Building a customer service culture in health care can be challenging if the practitioners themselves insist on categorizing and believing that everyone who seeks their services is actually a patient and will automatically defer to their authority and expertise. Seemingly simple things like being on time for appointments, greeting customers by name and inviting them to address you by your name (rather than role or title), and looking for opportunities to go the extra mile will send important and powerful signals to customer-oriented people that you are able to meet their needs.

Consumers: Around the world, in public and in private health systems, there is a growing and greater interest in fiscal accountability. Health services consume enormous resources for any society or government, and the need to seek value for money continues to grow. Importantly, governments everywhere are adopting the tone that they buy and pay for health services, and they are most interested in ensuring cost-effective use of limited resources. Individuals may also think of themselves as health care consumers, seeking the most inexpensive but effective support for their health needs. For example, many dermatological procedures (such as skin tag removal), some dental procedures (including teeth straightening and whitening), and most optometric interventions (e.g., buying glasses or contact lenses) have developed significant competition from diverse sources. On-line purchases of glasses, often manufactured abroad at a fraction of the cost of visiting your local optician, have significantly impacted the eye care professions. Dentists now find themselves competing with home-based interventions for tooth polishing and tooth whitening, and increasingly even for corrective appliances such as braces to straighten teeth. Much of this is driven by a desire to economize and save money, advances in technology that have now commodified what used to be professional work, and a decreasing belief in the value that professionals can bring to routine activities. When individuals think, feel, and behave as consumers, there is a strong desire to enhance competition among professionals in order to secure the highest quality product or service for the lowest price. Such competition can make professionals feel less valued and less invested in their role, and as a result, a fixation on the bottom line can adversely affect the morale of the health work-force. Still, the reality today and in the foreseeable future is that governments and individual members of the public will increasingly view themselves as consumers of health services.

There are several important drivers of this consumer movement. The first is the sad but real history of abuse of authority in the patient model. The consumer model completely inverts the power distance between the practitioner and the public, leav-ing the practitioner now as the one scrambling for attention. Second, as the general population continues to become more educated and gain greater access to informa-tion and technologies formerly only available to professionals, the work that health professionals do has become demystified and simplified for everyday use. Third, a more educated population is also healthier in general, and the resources that used to be focused on acute illnesses and accidents or traumas are being increasingly redeployed toward chronic conditions and initiatives to keep people well and healthy so they do not need acute or chronic medical care in the first place. A healthier, more educated population with unfettered access to information and technology will increasingly behave like consumers rather than patients, and this is a reality all prac-titioners need to consider.

4.3.1   Implications for Practitioners

The different needs and expectations of patients, clients, consumers, and customers raise important issues for all practitioners to consider. The first relates to ensuring that each individual practitioner is able to accurately assess and respond to the kind of person who comes to his or her office to seek care. People rarely present to practitioners saying, "Today I feel like a customer so just give me what I want," or "I'm really a patient today so make sure you attend to all my emotional and psychosocial needs fully." Instead, as part of the general health assessment every practitioner undertakes, it is important to identify personal strategies you can use to decipher what the individual wants, needs, and expects from you, and respond appropriately and accordingly. Sticking stubbornly to the notion that everyone who comes to see you is a patient can actually be counterproductive for both you and those whom you serve. With the best of intentions, you may actually inadvertently irritate and alienate people by appearing overly paternalistic or patronizing, resulting in your best efforts being rebuffed.

A potentially more challenging and complex issue may arise, however, when individuals feel they are customers, consumers, or clients while in your professional opinion you believe they should actually be patients. Consider the example where someone approaches a pharmacist, a physician, or a nurse and insists on receiving highly potent narcotic analgesics (such as morphine) due to lower back pain. This person may have "done the research" and "know what works for me," but as a practitioner, you have both a professional duty and an ethical obligation to help that person recognize the risks of opioid addiction and suggest alternatives they are not interested in hearing about. Similarly, consider a young mother who has "read everything" and knows that immunizations cause autism and therefore refuses to have her newborn child immunized. She is a customer and if you don't do what she says, well, she will just leave and never come back, which of course may further adversely impact the child. It is a challenging but essential balancing act. Without being paternalistic or a know-it-all, how can practitioners work constructively with people in situations where they consider themselves to be customers or consumers but when your professional and scientific judgment indicates they should be patients? Such situations occur with increasing frequency and point to the central importance of effective and empathic communication. We will explore these theories and techniques in greater detail in Chapters 5 and 6.

4.4 **Summary**

Understanding the psychology of those whom we serve is essential for success as a health professional. As outlined in this chapter, there are several key issues to consider that can support better communication and interactions. First, it is important to recognize that all human beings—including health care professionals!—are constantly working to balance emotional and cognitive responses to our environment. Current research in this area points to the central importance of emotions as a filtering mechanism for cognition. We perceive our world through an emotional filter before we are able to process it cognitively. This insight should help health care professionals recognize the importance of attending to the emotional needs of those whom we serve and to recognize in themselves situations where emotional filters may impair logical reasoning.

Second, it is essential to recognize that patients aren't always patients. As outlined in this chapter, there are at least four distinct roles that the same individual may hold at different times in their life: patient, client, customer, and consumer. Those who feel like patients need, want, and expect different things from health professionals than those who feel like consumers. Learning to accurately assess and interpret individuals' cues so that you can appropriately interact with them based on their individual and specific needs at the moment is important. Equally important will be developing skills to help you to manage challenging situations where individuals may need your support and care to transition between these roles, based on medical need.

4.5 Mind Map Chapter 4

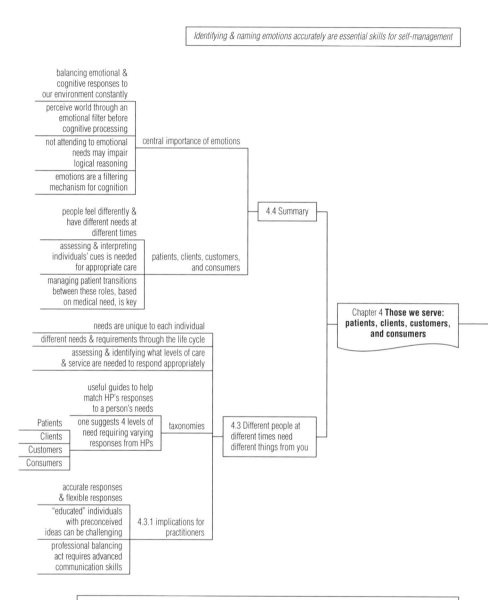

Mind Map for Those We Serve: Patients, Clients, Customers, and Consumers

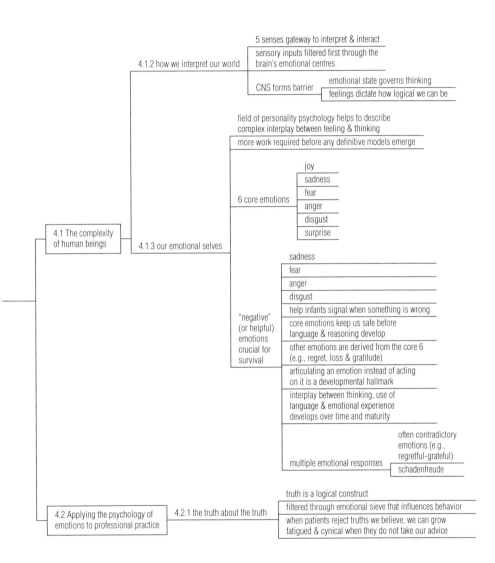

For Further Reading:

Austin Z, Gregory P, Martin J. Characterizing the professional relationships of community pharmacists. *Res Social Admin Pharm*. 2006;2(4):533–546.

Bridges A, Villalobos B, Anastasia E, Dueweke A, Gregus S, Cavell T. Need, access, and the reach of integrated care: a typology of patients. *Fam Syst Health*. 2017;35(2):193–206.

Charles C, Gafni A, Whelan T. Decision making in the physician-patient encounter: revisiting the shared treatment decision making model. *Soc Sci Med*. 1999;49:651–661.

Flynn K, Smith M, Vanness D. A typology of preferences for participation in healthcare decision making. *Soc Sci Med*. 2006;63:1158–1159.

Hadorn D. Kinds of patients. *J Med Philos*. 1997;22(6):567–587.

Kalanithi P. *When Breath Becomes Air*. New York: Random House; 2016.

Kenney C. *Transforming Health Care: Virginia Mason Medical Center's Pursuit of the Perfect Patient Experience*. New York: CRC Press; 2010.

Robins S. *Bird's Eye View: Stories of a Life Lived in Health Care*. Vancouver, Canada: Bird Communications; 2019.

5 | Introduction to Communication Theory (Part 1)

At the center of every relationship between practitioners and patients (or clients, consumers, or customers) is interpersonal communication—the act of transmitting and receiving both information and feelings in a reciprocal manner. Most of us are already highly experienced communicators who have developed our own theories and methods for communicating with others. In large part, these theories and methods will be connected to your emotional intelligence (see Chapter 2). Those with different emotional intelligences have different preferences and styles for communicating. Traditionally, communication theory has assumed there is a one-size-fits-all model or method for enhancing interpersonal relationships; as we have seen in Chapter 2 and Chapter 4, this assumption is likely flawed as there are significant individual differences among different people that must be taken into account when communicating. In this chapter, we will review foundational communication theories and apply them through the lens of emotional intelligence described in Chapter 2, and patient psychology discussed in Chapter 4.

5.1 A Basic Model for Interpersonal Communication

The term *interpersonal communication* refers to the transmitting and receiving of information and feelings between two individuals. These individuals could be a client and a professional, two professionals, or simply two friends sharing a coffee. When more individuals are added to the dynamic, the basic model for interpersonal communication still holds, but additional layers of complexity must be considered separately.

At its most basic, communication between two people involves transmission (i.e., sending) and receiving (i.e., collecting) of different kinds of information in a reciprocal manner. What kinds of information are sent in communication? Not simply words and facts but also feelings and emotions. Unfortunately, miscommunication can occur when the words, facts, feelings, and emotions we think we are sending are not being received by the other person in the way we intended. One reason for

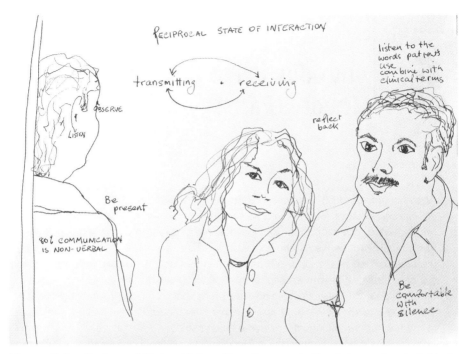

Figure 5.1.   Reciprocal State of Interaction. Communication between two individuals involves transmitting information and receiving information in a reciprocal manner.

such miscommunication is the reality that all interpersonal communication occurs in a broader environment that can influence the sender and the receiver. Think about a pharmacist attempting to have a delicate conversation with a client to discuss a new medication to treat a sensitive issue such as erectile dysfunction. If that conversation is occurring in a busy, commercially successful pharmacy across a countertop where other passersby may inadvertently overhear details, this environment can completely undermine both the pharmacist's and the client's best intentions to have a meaningful conversation. The client may be nervous and embarrassed that his personal issues are being overheard and the pharmacist, in an attempt to be discrete and helpful, may not be as clear and forthright as possible. Now, take those same two people in the same situation but change the environment. Imagine the pharmacist and the client are meeting in a separate, quiet room away from the hurly-burly of the store. The phone isn't ringing, other customers are not waiting in line, and there is no risk of being overheard or eavesdropped upon. The environment is immediately less stress provoking, which allows both the sender and receiver of information to be more focused on each other rather than on what is going on around them. In the interpersonal communication model, the environment is an important and independent variable that must always be considered, especially in health care. Issues of privacy, noise, and distractions can negatively influence a conversation unless these variables are managed beforehand.

A second key feature of the interpersonal communication model is its reciprocal nature. Senders and receivers are tethered to one another and are constantly and subtly changing roles throughout a conversation. A lecture is not interpersonal communication. If one person is simply reciting facts or downloading information onto another person, this is not a conversation. If a speaker is not paying attention to the verbal and nonverbal responses of the receiver, it is not communication or a conversation. Reciprocity means that, at the same time as information is being delivered, the sender is simultaneously receiving information that helps that sender confirm how the information being delivered is actually and really being received. Reciprocity also means that words are not the only thing being communicated; emotions and feelings are also integral to communication since (as we've seen in Chapter 4) emotion is the primary filter for cognition.

Although seemingly straightforward and sensible, the interpersonal communication model highlights important issues for health care professionals. Firstly, professionals and those who they serve are in a constant and reciprocal state of interaction with each acting as sender and receiver of information simultaneously. Secondly, this information consists not only of words and facts, but also of feelings and emotions, particularly since emotions are the primary filter for cognition. Thirdly, all of this is occurring within the context of an environment, which itself is an important independent variable influencing both sender and receiver. Suboptimal environments for communication—environments that are noisy, filled with distractions, or where privacy cannot be ensured—will undermine the health care professional's best efforts to communicate effectively.

5.2   Verbal and Nonverbal Communication

Human communication is incredibly rich—and complicated—because the information that is being sent and received between two people is dense and multifaceted. The most common way of describing the different facets of information is to differentiate between verbal and nonverbal communication. Verbal communication is focused on words and their meanings and nuances. Nonverbal communication is frequently described as everything else, including tone of voice, eye contact, sounds made that are not words (e.g., clearing your throat, saying "uh-huh" with a certain rhythm).

5.2.1   Verbal Communication: The Words We Choose to Use

As previously discussed in Chapter 4, human development is intimately connected to cognitive development, which is highly reliant on the evolution of language (vocabulary and words). The human capacity for language is incredible and one of the primary reasons why we are frequently described as social animals—biological entities who are highly reliant on ongoing social interactions with others, on par with our need for food and water.

If English is the first and only language you speak, it may not occur to you what privilege you have in the world. English is sometimes described as French spoken by Germans, reflecting the incredibly interesting and rich complexity of the language, as well as its unique flexibility in adapting to different circumstances and absorbing words, ideas, and concepts readily from other languages and cultures. As an English speaker, you may have traveled to other countries and realized how lucky you are that in so many countries of the world there is almost always someone who can speak some amount of English to help you as a tourist.

If English is your second (or third or fourth) language or if it is not your mother tongue and you only learned it later in life, you will have unique observations about the language. Compared to many other languages, it is relatively easy to start speaking English and quickly develop a passable level of conversation. The structure of English is very flexible; compared to other languages the grammatical rules are somewhat simpler, and there are many fewer issues of verb tenses and masculine, feminine, and neuter nouns. Although getting started with English may be relatively easy, becoming proficient and fluent in English can be extraordinarily frustrating and, after a certain age, perhaps impossible. The very flexibility and adaptability of the English language that seems to be a virtue is also maddening and frustrating because it all appears haphazard and unstandardized. English relies heavily on local variation and idiom. The kind of English spoken in the United Kingdom can appear completely unrelated to that spoken in the southern United States. Fluent English speakers use many shortcuts that can enhance the efficiency of a conversation, but can make the language appear unfriendly and impenetrable to those trying to learn it. Owing to its evolution from both Germanic and Romance language roots, there is a seemingly ridiculous number of nouns—at least two different words—to name almost everything.

5.2.1.2   What's the Right Word?

Verbal communication is critical in the interpersonal communication model. In the first instance, it involves selection of the most appropriate word to meet the needs of the audience with whom you are communicating. For example, for some clients who are experiencing gastrointestinal distress, it may be more appropriate to ask "Is your tummy sore?" than to ask about the stomach. In contrast, for some clients, it may be more appropriate to use anatomically correct and accurate terminology rather than try to sugar coat certain words. Some individuals may appreciate a practitioner using professional and forthright language such as "penis" or "vagina" rather than terms such as "down there" or "the lady bits." Importantly, every person you speak with will want and need something different from you in terms of verbal communication, and there is no one-size-fits-all model to help guide you. Some people may recommend reliance on external demographic characteristics to help guide you in terms of word choice. For example, those who may be less well-educated or who are recent immigrants may not appreciate or understand anatomically accurate terminology. It is generally advisable to avoid such stereotyping and instead treat each person as an individual rather than as a member of a predefined group. It is generally good practice to use appropriate medical and anatomic terminology in discussions with patients rather than risk using terms that may be misunderstood or that could actually undermine your credibility as a health care practitioner because these terms are either too juvenile or inappropriate. Of course, this is a balancing act. Rather than ask, "Are you experiencing significant gastrointestinal distress associated with reflux or esophagitis?" it would generally be preferable to ask "Do you have a stomach ache or heartburn?" which of course is also better than asking, "Is your tum-tum achy?" You do not want to overwhelm patients with terminology, but nor do you want to infantilize them by using childish vocabulary. Finding the middle ground of using appropriately complex and sufficiently mature words that are understood by the patient establishes the conversation as professional, rather than parental, in nature.

One common issue encountered by many health professionals is the use of technical jargon, acronyms, and other short forms that are immediately well understood by other professionals but may be unclear or problematic for patients. Consider, for example, the widely used abbreviation PRN on many prescriptions. Because health care professionals know PRN at the end of a prescription signifies "take as necessary" or "take as required," a prescription for lorazepam 1 mg po TID PRN can be translated as take one lorazepam tablet (1 mg) three times a day by mouth as necessary. Lorazepam is a medication that is widely used for the management of sleep problems and anxiety. The direction to the patient to "take one tablet (1 mg) three times a day by mouth" is clear enough, but what does "as necessary" mean to a patient? What are the circumstances that govern when it is necessary and when it is not? How is a patient supposed to know when "as necessary" triggers consumption of a tablet or not? Many physicians, nurses, pharmacists, and other health care professionals will simply convey the instruction "take it when you need to," which in most cases does not provide sufficient guidance to the patient to know what to do in a specific circumstance. Although the interpretation of the prescription direction is accurate and linguistically clear, it may not be sufficiently specific to be of help to a patient. Avoiding short forms and acronyms that health care professionals understand, but patients may not, is essential.

As we shall see shortly, nonverbal responses are frequently the best tool available to help you to redirect your word choices and reorient your verbal communication to better meet the needs of those you serve.

5.2.1.3   Word Intensity

A frustrating difficulty for many non–English speakers is the large number of synonyms that dominate the language. For most English speakers, different words that have the same general meaning can serve an important function. It can allow you to highlight the intensity of your emotional response using words rather than florid emotions themselves. Consider the following situation. A colleague has made an error that you have detected. Now think of how many different ways you could use words to communicate your discovery. You could say, "Hey, there's been a mistake," or "Hey, there's been an error," or "Hey, there's been a boo-boo," or "Hey there's a problem," or "Hey, we have a situation." If you are a native or fluent English speaker, you will immediately recognize that the specific word you select (mistake versus error versus boo-boo versus problem versus situation) is actually transmitting an enormous amount of important information. A boo-boo is trivial; when the Apollo space mission experienced major technical failures, the famous phrase "Houston, we have a problem" (not "Houston, we have an oopsie") was born. Native English speakers learn from an early age that these five different ways of saying the same thing (these five synonyms) are actually NOT equivalent. If your receiver does not understand your meaning because they do not understand the intensity of difference between "boo-boo" and "problem," much of what you are trying to communicate will be lost. There are many other words where intensity is conveyed through specific choices. Consider the differences between "disappointed," "frustrated," "irritated," "pissed off," "angry," and "furious." Depending on your comfort with the nuances of the English language, you will understand the different intensity of emotion that underlies the specific choice of word used in a given situation.

Of course, even among native English speakers, some of this nuance may be lost on occasion and not everyone will immediately understand the importance of the intensity of the word you choose. Again, careful attention to nonverbal cues transmitted by your intended recipient may allow you to assess how accurately your intentions have been transmitted and will allow you opportunities to recalibrate your delivery and potentially select alternative words to express your intentions.

5.2.1.4 *Direct and Indirect Verbal Communication*

As noted in Chapter 2, our emotional intelligence fundamentally influences not only our personalities and our interactions, but also our preferences in terms of communication. One important distinction in verbal communication linked to emotional intelligence is the difference between direct and indirect communication.

Direct communication is more typically favored by those who are strong accommodators and convergers. Direct communicators value efficiency and clarity of focus and as a result tend to use fewer words and appear more blunt in their style. Indirect communicators value long-term relationships and the importance of saving face and as a result tend to use many more words to express the same concept and tend to appear more gentle in their style. Direct communicators risk being seen as rude or aggressive, whereas indirect communicators risk coming across as confused or somewhat passive. Of course, there is no right way of communicating and in many cases it is difficult for those who are naturally inclined toward one form of communication to simply change to another. However, it is important to recognize the implications of direct and indirect styles on understanding by the receiver and, where necessary, recalibrate verbal communication in a way that is simply more helpful.

One key issue that distinguishes direct and indirect communicators is the way in which the word "you" gets used in conversations. Direct communicators tend to overuse the word "you," whereas indirect communicators may bend over backward to avoid using that same word. For indirect communicators, "you" sounds aggressive, demanding, domineering, and almost accusatory. For direct communicators, "you" may connote personal responsibility and self-control. Consider the following example. You discover a colleague has made an error. How would you prefer to be told about this: "Hey, you made a mistake" or "Hey, I see a mistake was made"? In this case, both are short sentences that more or less say the same thing; however, if you are an indirect communicator, you may bristle when you see the first sentence and immediately want to respond, "It wasn't my fault, it was because of [insert reason here]." The use of the word "you" by a direct communicator may automatically trigger a defensive response from an indirect communicator, which may ultimately lead to a disagreement, hurt feelings, or other emotional outcome rather than an attempt to fix the problem itself. Conversely, if a direct communicator hears you say, "Hey, I see a mistake was made," this person may naturally assume you're talking to someone else or that you don't think the mistake has anything to do with them. The intention of the indirect communicator may be to be polite, to not sound accusatory, and to give the other person a chance to save face, but in this case, the actual intention of the sentence might be lost on a direct communicator.

At first, this may appear to be a very subtle or nuanced problem, but on reflection, it may become clearer that this single, small three-letter word can actually produce a host of problems, situations, issues, and concerns if the communication between sender and receiver is misaligned.

5.2.1.5 *Open and Closed Statements*

Another important issue to consider in verbal communication is the balance of open and closed statements or questions. In general, closed statements or questions are those that can be answered with a simple "yes" or "no," whereas open statements or questions will require someone to elaborate or provide more details. There is no specific formula to help guide you in determining the balance of open and closed statements and questions to use in a conversation; however, your natural tendency to use or prefer one over the other is likely connected to your emotional intelligence. Divergers and assimilators typically favor or more naturally use open questions and statements, whereas convergers and accommodators typically favor or may more naturally use closed ones.

To help understand why this important, consider the difference between asking a patient, "How are you feeling" versus asking, "Do you feel depressed?" The first phrase—"How are you feeling?"—is an open-ended question. It cannot be answered with a simple "yes" or "no" and instead requires the receiver to actually describe or say more in order to appropriately respond. They may say, "Well, I've been having a hard time sleeping, and that's been making be feel tired all the time, like I have no energy to do anything." In contrast, the second phrase—"Do you feel depressed?"—is not as likely to trigger this kind of response. Instead, the receiver may simply respond "yes" or "probably" (if they are familiar with the common signs and symptoms of depression) or "no" or "I don't know" (if they do not recognize that lack of energy, difficulty sleeping, and constant fatigue may be symptoms of depression). Alternatively, consider the difference in the way a conversation will evolve if a health care professional asks, "Does it hurt?" versus "Tell me about your pain."

So which question is the right one to ask? Much of it will depend on the unique dynamic between practitioner and patient in this specific case, including their unique emotional intelligences. Some patients who are well informed, have previous experience with depression, and who themselves are direct communicators who prefer closed statements may appreciate being asked a blunt, direct diagnostic question like "Do you feel depressed?" More likely, however, a less experienced patient who may not want to hear the word "depression" just yet, or who honestly may not know that his symptoms are consistent with depression, may prefer the opportunity to provide more details, more context, and more words than simply "yes" or "no."

As discussed in Chapter 3, the difference between problem-oriented and story-oriented health professionals will also influence the choice of open- or closed-ended statements and questions. Recall that problem-oriented practitioners aim to enhance clarity and narrow focus by eliminating extraneous facts, and so these individuals may naturally gravitate to closed-ended questions as a tool to accomplish this objective. The risk, of course, is that this clarity and focus may occur prematurely and may result in inappropriately forcing a patient to believe depression is the cause when in fact more systematic questioning and ruling out of causes could be warranted. In contrast, story-oriented practitioners aim to get the biggest picture possible and want additional context and information to help them see connections and relationships among different aspects of a situation. As a result, they may gravitate to open-ended questions and prompts as a way of casting their net more broadly. The risk, of course, is that there is so much context and information that nothing ever gets decided or definitively diagnosed despite much time and effort spent asking questions and receiving answers.

The most skilled practitioners learn with time how to best balance open- and closed-ended questioning and statements within a conversation. Most often they find it is best to initially begin with open-ended questions to guide discussion, but for hypothesis testing and confirmation, closed-ended questioning may be preferred. In being both mindful and artful in segueing between open and closed questions and statements, it also makes the conversation feel and seem more natural and less formulaic, which in turn can be more comforting for a patient.

5.3 Nonverbal Communication

It is frequently noted that up to 80% of interpersonal communication is nonverbal in nature. Nonverbal communication consists of the information transmitted between senders and receivers that does not involve words; instead, it involves a wide array of obvious and less-than-obvious cues ranging from the tone of voice (sarcastic versus sincere), eye contact (direct versus indirect), body language and posture, verbal interjections that are not actually words (a nervous giggle or a vague "uh-huh"), among many other elements.

Why is nonverbal communication such an important part of human interactions? Recall from Chapter 4 the discussion regarding the power of emotional filters in shaping and directing cognition and thinking. Most psychologists believe that nonverbal communication is the language of emotion; we read and respond to nonverbal cues sent by others through this emotional filter, which in turn will directly influence and shape the way we literally hear the words being spoken. For example, if a nurse is instructing a patient on how to use a complex medication and says, "You're to take this medication five times a day. Will that be a problem?" and the patient replies "Five times a day? (gulp) Yeah, that won't be a problem!" much of the nurse's interpretation of the response will be focused on the tone and timing of the "(gulp) Yeah." If the tone and timing of those words is thoughtful and reflective, suggesting the patient is simply thinking about the question, then the nurse might confidently assume the statement that follows—"that won't be a problem"—is factually accurate and sincere. If, however, the sounds and words, "huh-yeah," are accompanied by a short, sharp inhalation, a snort, or a barely audible "phew" is noted, that could indicate a sarcastic tone. In such a case, the emotion the patient is trying to convey is, "Are you crazy and seriously asking me if taking a new medication five times a day is not going to be a problem? Of course it's going to be a problem!"

Depending on how attuned the nurse's emotional filters are to the nonverbal cues transmitted by this patient, very different outcomes may result. In many cases, patients do not wish to be seen as negative, demanding, or unwilling to follow instruction, so they may never use their words to clearly state when something is a problem. In such cases, patients may fear that appearing unwilling or demanding may result in a negative consequence or some kind of punishment later down the road from the professional. Rather than say the words clearly—"It will be a big problem for me to take this medication five times a day. I have a job with a long commute and children to take care of and I can't stop everything to remember to take a new medication every 5 hours!"—the patient may be *telegraphing* important information nonverbally hoping or expecting the professional is clever enough to decipher its meaning.

5.3.1   The Role of Telegraphing and Cues in Interpersonal Interactions

The power of nonverbal communication lies in its ability to transmit a large amount of important information about complex subjects—like emotions and emotional state—in a very condensed manner. Strong emotions, like anger or sadness, can cause receivers of communication to quickly change their behaviors and attitudes at a pace and in a way that simple words alone cannot. The process by which emotions and emotional states are conveyed between receivers and senders is sometimes described as *telegraphy*. This term is important because it suggests the receiver of emotional communication has an important job in deciphering accurately, clearly, and quickly the meaning and intention of the sender without relying on words alone.

Reflect in your own life on the difference in your responses to other people when they simply say "I'm angry" as opposed shouting "I'm angry." The addition of a louder voice and a strident tone conveys much more immediacy to the words themselves and will likely trigger a much more immediate response from you. When senders telegraph, they are providing receivers with cues (or clues) that must be interpreted in order to be effective.

Of course, herein lies the problem. In some cases, nonverbal miscommunication may arrive when telegraphed cues are misinterpreted, misunderstood, ignored, or simply overlooked. Some people may wonder (and actually ask), "Well, if your feelings are that important to you, why not SAY something rather than rely on telegraphing and cues and all that nonsense?" First, in many cases, a person telegraphing nonverbal cues may not yet even be consciously aware enough of their feelings to develop words and use vocabulary to describe them. Recall from Chapter 4 that human beings are hardwired to feel before they think, to experience emotion before logic. In some situations, a person may be experiencing a strong emotional response to something that has not yet been logically or cognitively processed to a sufficient degree to allow them to say how they are feeling. The only tool they have available for communication will therefore be nonverbal cues. Second, for a variety of cultural or sociologic reasons, there may be constraints or limits on what is socially acceptable to be said out loud. For example, if a friend were to seek your comments on a new outfit that had just been purchased and asked, "Well, what do you think?" in some cases you would have to be very brave (or extremely foolhardy) to say out loud exactly what you think. So, instead, we rely on nonverbal cues as a way of preventing conflict, easing the delivery of bad news, and maintaining good social relationships, all the while telegraphing nonverbally what we actually think by making neutral facial gestures and verbal interjections that on the one hand appear to say that you like the outfit, but most people will actually decipher accurately that intent as, "You've got to be kidding, I hope you kept the receipt!"

Learning to read telegraphed nonverbal cues sent by others is an incredibly difficult, complex, and never-ending job. Nonverbal cues themselves evolve over time and within small groups of friends and in communities. Sadly, there is no resource or encyclopedia of nonverbal cues that definitively lays out the significance of certain gestures or facial grimaces; deciphering nonverbal cues is something that must be learned but cannot be taught formally. For effective interpersonal communication, it is absolutely essential and consequently must be a focus of attention for all health care professionals.

5.3.2 Deciphering Nonverbal Cues in Interpersonal Communication

Learning to accurately interpret nonverbal cues begins with the simple act of observation, and a personal commitment to not overlook or ignore telegraphed communication between receiver and sender. If we remember that approximately 80%

of the information in interpersonal communication is nonverbal in nature, it suggests we must pay four times as much attention to it than to the actual words that are spoken!

Such observation is facilitated—and your ability to decipher vastly improved—through some basic principles associated with good quality communication between people.

Pay attention and avoid distraction. Many people complain that the quality of communication—and by extension, the quality of interpersonal relationships—has deteriorated in the last few years, mainly because of the environmental complexity within which human beings live and work. Regardless of your job or role in society, we are more distracted than ever. We obsess over mobile phones and text messages, we are constantly awaiting and expecting novelty and stimulation, and we have developed a culture of immediate gratification, which means that something as slow and old fashioned as a conversation between two people now appears boring and unnecessary. The intensity of distractions in daily life means that few of us pay sufficient attention to another person when they talk; instead, we all appear unusually anxious to end conversations abruptly and prematurely just in case something better and more interesting awaits us elsewhere. When we demonstrate the simple lack of courtesy associated with not paying attention to someone else, and when we allow distractions to interfere with communication, we cannot accurately decipher and interpret nonverbal cues. This is especially problematic as so much of our communication in the last few years has shifted toward electronically mediated formats across text messages, social media, and other platforms where there are no traditional nonverbal cues readily apparent. The art of interpreting telegraphed cues is a skill that requires constant practice and refinement and, as we increasingly avoid face-to-face communication in favor of other formats, it is a skill that is increasingly fragile.

Watch. Regardless of your professional field or education, all health care professionals must learn clinical skills associated with their role. For every health care professional, a common and core clinical skill is the ability to observe or to watch. Physically looking at patients (or clients, customers, or consumers) and drawing inferences from such observation is a crucial way of accurately deciphering nonverbal cues and enhancing the quality and impact of communication. We cannot watch patients if we are distracted by cell phones. We cannot observe patients if our nose in buried in a reference text or a patient's chart, or if we are staring at a computer screen updating an electronic health record. Keeping eyes on a patient in an appropriate and reasonable manner is an invaluable source of nonverbal information that is an essential complement to all the other data we are gathering.

Observing a patient and watching for nonverbal cues means paying attention to several key tells. To psychologists, tells are nonverbal cues that contain dense information that may or may not contradict verbal statements made at the exact same moment. For example, if you ask a patient, "Are you experiencing any pain right now?" and she says, "No, no, I'm fine," but you observe a facial grimace—closed and tight lips and sudden tight closing of the eyes—that may be a tell that the patient is *saying* one thing ("no, I'm fine") but is *actually experiencing* pain and for whatever reason (pride, not wanting to be a bother, fear of narcotic addiction) doesn't want to say so out loud.

Nonverbal tells are most frequently communicated through faces, posture, and gestures. An awareness of how nonverbal cues are transmitted physically and bodily through these regions is essential for truly effective communication.

Faces: The human face is an extraordinary tool for the expression of information. Importantly, for many of us, it is possible to use words to lie or dissemble, but faces will frequently betray the truth. There is good reason that the old expression, "Look me in the eyes and tell me the truth" has persisted for so long. Certain regions of the face are particularly important to be aware of: the eyes and the mouth (lips and tongue).

Eye contact is particularly important. In most Western cultures, direct eye contact usually is associated with truth telling, self-confidence, and openness. Lack of direct eye contact can in some cases suggest shame, avoidance, dissembling, or an attempt to trick others. It is essential, however, to recognize that this is not a universal nonverbal norm. For example, in many cultures, direct eye contact is considered vulgar and confrontational; people from such cultures may learn to avoid direct eye contact with others as a way of demonstrating respect and deference to authority. In this context, avoiding eye contact actually signifies respect rather than lying or evasiveness. Once again there is no one-size-fits-all rule or law that governs what appropriate eye contact means between individuals. As a health care professional, it is generally preferred if you nonverbally offer direct eye contact with a patient, but if they do not take you up on the offer, undertake some additional investigation to determine the reason. Is it cultural and simply the norm for this person, or does lack of direct eye contact constitute a form of nonverbal communication that is important for you to follow up further?

The area around the mouth is another important tell zone. Many people store psychological distress or tension in their lips; as a result, in difficult situations, many people's lips will tighten and tense up, literally becoming thinner than normal. Such so-called pursed lips can signify acute pain, a subconscious attempt to stop telling a lie, or general nervousness or anxiety about the direction of a conversation. This is usually not faked or able to be faked and is generally true across most cultures and communities. If pursed lips are observed, it may be an important nonverbal cue the patient is sending you that requires some kind of follow-up to gather further details. Another nonverbal tell involves a forced smile or a grimace. For example, if in a general health review, a practitioner asks a patient a question about his sexual functioning, and the patient replies, "Everything's good in that department, no worries at all for me!" but puts forth a short, unsustainable, and seemingly inauthentic smile, that could be a sign that there is a problem but the patient is embarrassed or reluctant to discuss it further. A forced or fake smile does not mean the patient is happy; just the opposite is true. Another tell with the forced smile is the lack of involvement of the area around the upper cheeks and eyes; a true smile involves large regions of the face that is conspicuous to an observer, whereas a forced smile is tightly limited only to the lips. The tongue and an open mouth may signify another kind of tell that is important. Constantly licking one's lips and a hyperactive and darting tongue usually is associated with some kind of nervousness that may require a follow-up. In some cases, this behavior may also be associated with side effects of certain medications or the evolution of a medical condition. In any of these circumstances, this unusual behavior can only be followed up on if the practitioner is actively watching the patient and notices it.

A third important region of the face to be aware of is the area around the eyebrows and the forehead. This area serves as the roof of the face and so is essential in actually shaping how one's face appears to another. A furrowed brow (i.e., forehead region that was once smooth but suddenly becomes abruptly wrinkly or wavy), particularly when accompanied by rapid blinking of the eyes, is frequently an attempt to stifle or hold back tears. A patient exhibiting this behavior while simultaneously saying, "Everything is good!" is nonverbally telling you "Everything is not good, so please, ask me more and help me."

Many psychologists have dedicated their careers to deciphering the nonverbal cues telegraphed by faces, and volumes have been written on this subject. Of course, we are not able to cover all these details in this book. Importantly, as a functioning human being, you have been writing your own book on this subject since you were old enough to start communicating with other human beings. The key is not to look for a comprehensive listing of all possible facial tells but instead to take the time to actively observe and carefully watch patients and other people you work with to ensure alignment between what they are saying (the words they are using) and the nonverbal tells they are communicating. If you have doubts, ask more questions and find alternative ways of following up, but do not simply ignore or overlook this important communication.

Gestures: Gestures typically involve hands and arms, and are an essential shortcut that has developed to facilitate interpersonal communication. Some gestures are deliberate and conscious and simply used to replace words, a convenient way of expressing a lot of information quickly. Think, for example, of the thumbs-up gesture frequently used to nonverbally say "Great!" or "I'm good!" or "Congratulations, I'm so proud of you!" Of course, that gesture may only make sense in some cultures and contexts; in some parts of the world, the thumbs-up gesture is both incredibly rude and quite provocative and thus can be easily misunderstood. Some other gestures are subconscious and can act as important tells about a person's internal emotional state before they are actually able or ready to use words to describe it. Think, for example, of tightened or clenched fists in a conversation, which will usually signify at best disagreement or at worst a readiness or willingness to fight. Some gestures can be emotionally triggering because they appear highly dismissive and disparaging. Consider someone's natural inclination when saying the word "stop" to add an additional gesture of an upturned, outward-facing palm, sometimes referred to as showing the hand. In some cultures and communities, this gesture is natural and immediately understood as a simple accompaniment or replacement to the words "stop," or "slow down," or "hold on." In other cases, this gesture looks rude and dismissive, as though one person is treating the other as a child, and as a result, it can produce a strong emotional and negative response.

Other gestures may serve as important tells. For example, nervousness and tension can sometimes manifest in rubbing of palms or hands (as though a person is trying to rub away excessive nervous sweating) or rubbing of fingers against the palm of the same hand as though the person is subconsciously trying to avoid making a fist. Other gestures (e.g., drumming fingers on a table top) may indicate boredom and impatience.

Importantly, among all nonverbal cues, gesturing may be the one that is most closely linked to culture, socialization, and upbringing rather than emotional state. Some cultures and some people are simply more manually demonstrative than others. For some people, talking with their hands is perfectly natural and normal, and those who do not do this can come across as boring or aloof. For others, talking with their hands may appear childish or alarming, or a sign of not being well-educated. The associations we make with gestures can inaccurately and unfairly stereotype people and can result in us missing out on the actual significance and meaning of what these gestures are trying to convey.

Posture: Posture is another bodily form of nonverbal communication that refers to the uprightness of stance and the way in which the person's body occupies the space around it. Posture is a challenging nonverbal to decipher at times, especially for health care professionals, because many biological and medical processes, such as simple natural aging, influence posture directly. Traditionally, a good posture has been associated with a long, firm back that supports an open ribcage and chest. Such a posture is usually associated with health, honesty, and openness. A hyperextended posture is one in which an individual is consciously or subconsciously trying to be taller than they actually are, and it is usually associated with a state of hypervigilance associated with fear, anxiety, or sense of danger. Conversely, a slouching posture can sometimes be interpreted as an absence of interest, disrespect, or a lack of self-confidence. Although such traditional interpretations may be appropriate in situations where an individual has both muscle control and tone that allows for self-regulation, of course with age and in the presence of certain musculoskeletal conditions, posture can be a difficult nonverbal cue to decipher if indeed posture is even being used as a nonverbal cue. Misinterpreting posture as a cue when in fact it is something that is not controllable by the sender can lead to misunderstanding.

Listening. It may seem peculiar to include this action in a section focused on nonverbal communication, given that listening typically involves words. There are an incredibly diverse and large number of nonverbal speaking tells that transmit important information in any conversation, including tone, insertions, volume, and pace.

Tone: Among the most important aural tells, tone refers to not what is said but the way in which it is said. Think of a simple phrase such as "Hey, buddy!" Those words, said with a friendly tone, can mean warmth, affection, and openness. The exact same words said in a pinched tone are sarcastic. Those words said in a menacing tone can sound threatening. In part this may relate to the musical pitch of the voice saying these words: a friendly tone is generally higher than a menacing tone that may have a rumbling quality to it. Tone is among the most frequent causes of conflict and misalignment in nonverbal communication. A sarcastic tone of voice can completely undermine whatever words are being used. One of the greatest skills great leaders have is to be able to say difficult or even hurtful words in a tone that is reassuring and supportive, thereby reducing the sting of the words themselves. Tone is also interesting because it is among the most instantaneous things we respond to in the most emotional ways. For example, if a friend or parent says to you, "I can't believe you did that" in a tone that suggests they are really saying, "Wow you're stupid," we cannot help but react strongly, emotionally, negatively, and defensively. The exact same words spoken in a tone that is more associated with disappointment (rather than dismissiveness) will prompt a much different response. In many cases, tone is something that can be controlled by the speaker or sender, although it does require significant thought and intention to do so. In this way, tone may not necessarily be a tell in the way other nonverbal cues may be. Attentiveness to others' tone is important but may be challenging because it is sometimes difficult for us to logically and calmly analyze a sarcastic or dismissive tone aimed at us without becoming emotional and defensive ourselves.

Insertions: Insertions represent a somewhat unique but important kind of non-verbal communication insofar as they are actually words (of a sort) but are not considered verbal communication. Classic insertions include sounds such as "um," "huh," "uh-huh," or even sounds like heavy sighs or sharp expirations of air similar to "phew." Despite being short and small bursts of semiverbal energy, such insertions convey large amounts of important nonverbal communication. Consider the following situation. A physical therapist is instructing a patient on a series of exercises to be undertaken to strengthen the quadriceps muscles, to reduce pain, and to enhance joint mobility. These are somewhat complex exercises that must be done several times a day at home, and will cause some inconvenience, require effort and commit-ment, and may cause some mild pain initially. However, in order to achieve the nec-essary muscle strengthening, these must be done regularly. If directly asked, most patients would say, "Sure, I understand this is important. Of course I'll do as I'm told because you're the expert." The patient, however, may have reservations about their capacity or even their desire to comply with the exercises, and these reservations will rarely manifest or express themselves in the form of a clear sentence such as "Are you kidding me? I don't have time for this!" Instead, they may subconsciously, or consciously, use insertions such as "uh-huh," "yup," or "riiiiight" in a tone and manner that actually means what they are thinking. Insertions are frequently overlooked or ignored because they fall in a middle ground between being verbal and nonverbal communication simultaneously; however, they are an essential source of information in better understanding what a patient or another person is really thinking and most likely to do.

Volume: In most cultures, the volume of one's voice corresponds to the intensity or level of emotional arousal. The louder the volume, the more intense the emotion that is being conveyed. This generalization, however, must be understood in the context that individuals have a baseline, normal, or natural volume that differs widely based on personal characteristics, culture, and socialization. In some cultures and communities, this baseline volume may be quite loud compared to others, and as a result, a normal speaking volume may be misinterpreted within a different culture as being angry. Conversely, in some cultures or communities where the baseline volume may be relatively low or quiet, an increase in volume corresponding to increasing intensity of emotion may literally not even be heard. Similarly, some individuals have a volume pattern that might seem quite paradoxical to others. Some people get quieter, but more intense in their eye contact or more deliberate in the articulation of their words, as they become angrier. As with so many other facets of nonverbal communication, it is not possible to develop a one-size-fits-all list of the meaning behind a particular nonverbal attribute like volume. Instead, it requires us to consider each individual as a unique person and better learn their own individual and unique nonverbal characteristics in order to more accurately and appropriately decipher the cues and tells they are transmitting.

There are of course many more paragraphs that could be written regarding specific attributes of listening attentively to nonverbal cues, but space here does not permit further discussion. As was noted in the previous discussion on observing faces, success in accurately deciphering telegraphed cues through listening is very reliant on the simple but important act of actually listening attentively in the first place and consciously deciding not to overlook or ignore cues being sent your way.

Be present. Avoiding distractions, watching, and listening are of course all essential tools for accurately deciphering nonverbal cues. As we have now seen, however, observing and not ignoring or overlooking, although essential, are not sufficient to truly understand telegraphed nonverbal cues. There are so many individual and cultural nuances and differences in nonverbal communication that more than simple observation is required. Active engagement and thinking about the meaning of the nonverbal cues being transmitted are equally or more essential. It is perfectly natural to hope or expect a book such as this to provide a comprehensive list of nonverbal cues and their meanings that could be referred to with confidence to help you to discern what people are saying when they are not using words. Alas, no such list is possible and no such list would be helpful. Deciphering nonverbal cues appropriately and accurately requires a psychological state of engagement with another person, sometimes simply described as being present.

What does it mean to be present in a conversation? Beyond avoiding distraction, watching, and listening, it means actively and cheerfully trying to find meaning in nonverbal cues for no other reason than to enhance the quality of a conversation. It is a psychological state of curiosity and openness characterized by altruism and a genuine desire to form a connection with the other person. It is this internal psychological state of openness and engagement—not a textbook or a list—that will help you to decipher telegraphed nonverbal cues.

Presence should not and cannot be faked. If you are preoccupied or disinterested for whatever reason, you will simply not have the psychological energy and reserves available to translate nonverbal cues into understanding. You will not be able to avoid the temptation to seek shortcuts, conveniently overlook or ignore nonverbal cues that require too much thinking, and prematurely end conversations that are getting troublesome. Of course, it is not humanly possible to be present in every conversation; you are also a human being and have your own issues and concerns to deal with that cannot help but interfere with your ability to be present for others.

The psychological power of presence in enhancing interpersonal communication is substantial. As we will see in Chapter 6, it is also the foundation of one of the most important concepts in health care: empathy.

5.4 **Summary**

The psychology of communication is both fascinating for us as human beings and an essential component of what makes for a successful health care professional. All human beings are amateur psychologists or detectives when it comes to communication theory. We spend our whole lives learning, developing, testing, refining, and applying such theories in all our interactions with others. Certain foundational principles of communication theory—such as receivers, senders, and the environment, and the differences between verbal and nonverbal communication—are essential for all successful human interactions.

5.5   Mind Map Chapter 5

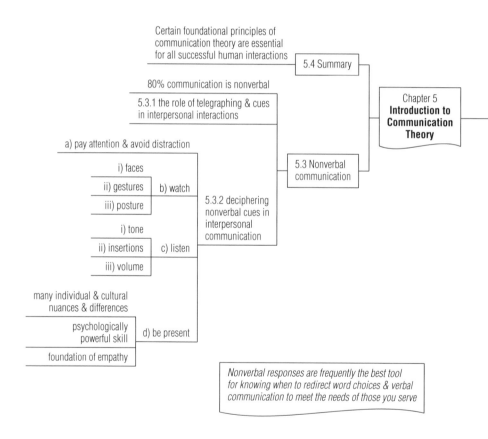

Considering & applying foundational communication theories through the lens of emotional intelligence (Chapter 2) & patient psychology (Chapter 4)

Certain foundational principles of communication theory are essential for all successful human interactions

5.4 Summary

Chapter 5
Introduction to Communication Theory

80% communication is nonverbal

5.3.1 the role of telegraphing & cues in interpersonal interactions

a) pay attention & avoid distraction

5.3 Nonverbal communication

i) faces

ii) gestures   b) watch

iii) posture

5.3.2 deciphering nonverbal cues in interpersonal communication

i) tone

ii) insertions   c) listen

iii) volume

many individual & cultural nuances & differences

psychologically powerful skill   d) be present

foundation of empathy

Nonverbal responses are frequently the best tool for knowing when to redirect word choices & verbal communication to meet the needs of those you serve

Mind Map for Introduction to Communication Theory

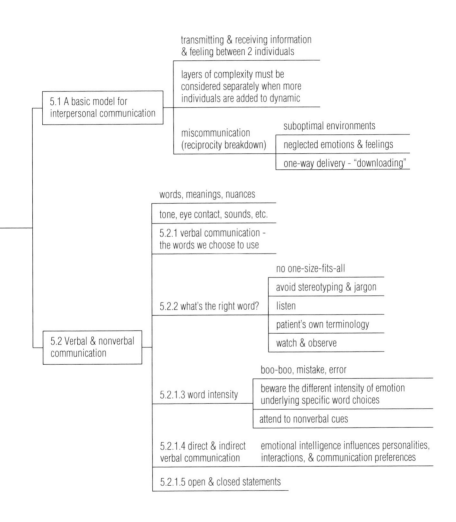

transmitting & receiving information
& feeling between 2 individuals

layers of complexity must be
considered separately when more
individuals are added to dynamic

5.1 A basic model for
interpersonal communication

miscommunication
(reciprocity breakdown)

suboptimal environments

neglected emotions & feelings

one-way delivery - "downloading"

words, meanings, nuances

tone, eye contact, sounds, etc.

5.2.1 verbal communication -
the words we choose to use

5.2 Verbal & nonverbal
communication

5.2.2 what's the right word?

no one-size-fits-all

avoid stereotyping & jargon

listen

patient's own terminology

watch & observe

5.2.1.3 word intensity

boo-boo, mistake, error

beware the different intensity of emotion
underlying specific word choices

attend to nonverbal cues

5.2.1.4 direct & indirect
verbal communication

emotional intelligence influences personalities,
interactions, & communication preferences

5.2.1.5 open & closed statements

For Further Reading:

Berry D, ed. *Health Communication: Theory and Practice.* Milton Keynes, UK: Open University Press; 2006.

Blanchette I, Richards A. Reasoning about emotional and neutral materials: is logic affected by emotions? *Psychol Sci.* 2004;15(11):745–752.

Bylund C, Peterson E, Cameron K. A practitioner's guide to interpersonal communication theory: an overview and exploration of selected theories. *Patient Educ Couns.* 2013;87(3): 261–267.

Duggan A. Understanding interpersonal communication processes across health contexts: advances in the last decade and challenges for the next decade. *J Health Commun.* 2006;11(1):93–108.

Gwyn R. Communicating health and illness. London: Sage Publications; 2002.

Jung N, Wranke C, Hamburger K, Knauff M. How emotions affect logical reasoning: evidence from experiments with mood-manipulated participants, spider phobics, and people with exam anxiety. *Front Psychol.* 2014;5:570.

Mitchell M, Brown K, Morris-Villagran M, Villagran P. The effects of anger, sadness, and happiness on persuasive message processing: a test of the negative state relief model. *Commun Monogr.* 2001;68:347–359.

Parrott R. Emphasizing communication in health communication. *J Commun.* 2004;54:751–787.

Ruben B. Communication theory and health communication practice. *Health Commun.* 2016;31:1–11.

Street R, Makoul G, Arora N, Epstein R. How does communication heal? Pathways linking clinician-patient communication to health outcomes. *Patient Educ Couns.* 2009;74(3): 295–301.

CHAPTER

6 | Introduction to Communication Theory (Part 2)

It is essential for health care professionals to understand the interplay between human psychology and interpersonal communication. As we have seen in the previous chapters, psychology determines a great deal of how communication is sent and received, and in turn, communication shapes beliefs, behaviors, and attitudes. In this chapter, we will review foundational psychological theories in order to provide you with a more robust understanding of how to communicate more effectively, particularly in difficult situations.

6.1   The Johari Window

One of the most important theories in psychology—and communication theory—is the Johari Window. This theory provides important insights into the nature of human consciousness but also provides practical strategies for health care professionals to more effectively connect and communicate with patients. It also helps us to better understand a term that is frequently used by health care professionals but sometimes difficult to actually describe or apply: *empathy*.

The Johari Window is an example of a psychological model that intersects with communication theory. It is a model that has been derived over many years using observational methods and, consequently, is difficult to test or prove using traditional scientific methods such as randomized controlled double-blinded studies. As with many theories and models in psychology, this particular model provides a framework for understanding one of the most complicated things in the universe: the human psyche.

The psyche is a difficult concept to define and explain, but perhaps is best thought of as the psychological self that is at the foundation of all human beings. The psyche can be viewed as consisting of distinct yet interconnected halves—aspects that we are consciously aware of and therefore have some control over, and elements that we are only barely conscious of or sometimes entirely unaware of, which consequently may be beyond our control. You may wonder if this division corresponds to the division previously described in Chapter 4 as emotion versus logic or thinking versus feeling. The Johari Window is somewhat more complex than simply that

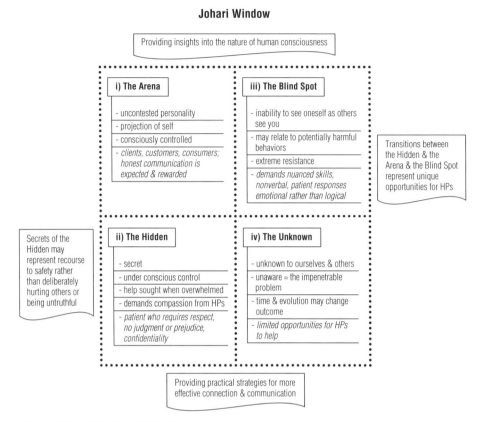

Figure 6.1.   The Johari Window.

division and provides a more nuanced—and therefore more complex, more interesting, and as a result likely more accurate—version of what it means to be human and how the psyche influences our lives.

The Johari Window proposes that the psyche is divided into four distinct quadrants, as depicted in Figure 6.1. Each of these quadrants describes a different facet of the psyche. Although the figure is symmetrically presented, this does not necessarily imply that our psyche is divided into neat and tidy quarters, with each facet representing 25% of who we are. This may be accurate in some cases and circumstances but is not universally applicable to each of us. The four quadrants of the Johari Window are the Arena, the Hidden, the Blind Spot, and the Unknown (or the Unconscious). Let's look at each of these components separately.

The Arena: The Arena can be best described as the portion of our psyche in which what the world knows about us, we equally know about ourselves. The Arena relates to the aspects of our personalities and selves that are uncontested and generally agreed to by everyone. As we all know from our day-to-day experiences, all human beings present a certain face to the rest of the world. Most of us have a desire to be liked, respected, or approved of by others, and to put our "best foot forward"

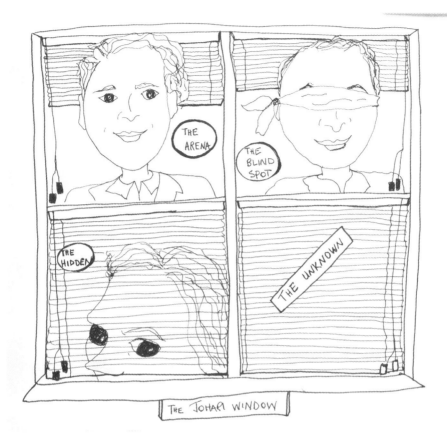

in the world in order to get what we want and simply make our lives easier. The Arena is that part of our psyche over which we have the greatest control. This does not necessarily mean we are constantly making minute-to-minute decisions about what we say and what we present; over time, the face we present to the rest of the world becomes somewhat automatized and routinized, even though we may have once made many conscious decisions in shaping it initially. For example, a person who views himself as somewhat unexceptional academically or athletically, or has self-doubt regarding appearance or body image, may consciously choose to project another image to distract everyone else's attention from these self-perceived short-comings. Such a person may choose to become "the funny one"—the person who is always cracking jokes, always smiling, and always jovial. Such a projection into the Arena consumes some psychological energy and requires conscious effort at first. Over time, however, it becomes easier as the rest of the world grows to expect the jokes and sense of humor, and the person and all those around that person agree that this is one funny guy! It is important to note that the Arena is NOT some kind of fake self or some sort of act that is foisted on the rest of the world. Over time, the projection of self into the Arena becomes who you are and who everyone else knows you to be. The Arena is what is generally described by others as personality . . . for good or for bad. At times, of course, the projection into the Arena may involve seemingly negative attributes as well. A person who is considered unusually physically attractive may grow lazy and over-rely on physical attractiveness as their projection at the expense of cultivating other projections into the Arena. Alternatively, someone who simply happens to be smarter or bigger, or faster, or more talented than others may overcultivate that projection into the Arena and risks being stereotyped by others as "a nerd", a "jock", or a "band geek."

Because the Arena is the part of the psyche that is most readily controlled by us consciously, there are seemingly endless self-help and popular psychology books that focus on "changing yourself, changing your life." This is not unreasonable. Each of us has power to change our projection into the Arena, but it does require conscious effort and psychological energy. Importantly, however, as we shall soon see, this is only part of the story of our psyche; there are several other aspects of our psyche that may be much more resistant to conscious influence or of which we may simply be unaware.

The Hidden: The Hidden is that part of our psyche that is known only to ourselves and, consequently, kept hidden and out of sight to the rest of the world. As human beings, all of us are aware that there are parts of ourselves we want no one else to know about—thoughts we are embarrassed about or behaviors we may be ashamed of it they were known by others. Frequently, many of these thoughts and behaviors may have a sexual aspect. The Hidden corresponds to your "little secrets," the things you know very well about yourself that you would never tell another person, including your closest friends. At first glance, this may appear negative or problematic. In today's environment of reality television, there is a strong social bias toward "radical transparency," "having no secrets," and "letting it all hang out." According to the Johari Window, not only is this not possible, but it is arguably not desirable. For society to function safely, and for individual relationships to be sustainable, it is simply not possible to be 100% honest with everyone all the time. The Hidden serves as the repository of those thoughts, behaviors, and attitudes that we are fully aware of but that we have consciously chosen to suppress from public view.

Because the Hidden is generally under conscious control, most human beings find a way of reconciling this notion of the "secrets and lies" we all hold. For example, an individual who lives in a particularly conservative culture or community but who has strong homosexual impulses or feelings may simply not feel safe disclosing the truth to others. Such a person may consciously choose to live an outwardly conventional life involving heterosexual marriage, yet "on the side" is fulfilling secret desires. Although the ethics of this kind of double life, and its long-term sustainability, are different matters entirely, from a psychological perspective, the Johari Window helps us to understand how this is possible and why this may be perceived as necessary.

In this way, the Hidden can sometimes be seen as a kind of safety valve; being under conscious control, an individual can choose the time and circumstances under which secrets (and sometimes lies) can be brought forward into the Arena. Except of course when sometimes they can't, because as we all know, there are situations where the most deeply buried secrets may accidently erupt into public view (or project into the Arena) and this can cause enormous difficulty for self and others.

Importantly, the notion that the Hidden refers to the secrets only known by the self has important implications for health care professionals. Owing to their unique role and status in society—and legal, professional, and ethical obligations to maintain confidentiality—many people will seek out health care professionals to unburden themselves when the secrets of the Hidden become overwhelming. Some professionals—for example, general practitioners, psychotherapists, and social workers—are highly trained for this kind of situation and it is a central part of their role. Other professionals—for example, pharmacists, physiotherapists, or dentists—may not think of themselves in such a way, yet may find themselves in situations where patients who see them for seemingly technical or procedural issues suddenly disclose information that is uncomfortable. In such situations, these professionals may think (or even say), "I'm not a social worker. You should go find one and let me do my job instead." Of course, the reality is that, as a health care professional, all of us at certain times will need to develop the compassion and communication skills generally associated with a profession like social work in order to help a patient in real time, even if this makes us feel uncomfortable as we are doing so.

The Blind Spot: The Blind Spot exists at the intersection of the things the rest of the world knows about us that we, in fact, do not even know about ourselves. Think, for example, of the plight of some middle-aged men. Once, in their youth, they may have had a thick and lustrous full head of hair. With time (and hormonal fluctuations) some men go bald or experience thinning hair. Although many men accept this gracefully as an inevitable part of aging (and some go so far as to fully embrace it by actively shaving themselves bald to keep ahead of it), there are some men who do not or cannot accept such reality and instead engage in the act of the comb-over. The comb-over is a hair style in which remaining wisps of hair are arranged in a manner that, when observed front on in a mirror, gives the appearance of not going bald, but from every other direction and by every other observer signifies a balding middle-aged man's desire to fruitlessly and vainly cling on to an illusion of masculine virility. For most engaged in comb-overs, there is no self-awareness that baldness is real or a problem; further, there is a firm belief that the way I look in the mirror is exactly the way everyone else sees me. In reality, of course, this is the definition of a blind spot: the inability to see oneself as others see you.

Of course, some Blind Spot issues are much more impactful and problematic than the trivial and somewhat amusing issue of the comb-over. In some cultures and communities, the issue of homosexuality is so forbidden and such a taboo that, in such cases, an individual experiencing same-sex attractions or inclinations may not even have a vocabulary or words to explain these feelings and, consequently, doesn't even know they are gay or lesbian. Through their words, actions, and behaviors projected into the Arena, it may be painfully and tragically obvious to everyone else.

Another example of the importance of the Blind Spot for health care professionals may relate to certain potentially harmful lifestyle behaviors. Some individuals may have no awareness of the longer term potential medical complications associated with high blood pressure, obesity, or smoking. Despite decades of public health campaigns and education, they may have no conscious awareness that their behaviors may shorten their life, even if everyone else around them knows this. Because the Blind Spot is not subject to conscious control, it becomes extraordinarily challenging for a health professional or family member to help in such a situation. Simply telling or lecturing someone will have very limited influence in the Blind Spot until the person comes to conscious awareness on their own. Indeed, pushing too hard in the Blind Spot by nagging and lecturing can actually worsen the situation because it may trigger defensive responses by the person to specifically safeguard an existing worldview. For example, telling conservative parents who have no mental model or understanding of homosexuality (because in their culture, it doesn't exist) that their child may be gay, lesbian, or bisexual and offering education, counseling, and support can spectacularly backfire if it provokes a circle-the-wagons response in which the messenger of such news is then diminished or vilified.

The Blind Spot helps us to understand some of the enormous complexity associated with human behaviors, particularly when people engage in certain actions that to everyone else may appear deliberately self-injurious, yet they persist in acting this way. Within the Blind Spot, there is extreme resistance to simple conversations or friendly advice, and in some cases there may be very limited options available to help support change.

The Unknown (or the Unconscious): In some ways perhaps the most important yet mysterious facet of the psyche, the Unconscious represents the part of ourselves that is both unknown to ourselves and unknown to the rest of the world, yet it is real and has a demonstrable impact on thoughts, behaviors, and actions. The power of the unconscious lies in its unpredictability. By definition, it is not under conscious control, and because the rest of the world is unaware of it as well, there are few if any options for dealing with unconsciousness leading to negative behaviors. The Unknown is an extraordinarily challenging yet very important aspect of the human psyche. On the one hand, it is perhaps the place where some of our problematic but rarely challenged stereotypes of others may reside. For example, individual prejudice against certain groups of people becomes particularly toxic and overwhelming when it is matched by societal unawareness that this is a problem. Within a health context, the Unknown represents an almost impenetrable problem: If neither the patient, her family, her community, nor her health care providers know something is a problem, how can it be fixed?

Importantly, although the Unknown can seem to be a complete black hole impervious to the light of awareness, with time, change is possible. Years ago, homosexuality was thought to be a disease, a victim of the Unknown. Today, depending on the individual, her community, and society, it may be in the Arena, the Hidden, or the Blind Spot. The Unknown may not be as fixed and unchangeable as it appears at first glance, and with time, evolution of this sort may be possible.

6.1.2   How Can Understanding the Johari Window Support Better Communication with Patients?

The value of understanding the Johari Window as an important psychological theory lies not only in providing a framework for assessing an individual's behavioral choices, but in also providing a framework for helping direct and manage interpersonal communication between the health care professional and the patient. In recognizing the segmented nature of our psyches, and in acknowledging the balance between conscious control and unconscious unawareness, health professionals may have unique opportunities to engage with patients in highly meaningful ways to promote better health outcomes.

The Arena represents the most straightforward opportunity for communication. In this quadrant, little is contested or hidden, and consequently, honest and open communication is both anticipated and rewarded. Interestingly, the open nature of the Arena may produce a paradoxical shift in the nature of practitioner–patient relationships. When health discussions occur in the Arena, individuals may not perceive of themselves as patients but instead as clients, customers, or consumers. As we have seen in Chapter 4, such a shift will require a change in communication style and an intent to reach the individual where they are, not where the health professional wants or wishes them to be.

The Hidden represents unique challenges and opportunities for health care professionals. The unique social status of practitioners, coupled with widely known requirements around maintaining confidentiality of disclosed and shared information, may mean that health care professionals are the first people an individual may consult as they contemplate their trajectory between the Hidden and the Arena. This represents an enormously sensitive, delicate, and vulnerable time for an individual, who in this case may be more likely to think of themselves as a patient rather than as a client, customer, or consumer. With this vulnerability comes the potential for abuse of power by the professional who may be feared. In such a moment, there are enormously important requirements for practitioners for a communications style characterized by respect, warmth, and affirmation. No matter how shocking, surprising, or potentially unethical or illegal the secret is in the Hidden, it is incumbent upon the health care professional—in the first instance at least—to demonstrate respect, to gather information nonjudgmentally and without prejudice, and to reserve judgment for a later time. Leaping too quickly to conclusions or judgment, or allowing personal bias to interfere with clinical compassion or care, will sabotage the relationship with the patient and undermine future shifts between the Hidden and the Arena. The reality, however, is also that, in some instances, health care professionals may learn of details in the Hidden that do indeed warrant some kind of legal intervention, and that the duty for such intervention may override other patient-focused considerations (e.g., in the case of child abuse). In such situations, your relevant legal and ethical obligations regarding mandatory reporting and confidentiality associated with your profession and described in your profession's code of ethics should be followed.

The nature of the Blind Spot suggests the greatest opportunities for positive intervention from health care professionals, but also demands the most sophisticated and nuanced form of communication to prevent emergence of defensive responses. Approaching a patient (who may not self-identify as a patient in the Blind Spot) will require careful use of open-ended questions, a nonjudgmental style, and a carefully crafted sense of priorities rather than attempting to solve every problem at once. Within the Blind Spot, there is limited value (if any) to lecturing, telling, or threatening. Saying, "Listen, I'm the health care professional and I know what's best—you have no idea what risk your facing" will be both offensive and unproductive in most cases. Instead, helping the patient to bring to full consciousness the issue you (and everyone else) knows about but that they are currently unaware of requires a gradual give and take along with time, focus, and attention. The journey from Blind Spot to Arena can be long and does not fit neatly into a 4-minute appointment time slot. It can take months or years to make this transition along with patience (and a strong sense of priorities as to what is most important). The practitioner must carefully monitor and effectively respond to nonverbal cues transmitted by patients as this process evolves. The unconscious nature of the Blind Spot means that many responses will be nonverbal in nature and may frequently trend toward the emotional rather than the verbal or logical. Attentiveness to faces, gestures, and tone can provide important clues as to how the patient is receiving the communication transmitted by the professional (see Chapter 5).

Because the Unconscious is, by definition, unknown to both practitioner and patient, there are limited communication interventions (if any) to support development in this area. The reality is that there are, of course, limits to what health professionals are able to do and, sometimes, sadly and tragically, awful things may happen where everyone, even the patient, is unaware.

Reflecting on your patients—and clients, customers, and consumers—through the lens of the Johari Window can help you to better understand and communicate with them. Key lessons from the Johari Window include the following: Much of what influences our behavior as human beings is actually unconscious or unknown to ourselves; the secrets of the Hidden may be important and represent recourse to safety rather than any attempt to deliberately hurt others or lie; the transitions between the Hidden and the Arena and the Hidden and the Blind Spot represent unique challenges and opportunities for health care professionals; and despite best hopes and intentions, there are limits to what practitioners can actually do for patients. The existence of the Unknown as a quadrant of the Johari Window highlights areas of the psyche that are off-limits to everyone.

6.2 The Transtheoretical Model for Change

The work of health care professionals, although important, is frequently challenging and sometimes frustrating. In part, this challenge and frustration is a function of the reality that health care professionals—regardless of their professional role or scope of practice—spend a lot of their time asking people to cheerfully and consistently make big changes in their lives. For example, nurses frequently suggest to patients they quit smoking in order to help improve their health. Do these nurses have any idea how hard this is to actually do? Doctors frequently insist to their patients they need to lose weight. Do they realize that in most cases patients already know this and if it were that easy, the weight would already be gone? Pharmacists frequently educate patients about how to manage complex (and sometimes seemingly simple) medication regimens. Don't they realize that their directions to "take one tablet three times a day without food, spaced out at least 1 to 2 hours from any antacids or calcium-containing vitamin pills" are incredibly and impossibly complicated to figure out once the patient goes home? Dentists ask us to floss regularly, physiotherapists give us complex and sweat-inducing exercises to follow, etc.

As anyone who has actually received care from a practitioner will tell you, knowing the reasons behind and understanding the importance of changing personal behaviors does not automatically result in those behaviors being changed. The Transtheoretical Model for Change proposed by Prochaska et al. is one of the most enduring theories in health professions education, and it not only helps us to understand how change occurs and why it is difficult but also what specific communication strategies may be most effective in helping to motivate and support patients through a change process. The five stages of this model are (1) precontemplation, (2) contemplation, (3) preparation, (4) action, and (5) maintenance. Let's examine each of these stages of change experienced by patients—and implications for health care practitioners—in further detail.

Precontemplation: In this stage, individuals do not self-identify as patients, and may not even self-identify as consumers. Instead, they have little or no awareness that there is any problem that requires any change on their part. In precontemplation, individuals respond to a subjective sense of equilibrium or well-being; they are not necessarily denying the existence of a health-related problem but instead are unaware something in fact is a problem. Consider many middle-aged individuals who lead busy and productive lives but experience little or no impairment of daily activities due to health concerns. They feel fine, they can do whatever they want to do, and they only go visit a nurse practitioner or family doctor once a year for a checkup because their spouse or partner badgers them to do so. One day, at such an annual check, the practitioner announces, "Yup, your blood pressure is too high. We've been seeing it go up the last few years but didn't do anything about it, but now we need to put you on medications to treat it." To an individual in precontemplation, this is a lot of new information coming at them too quickly. High blood pressure—*but I feel fine!* Medications—*that's going to be way too complicated in my already busy life, and besides, I don't want to be the kind of person who has to take drugs every day!* And treatment—*you think I'm sick, but I feel fine!* No matter how medically accurate the medical diagnosis and treatment plan may be, this is a lot of information to dump on a person when, 10 minutes earlier before they walked in your office, they were feeling fine and thinking nothing was wrong.

In precontemplation, individuals are unaware there is a problem, so the language of "don't worry, we can fix this problem you have" literally makes no sense to them. People in precontemplation are not necessarily able to cognitively process what you're telling them, in part because all of this news is primarily being processed emotionally, and part of this emotional processing is the time required to realize and acknowledge, "Oh, you're actually talking about ME."

Many well-intentioned health care professionals make communication errors that can be problematic when they assume telling a patient who is in precontemplation that something is important. If a person is truly in precontemplation with respect to behavioral change, telling (or advising, or warning) may actually backfire because the person isn't yet ready to hear a message and will consequently ignore you, or worse, never come back to see you. Strange though it may seem, for a client in pre-contemplation, the focus for the practitioner should be on simply keeping the lines of communication open, and letting the client know you are available, rather than trying to foist something new on them or cajole them into making a change they are psychologically unprepared to make.

Most of the signs and symptoms of precontemplation are nonverbal and emotional in nature; no one will say, "Hey Doc, I'm in precontemplation so you are getting way ahead of me here . . . just give it a rest about this blood pressure thing for now and maybe in a few months we'll get together again and discuss further." Instead, through facial responses, hand gestures, and tone of voice, many clients will transmit their precontemplative state, and it is up to the practitioner to appropriately pick up on these cues and respond effectively.

Some practitioners may be concerned about the ethics of simply going along with a client and ignoring medically important issues just to maintain a positive relationship. Some may argue that untreated hypertension (sometimes called "the Silent Killer") demands a more forceful response and intervention from the health care professional. According to the Transtheoretical Model, this well-intentioned sentiment is fundamentally misguided at best and will break the practitioner–client relationship at worst. Recall from Chapter 1 that health care delivery only works when practitioners and clients are actually connected with one another; if a person is in precontemplation and a practitioner comes across too strongly, forcefully, or heavy handed, there is a high probability the relationship and connection will break, and the individual will simply withdraw from receiving health care of any kind because the experience has been so negative for them. In precontemplation, the focus is on maintaining the relationship and keeping the door open for further conversation when the time is right. Trying to solve someone else's problem when that someone else doesn't even know they have a problem is rarely successful.

Contemplation: The shift between precontemplation and contemplation is both subtle and important. In the contemplation stage of the model, individuals are growing into an awareness that they themselves have some kind of problem. They may not yet be willing or able to fully describe it, acknowledge its full extent, or completely accept it, but the self-awareness that there may be "something I need to fix" opens the door to thinking about changing personal behaviors. The bubble of contemplation can be very fragile. If at this stage a practitioner or family member pushes too hard or becomes too forceful, a person can easily slide back into precontemplation and slam the door shut on further discussion or behavioral change.

In contemplation, there are very specific communication interventions that have demonstrable superiority in helping to motivate individuals in a more productive manner toward change. For example, rather than saying, "You have high blood pressure and as a result you need to lose 20 to 25 lbs in the next 3 months to stay healthy and avoid medications . . . let's see how that goes," it may be more productive to use less directive (you-oriented sentences) and instead speak in generalities. For example, saying, "Lots of people in this age bracket have higher than desired blood pressure. For many of these people, there is a desire to avoid medications. The first step in seeing if that's possible is to try to lose some weight." In this sentence, the word "you" is not actually used, and as a result, the sentence is less threatening and provocative. The second approach does not provide specific details such as the amount of weight to be lost or the expected time frame and is consequently less overwhelming and daunting for the patient. Key elements to communication with patients who are in the contemplation stage include the following concepts: (1) Acknowledge that patients are ready to learn more BUT not necessarily ready to commit to a decision or a behavior. (2) Avoid use of direct sentences involving the word "you" because this may come across as overly demanding and intimidating and may cause patients to revert back to precontemplation. Instead, use indirect sentences or phrases, or focus on what other people do or think to make the situation less immediate for the patient. (3) Be cautious about overloading a patient with facts and figures and overwhelming them with detailed expectations. General comments and statements are useful to provide further food for thought, but too much of this can be counterproductive. (4) Similar to the precontemplation stage, an important goal of communication with the patient in contemplation involves ensuring the door remains open to future conversations and the patient feels the relationship with the practitioner is strong. This can be accomplished by letting the patient know you'd be happy to speak more about this when the patient is available or ready, and signal that further information is available. (5) Provide patients with opportunities to do their own research in private to learn more, by signposting resources online or in other public places such as health clinics. This allows the patient to gradually move from contemplation to the next stage (preparation) in their own time and away without feeling they are being monitored or watched.

Preparation: In the preparation stage of change, patients have moved from lack of awareness regarding a problem to openness to acknowledging and learning more. In preparation, patients have learned enough and accepted it to recognize that real behavioral change is likely necessary. At this stage, the recognition of necessity may still not be enough to actually produce sustainable change over time; "the spirit may be strong but the flesh continues to be weak." In preparation, patients know the right thing to do but may lack the self-confidence, tools, or support to actually make changes that last. As a result, many patients benefit from a preparation period in which they can actually take incremental steps (i.e., baby steps) on their pathway to change in private and at their own pace, so in case they do not succeed they are able to save face and not lose respect in front of others. In this way, precontemplation and contemplation can be likened to the Blind Spot, whereas in preparation, the patient is shifting toward the Hidden, using the Johari Window model.

What can health care professionals do to provide support and guidance during preparation? First, they must recognize that, as with the previous two stages, time and patience are required. Praise and positive reinforcement are essential at this time, but practitioners need to be cautious about anything that sounds like or resembles criticism. For example, if a patient is considering losing weight, the first time they try a diet, there is a likelihood it will not be successful (i.e., no or very little weight will be lost, or if weight is lost, it will be regained relatively quickly). This does not represent failure; instead, it represents an important learning curve that is a part of a change process. Preparation represents the early stages of that learning curve, where patients will be particularly susceptible to criticism or being made fun of because they lack will power or stamina. Supporting the patient's decision to take these initial baby steps within the Hidden and out of sight from family and friends can help build a strong bond and strengthen the relationship between patient and practitioner. It also gives the patient the time and space they need in order to actually unlearn old behaviors and patterns and relearn new, healthier ones instead.

Action: The fourth stage of the process of change represents an important milestone. In the action stage, patients are able and willing to make a public declaration to change. The importance of publicly stating "I'm going to lose weight," "I'm going to stop smoking," or "I will run a 10K race by the end of the year" is significant. In publicly declaring a commitment to change, individuals begin to mobilize their family, friends, and communities to be part of the process. Unlike a caring practitioner, who in the preparation stage understands the importance of positive reinforcement rather than criticism and gives the patient space to learn to change privately, a public declaration opens the patient to a degree of scrutiny and potential vulnerability. Some friends and family may not be very gentle and considerate if the patient fails to live up to the commitments made.

Although this may sound cruel, this vulnerability and the fear of public failure is actually part of the psychological energy that may fuel success during action. Any major change is hard and requires overcoming inertia and years (sometimes decades) of well-rehearsed behaviors. In the action phase, patients have acquired sufficient self-confidence to believe they have the skills needed to succeed in the declared change, and the fear of mockery or disappointing others may be an important part of what keeps them trying to change even when they are getting tired. Of course, health care professionals must never engage in mockery or express this kind of disappointment in patients who struggle in the action stage. In maintaining a stance of positive reinforcement and support, practitioners can become even more connected to patients and even more trusted by being the good cop, while friends and families with well-established histories can assume more of the bad cop role in motivating change.

At a certain point in the action phase, a patient's psychology will start to shift. The initial effort required to, for example, make healthier eating choices or stop smoking consumes enormous cognitive and emotional energy. Over time, the effort to sustain this becomes less effortful. Although it may never become easy or second nature, it likely will become more automatic or more routine, and as a result, the patient grows more comfortable with this change. The praise (or at least absence of mockery or criticism) that comes with this success further adds psychological fuel to sustain the change initiative, and it all simply becomes easier to maintain over time.

Maintenance: The final stage of the Transtheoretical Model is maintenance, the point where the time, energy, and effort required to change a behavior becomes rewarded by the behavior becoming incorporated into day-to-day life with a minimum amount of additional effort or exertion. In maintenance, there is always a continuing risk that old behaviors may reemerge, particularly if there is a life stress or other particularly difficult situation. By this point, however, most individuals will have learned to self-identify risk factors for relapse into old behavior and will develop coping strategies to help prevent this from happening. At this stage, health professionals can be most beneficial by acting as an external set of eyes and ears to alert the patient to any small changes of behavior signaling reversion to old habits before these become too serious, and to continue to offer praise, support, and encouragement as appropriate.

The Transtheoretical Model has most frequently been used by health care professionals in helping to structure a series of conversations with patients attempting to undertake difficult lifestyle modifications such as quitting smoking or losing weight. Although it is presented as a tidy and sequential process, the reality is of course that it can be much messier. People may frequently slide back and forth across these stages rather than progress in a forward, stepwise fashion. The Transtheoretical Model uniquely helps structure communication with patients by emphasizing different forms and styles of communication at different stages of the process. Knowing when it is best to say nothing (or very little) and when it is appropriate to be more direct in a conversation can be very helpful for support practitioners to better help their patients. This model also highlights the importance of effective communication, and the consequences of getting it wrong. For example, being overly directive in communication and using "you" statements while someone is in contemplation may unintentionally irritate patients who may respond by simply walking away from the practitioner and not returning. In contrast, some well-placed indirect statements and questions followed by a genuine invitation to stay connected with one another can, in the weeks and months ahead, produce not only a stronger practitioner–patient relationship, but ultimately can help a patient succeed on their own in changing behaviors.

6.3   Communication in Social Media: More of the Same or Fundamentally Different?

Throughout this chapter and the previous ones, there has been an implicit assumption that interpersonal communication involves interactions between two individuals within a physically connected space; that is, communication involves face-to-face interactions such as talking with one another. Although this has historically been the dominant way in which practitioners and patients have interacted and health care teams have operated, in many settings, alternative forms of communication are becoming more common and will likely become ever more routine in the future. Among these alternative forms of communication are those involving commercially available (and ever-changing) platforms such as Facebook or Instagram, use of text-heavy systems that may or may not include emoticons, and use of digitally mediated communication vehicles such as telemedicine or videoconferencing.

The evolution of social media communication in health care is nowhere near complete, and rapid acceleration in technologies is to be anticipated in the years ahead. As a result, it is difficult to make definitive and generalizable statements regarding communication in a technologically mediated world, but several trends appear to be emerging.

Technology and social media do not necessarily replace old-school, face-to-face communication, but instead extend it for the purpose of convenience. Busy health care providers cannot possibly meet with every patient who needs their attention at the time it is required. A significant advantage of technology and social media is the ability to reach more people in a more convenient manner and provide quicker consultations as appropriate. Importantly, current experience suggests that the use of technology in health care is most effective when it builds on a preexisting, face-to-face relationship rather than replacing it completely. Especially when individuals self-identify as patients, there is significant psychological value and comfort associated with having met, shaken hands, and physically seen a health care professional in person first and at least once or twice after. Once a foundation of face-to-face communication has been established, it may be easier to use different technologies to extend it. Health care relationships that only exist in a virtual space may not be as satisfying or effective for either the patient or the practitioner, although at times it simply may be the only option available. Where the option exists, finding opportunities to initially connect with patients (or other health care professionals) in person can rapidly enhance the efficiency of subsequent online or digital interactions by accelerating the development of the all important relationship required to build trust.

Digitally mediated communication will never disappear. As is well known, there is a permanence associated with many forms of digitally or technologically mediated communication that introduces important opportunities and challenges for practitioners. On the one hand, social media may allow patients to review communication many times, at their own pace and in their own way, and in the process, can facilitate greater learning and understanding without actually consuming more of the practitioner's time. On the other hand, the permanence or semipermanence associated with technologically mediated conversation may intimidate some practitioners who find themselves always worrying about saying the wrong thing and there being a permanent record of it. The professional and legal risk issues have not been fully determined either by the courts or within professions, and as this understanding evolves, technology continues to become more sophisticated.

Privacy, confidentiality, and security become exponentially more complicated within technologically mediated communication environments. The skills to manage this are generally beyond those of most clinically trained practitioners. Communicating by email, Skype, Zoom, Instagram, Twitter, or WhatsApp (and whatever platforms will evolve in the years ahead that will replace them) may seem simple, free, and easy, but for health professionals, there are enormous implications with respect to the content of medically sensitive personal health information and context-specific advice or information provided to patients or shared within a health care team. Maintaining a secure communication chain and ensuring that only those who are legally, ethically, and professionally able to access information do so becomes an important consideration. For example, if a health care professional is contacted by email by patient Katie McHilbo, but the email address provided is katie&anthony@gspace.com

(as is common for some couples), is this email address private and secure? Is it legal, ethical, and professional to disclose personal medical information to this email address? You could claim, "Well, she contacted me using this email address and all I did was respond!" Or is there an expectation that the health professional gain explicit consent from Katie (the patient) to use the provided email and that the patient should state they understand confidential information may be transmitted this way? This is an evolving legal area of practice, but in the mean time, practitioners must make decisions everyday as to whether it is safe and appropriate to respond to patient's emails, text messages, and other social media and what the consequences may be from a professional and ethical perspective.

In the absence of nonverbal cues, human communication is fundamentally altered. Although some digital forms of communication (e.g., Skype, videoconferencing) allow individuals to see and hear one another, other forms of communication (e.g., texting, email) are predominantly written with or without the addition of emotional signifiers called emoticons. Over the course of human evolution, this is an extraordinary development. As described in Chapters 4 and 5, the psychology of human communication relies heavily on both verbal and nonverbal cues, and when one of these cues (representing perhaps 80% of the information transmitted between receiver and sender) are removed, it is not clear what implications exist for human relationships and accurate understanding of the content transmitted. You likely have experienced this issue yourself, such as an offhand comment intended as humorous or sarcastic being misinterpreted when it is a text message or email because the nonverbal cues we use to signify humor or sarcasm aren't available. Even when emoticons such as "☺" are included, it can be hard to decipher the intensity of an emoticon versus the intensity of a nonverbal cue. In such environments, literalism tends to prevail, and technologically mediated communication can take on an almost legalistic tone of "well, you SAID this . . . " versus "well, I MEANT that . . . ." Worse, without nonverbal cues, it is difficult for emotional filters to fully engage, and the opportunity to build meaningful trusting relationships between human beings may be directly impeded or not.

Although the convenience and appeal of technologically mediated communication is a large part of what has made it so popular, other aspects of this evolving form of interpersonal relationships have raised unanswered questions.

In theory, technologically mediated communication facilitates the expression by a larger number of more diverse voices by reducing traditional barriers that in the past may have held back individuals and communities from fully participating in discussions. Although this may be true, it is equally apparent that, in many cases, technologically mediated communication has also generated an echo chamber effect in which individuals seek out communication and interpersonal relationships mainly with people who think and resemble them already. Rather than use the power of technology to meet new people with different perspectives and ideas, online communication has become a way of reinforcing, rather than challenging, individual beliefs and thoughts. As a result, amplification, rather than critical analysis, of ideas may be leading to increased polarization and isolation rather than true community building.

Psychologists have described the power of variable intermittent rewards (VIRs) as one of the most influential forces shaping human behavior. As we know, rewarding certain kinds of behaviors increases the likelihood that that behavior will occur in the future, whereas use of punishing behaviors decreases the likelihood of recurrence. For example, if a parent wants to incentivize a child to clean her room, providing gold stars, lavish praise, or a financial reward is one way to accomplish this aim, but alternatively, punishing the child for NOT cleaning her room (by withholding computer privileges, not allowing her to go out with her friends, or criticizing her) may also be used. VIRs are rewards that are unpredictable and do not follow a schedule, thereby forcing the person seeking the reward to believe something better is always just around the corner, so that person keeps on behaving and performing in a way that might trigger the next big reward. VIRs have been studied extensively in the context of casinos and slot machines, and why gambling has such an addictive quality. VIRs seduce gamblers into believing the next big payout is coming up so gamblers keep feeding the machine awaiting that outcome. Increasingly, psychologists have noted that many social media platforms operate in a similar manner. The chronic need to check Facebook or Instagram, or the constant desire to swipe right on online dating sites, points to the problem of FOMO (fear of missing out on the next big thing), which drives a craving for constantly checking websites. Worse, over time, this behavior may produce a state where happiness in the moment and contentment with what one has now becomes difficult or impossible to achieve because of FOMO. The implications of these observations, especially on younger people who have only ever known a world immersed in technology, are not entirely understood.

Induced demand is a term that describes the insatiability of human needs. It was initially described by transit planners, who noted that every time a new road was built or an old road was expanded, within a few years traffic would build up to the point where further expansion was once again necessary, but to the point where there was literally no more space to build new roads. By making a road better and easier to drive on, they were encouraging more and more people to drive on it, which in turn lead to oversaturation. Within technologically mediated communication, a similar pattern of induced demand has been observed: The faster you respond to other people's emails and texts, the faster they expect you to respond to the next one . . . and the greater the disappointment when you don't. Induced demand places inordinate pressure on individuals to be constantly tethered to their phones and computers to the point of sacrificing weekends, evenings, holidays, family time, and especially, face-to-face interpersonal communication and relationships in order to attend to the next text, email, or Facebook posting that comes along. Paradoxically, tools that were supposed to enhance human communication now have become a barrier to the face-to-face relationship building that nurtures and grows interpersonal connections. Health care professionals who facilitate patient communication through electronic means must be especially careful of this problem of induced demand and the potential impact it could have on their personal and family lives, as well as eventually serving as a substitute or replacement for what should be a face-to-face professional relationship.

6.4 Summary

In Chapters 5 and 6, we reviewed important aspects of communication theory that are useful for health care professionals working in teams. Of course, there are many more models and theories that have been studied; it is simply not possible to present all relevant theories here. Introducing yourself to these communication theories is an important first step in understanding some of the psychological underpinnings of interpersonal relationships, and this in turn can help you to better understand, predict, and manage the complex relationships that will occur in your practice.

6.5 Mind Map Chapter 6

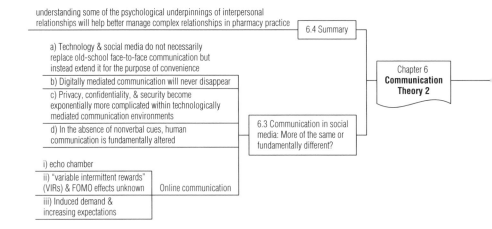

understanding some of the psychological underpinnings of interpersonal
relationships will help better manage complex relationships in pharmacy practice

6.4 Summary

Chapter 6
**Communication
Theory 2**

a) Technology & social media do not necessarily
replace old-school face-to-face communication but
instead extend it for the purpose of convenience

b) Digitally mediated communication will never disappear

c) Privacy, confidentiality, & security become
exponentially more complicated within technologically
mediated communication environments

d) In the absence of nonverbal cues, human
communication is fundamentally altered

6.3 Communication in social
media: More of the same or
fundamentally different?

i) echo chamber

ii) "variable intermittent rewards"
(VIRs) & FOMO effects unknown   Online communication

iii) Induced demand &
increasing expectations

Mind Map for Team Psychology

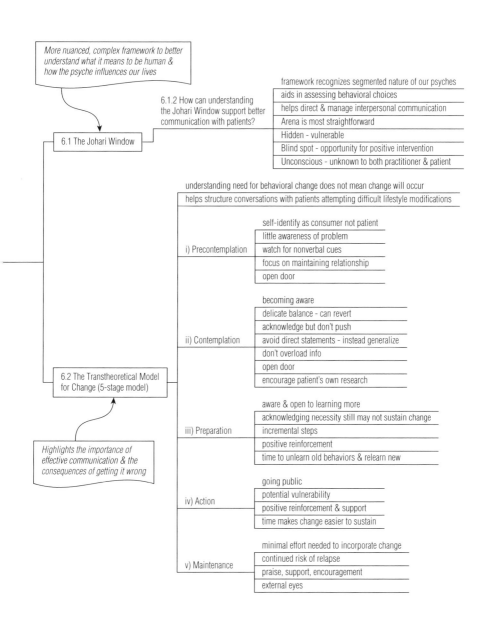

More nuanced, complex framework to better understand what it means to be human & how the psyche influences our lives

6.1 The Johari Window

6.1.2 How can understanding the Johari Window support better communication with patients?

framework recognizes segmented nature of our psyches
aids in assessing behavioral choices
helps direct & manage interpersonal communication
Arena is most straightforward
Hidden - vulnerable
Blind spot - opportunity for positive intervention
Unconscious - unknown to both practitioner & patient

6.2 The Transtheoretical Model for Change (5-stage model)

Highlights the importance of effective communication & the consequences of getting it wrong

understanding need for behavioral change does not mean change will occur
helps structure conversations with patients attempting difficult lifestyle modifications

i) Precontemplation
self-identify as consumer not patient
little awareness of problem
watch for nonverbal cues
focus on maintaining relationship
open door

ii) Contemplation
becoming aware
delicate balance - can revert
acknowledge but don't push
avoid direct statements - instead generalize
don't overload info
open door
encourage patient's own research

iii) Preparation
aware & open to learning more
acknowledging necessity still may not sustain change
incremental steps
positive reinforcement
time to unlearn old behaviors & relearn new

iv) Action
going public
potential vulnerability
positive reinforcement & support
time makes change easier to sustain

v) Maintenance
minimal effort needed to incorporate change
continued risk of relapse
praise, support, encouragement
external eyes

For Further Reading:

Antheunis M, Tates K, Nieboer T. Patients' and health professionals' use of social media in health care: motives, barriers and expectations. *Patient Educ Couns.* 2013;92:426–431.

Berland A. Using the Johari Window to explore patient and provider perspectives. *Int J Health Gov.* 2017;22(1):47–51.

Moorhead S, Hazlett D, Harrison L, Carooll J, Irwin A, Hoving C. A new dimension of health care: systematic review of the uses, benefits, and limitations of social media for health communication. *J Med Int Res.* 2013;15(4):e85.

Prochaska J, Velicer W. The transtheoretical model of health behavior change. *Am J Health Promot.* 1997;12(1):38–48.

Ramani, S, Könings, K, Mann K, van der Vleuten C. Uncovering the unknown: a grounded theory study exploring the impact of self-awareness on the culture of feedback in residency education. *Med Teacher.* 2017;39(10):1065–1073.

Saxena P. Johari Window: an effective model for improving interpersonal communication and managerial effectiveness. *SIT J Manag.* 2015;5(2):134–146.

Verklan M. Johari Window: a model for communicating to each other. *J Perinat Neonatal Nurs.* 2007;21(2):173–174.

Whitelaw S, Baldwin S, Bunton R, Flynn D. The status of evidence and outcomes in stages of change research. *Health Educ Res.* 2000;15(6):707–718.

7 | Communication Skills

Understanding psychological and communication theories can be an important and helpful first step in building your practical and clinical skills as a health care professional. Knowing the reasons WHY certain communication strategies work—or do not work—can help you to better plan conversations and anticipate how they may evolve. Knowledge of these theories can also help you to reflect on your relationships with patients, clients, customers, and consumers, as well as your colleagues, and identify opportunities to improve them.

In this chapter, we will focus on application of these theories to support development of communication skills. Many people may feel they are already skilled communicators, but of course, there is always room for improvement. Others may feel they have good skills as a communicator in everyday life, but the context of health care work and collaborative interprofessional teams is quite different than a sports team or community orchestra; although the context may be different, many of the skills we will discuss in this chapter are applicable in any interpersonal setting. Still others may be concerned that they simply lack the necessary communication skills to function effectively as a health care professional or interprofessional team member, or somehow cannot learn them. Although it may be true that communication may come more easily to some people than to others, communication is also a skill that can be learned and improved through rehearsal, reflection, and application.

7.1 Effective Listening: The Cornerstone of Communication

Recall from Chapter 5 the model of interpersonal communication involving senders, receivers, and the environment around them, and the idea that communication involves the reciprocal transmitting and interpreting of information. This model prioritizes the notion that both sender and receiver are connected to one another and are constantly delivering and receiving information (e.g., verbal and nonverbal, factual and emotional) to and from one another. Central to this process is *effective listening*.

This term is somewhat imprecise because it suggests that the hearing of words is all that is important. Effective listening is about much more than simply words, although words are an important aspect of it. Instead, effective listening is a general term that encapsulates the importance of noticing and paying attention to everything that is going on during an interaction with someone else: words, facial grimaces, hand gestures, tone of voice, body language, etc.

Every interpersonal interaction is a give-and-take dynamic, with one person saying or doing something and the other person responding in some way in a reciprocal and iterative fashion. Many unfortunate miscommunications occur because individuals simply do not pay sufficient attention to the other person, misread, or deliberately ignore important verbal or nonverbal information being transmitted. Effective listening is the opposite of this. It is a technique that focuses our attention on all information being transmitted. Effective listening opens up the possibility of effective responding—responses that take into full account all the information you have absorbed in a conversation.

There are four important kinds of responses that demonstrate different levels of effective listening and different intensities of engagement with another person: summarizing, paraphrasing, reflecting, and empathizing. Let's consider each of these in more detail.

Summarizing is a communication technique used to confirm understanding of the facts of a situation. When we summarize, we are focused substantially on the facts of what we have heard rather than any nonverbal communications or feelings. When we summarize, we most typically use the person's own words in a way that allows them to hear back what they have said with minimal amounts of interpretation or distillation by the receiver. Frequent summarizing, therefore, is an important technique to prevent small misconceptions or errors from snowballing into larger problems. Importantly, when we summarize effectively, we send a signal to the other person that they have been listened to, and this signal is an important way of indicating we are open and want the conversation to continue.

Paraphrasing is a communication technique to convey back to the other person what was said by using different words than those used in the first place. Paraphrasing requires a type of intellectual effort and commitment; instead of just repeating things back, paraphrasing indicates you have actually taken the time and trouble to think about what a person has said and are trying to confirm your own understanding of it by using your own words. Paraphrasing is a more cognitively complicated activity than summarizing and can be used as a way of distilling or focusing complex details in a more digestible or refined manner. When we paraphrase effectively, we send a signal to the other person that not only have they been listened to but they have also been heard. This is an important distinction; even though the words "listened" and "heard" may sound synonymous, we can all relate to situations where someone has clearly listened (i.e., they know what we have said) but equally clearly have not heard us (i.e., actually got the meaning of what they have heard).

Reflecting is a communication technique that takes into account both facts and feelings and is an attempt to convey back to the individual the essence of what was communicated and transmitted both verbally and nonverbally. Reflecting includes both content and facts as well as the nonverbal cues (e.g., emotions, gestures, body language) associated with that communication. It is most typically associated with the use of a kind of summarizing emotional term to let the individual know you are actively trying to integrate both the facts and the emotional response to those facts. When we effectively reflect in a conversation, we send a signal to the other person that not only have we listened and heard but we have also actually understood the significance and impact of the situation. Importantly, failure to reflect appropriately in some situations can equally send an important signal to someone that you are not really that interested in them and have not really been paying that much attention, despite what you might be saying to them.

Empathizing is a communication technique that requires you to use all your verbal and nonverbal communication skills to demonstrate to the other person that you have listened, you have heard, you have understood, and that you acknowledge what that person is experiencing. It is the most complex level of interpersonal interaction and is considered the highest form of communication because it sends a strong signal that you are genuinely interested in the other person, you are focusing both your logical and emotional self on that other person, and you are bringing all your best resources to this conversation in an honest an open manner.

To help illustrate these different levels and intensities of response, consider the following case:

> A 39-year-old patient has been experiencing difficulty sleeping, low-grade fever (100.4–101°F) alternating with chills, muscle pain, and mild nausea. It's not entirely clear what the problem is, but there has been a "bug" going around the office lately and everyone seems to be getting some kind of antibiotic prescription for this, and for everyone else at the office, this seems to work after about 4 or 5 days. The patient goes to an ambulatory primary health care clinic looking for relief and is given a prescription for an antibiotic after an assessment by one of the team members. As the appointment is about to end, the patient—looking down with slightly slumped shoulders and a defeated tone of voice—says, "I don't know if I should even bother taking these pills. I mean, the last time I came here, you people gave me something just like this, I got a huge rash all over my body, had to call an ambulance to take me to the emergency department. Do you know how expensive that was? And nobody even cared afterward."

Take a moment and carefully reread that previous paragraph. Think about the words that the patient has said and think about the description of the nonverbal cues that accompanied it. And of course remember that this whole case is playing out in a busy ambulatory primary care clinic where there are other patients waiting to be seen, charts to be completed, colleagues who want your expertise, and a hundred other distractions around you.

The reality is, situations like this occur all the time, and smart, nice, well-intentioned health care professionals have to respond in real time, in seconds, when complex verbal and nonverbal communication is being transmitted by patients. What would you do in this situation, and what would most practitioners do? The reality, unfortunately, is that the frantic pace of most primary care settings means that even well-intentioned health care professionals will receive this communication and may immediately think, "Oh crap. I don't have time to deal with this!" And, as a result, may say something like, "There, there. It'll all be better for you soon, just take the medication and you'll be your old self in a few days' time!"

As you review what this patient has said and what they have communicated nonverbally, it is probably obvious to you that there is a lot more going on with this patient than meets the eye. Why did the patient have to call an ambulance to go to the emergency department? Was there no one else (a friend, a family member, a neighbor) close enough geographically and emotionally to help him? What is the patient implying or trying to say when, in a defeated tone of voice, he complains, "nobody even cared afterward"? What emotional information is being conveyed by the slumped shoulders and the downward gaze? Is this really about an infection of some sort anyway? The symptoms are vague and nonspecific enough as to be many other things.

Primary care is complex, but in this one case scenario, we see that the practitioner is facing an important choice. The patient has communicated, verbally and nonverbally, a lot of information, and now is waiting to see if the practitioner listened, heard, understood, and acknowledged what has been transmitted. Let's look at what kinds of responses may be possible in this situation and evaluate what might be the best path forward.

A *summarizing response* to this patient's comment might be something like, "Are you thinking you might have an allergic response to this medication? If that's the case we can certainly arrange for you to have some allergy testing done." In reviewing what the patient said, it is factually correct that the patient described a situation involving a serious allergic response to a previous medication requiring a hospital visit. The patient has also stated no one cared, which could be interpreted as meaning no health professional was concerned enough to verify the safety and appropriateness of the medication and ensure he had no allergic responses.

In this situation is a summarizing response correct or incorrect? The answer of course is "it depends." On the one hand, such a statement delivered by the health care professional right after the patient has made his comment does signal to that patient that he has been listened to. This summarizing statement is clearly superior to an insincere throwaway comment like, "Yeah, don't worry about it." However, this summarizing statement seems somewhat incomplete and not particularly responsive to what the patient is saying, and what he is meaning to say beyond the simple words. The summarizing statement does not address the nonverbal communication (e.g., defeated tone of voice, looking downward).

Although a summarizing statement is not necessarily wrong here, it is clearly not very right either. At best, we can say a summarizing statement such as this is not inappropriate and may, perhaps, open the door to another statement from the patient, which in turn could provide the health care professional with yet another chance to prove she is really interested in what the patient is saying. More likely, however, if the patient heard the professional suggest allergy testing following the statement he had made, the patient would likely think, "Hmm, I guess you really don't care, and you are just trying to fob me off to someone else. So, thanks but no thanks."

Another potential trap with this particular summarizing statement (and summarizing statements in general) is that they can appear to the patient to be offering a solution when there hasn't yet been an agreement on what the problem actually is. Most of us have had the experience of speaking to a well-intentioned friend or family member, and complaining about something that happened at school or at work. For example, you might say, "I can't believe how hard this course I'm taking is! I really think the teacher has it in for me and there's no way I'm going to be able to pass." If in response to that statement your friend responds, "Well why don't you go talk to the teacher and get some advice on how to prepare for the tests? That way the teacher will get to know you better, see you're trying hard, and he'll probably like you more so you'll do better in the course!" Such a facile response, no matter how well intentioned, can sometimes be profoundly irritating and can actually undermine the quality of a relationship. First, a summarizing response like this that offers a neatly packaged solution to a complex problem may appear presumptuous. It suggests: "I know better than you, I can solve your problems, I'm therefore better and smarter than you." In almost all cases, that is never the actual intention of what the friend or family member is trying to say in this case, but sadly it may come across that way. Secondly, jumping to a solution to someone else's problem may not even be why they are speaking to the friend or family member in the first place. Many times, people just need to vent. They need to simply blow off steam in a safe place with a trusted friend or family member. They are not looking for you to solve their problems, they are simply looking for you to listen and hear them. By summarizing and problem-solving, this friend or family member is actually not helping. They are coming across as a bossy know-it-all. If the answer to my problem was really that simple that after one brief sentence you were able to solve it, don't you think I would have already figured that out? Third, a summarizing statement like this sends a strong nonverbal signal that the friend or family member doesn't have the time or interest to focus on you right now, they just want to fix the problem and move on rather than take the time to truly listen and care about what is going on.

If you spend any time listening to and observing health care professionals, particularly problem-oriented health care professionals and those with an emotional intelligence style that trends toward converger or accommodator, you will note that summarizing statements are used with remarkable (and perhaps inappropriate) frequency. Why? They work, at least in the short term. They give the appearance of managing problems and helping people, and most frequently in response to a summarizing statement such as the one in the example above, the patient will often say, "Gee, thanks" and walk away. However, in reality, despite saying "Gee, thanks," what they really may be thinking is, "You don't really have the time or interest to focus on what I need from you right now, so what's the point of me staying and trying to connect with you anymore? I guess I was right all along. Nobody really cares, do they?"

Recall what the patient in our case scenario example said at the end of the appointment: "I don't know if I should even bother taking these pills. I mean, the last time I came here, you people gave me something just like this, I got a huge rash all over my body, had to call an ambulance to take me to the emergency department. Do you know how expensive that was? And nobody even cared afterward." A *paraphrasing response* to this statement might be something like, "You're worried something like this may happen again and if it does it will cost you a lot of money for another ambulance trip? Okay, if you have any problems with this medication, call our 24-hour service at this number and they will make sure you get to the hospital at no cost to you."

How does this paraphrasing response differ from the summarizing response? First, it includes one very important word: worried. By including this word, which describes the emotional state of the patient, the health care professional has signaled that she has not only listened but that she has heard what the patient said. What she has heard involves both words and feelings, verbal and nonverbal cues. With the inclusion of this single emotional word, the paraphrasing response achieves a higher level of communication than the summarizing statement. Is this the right response in this case?

Although it is certainly better than a summarizing response, it still feels incomplete and inadequate. First, similar to the summarizing statement, there is a rush to solve the problem before we've actually confirmed with the patient what the problem is. It is fobbing the patient off on someone else—in this case, a 24-hour telephone service—rather than taking the time and giving the attention needed in the here and now to help the patient. Second, although the use of the emotional term *worried* is a good thing, it is still framing the problem as a cognitive rather than emotional issue. Is the patient REALLY worried about another allergic reaction? Although this may be part of it, the defeated tone of voice, the drooped shoulders, and the downward gaze suggest there is much more than just this going on, and a 24-hour telephone line in case of allergic reaction isn't going to address that.

Paraphrasing statements, in general, are superior to summarizing statements but may not be sufficient to address what patients really need and want. They still invoke a kind of premature closure on a discussion by leaping to a solution, but they do have the advantage of at least demonstrating to the patient that you have heard them, insofar as you indicate that you have actually noticed there was an emotional response. This alone may be enough of an opening for a patient to stick with you and not walk away immediately, or it may not be enough, depending on the individual patient and his circumstances.

Paraphrasing statements feel and seem riskier than summarizing statements to some health care professionals, which is why you will hear and observe them used with much less frequency. Why? Some health care professionals will say, "I don't have time to open that Pandora's box," or "I'm not a social worker, I don't have the expertise to deal with all this emotional stuff." Although on the surface this may be true, the reality is that if this is the reason you are not using paraphrasing statements when the opportunity arises, you may be putting your own needs and wants ahead of the patient's best interests.

In other circumstances, individuals may feel that, despite every best intention and every strenuous effort, a paraphrasing statement is all they can offer at the present time. This too is a reality of practice; sometimes we really do not have the personal resources or professional capacity to go beyond this kind of statement, and if so, we and our patients must try to do the best we can under the circumstances. Importantly, we also have to acknowledge when this is actually the case, and when we are simply using this excuse as a convenient way to not feel guilty for not trying harder.

A *reflective statement* is a yet higher form of communication that focuses more fully on the emotional and nonverbal cues sent by the patient. Reflective statements may not come easily or naturally to many scientifically oriented health care professionals, and some people feel awkward or shy about using them, thinking they are invading a patient's privacy or trying to get too close to them. An example of a reflective statement or response to the patient's comment in our case scenario might be, "I can see the idea of all this is upsetting you, especially based on what you've experienced in the past. Can you tell me a little bit more about what happened that last time and let's see if we can find a way to make sure it won't happen again." How does this reflective statement differ from the previous summarizing and paraphrasing statements? First, similar to the paraphrasing statement, there is inclusion of an emotional word, in this case "upsetting," and in the case of the paraphrasing response above, "worrying." "Upsetting" is generally a more emotionally intense word than "worrying," so by using this in the reflective statement, the health care professional is signaling that they have not only listened and heard, but they have actually truly understood the impact of the previous experience on this patient. Second, this reflective statement doesn't seek to solve the problem immediately by fobbing it off on to someone else (like a 24-hour telephone line). Instead, the professional in this case is providing an opportunity for the patient to talk some more and share more details for the expressed purpose of trying to figure out how to make sure it doesn't happen again. Third, this reflective statement states this is OUR problem (not your problem) and that WE will try to find a way to make sure it won't happen again (as opposed to someone else will help you with that). This careful wording in the reflective response is crucial because it helps to establish a personal and emotional bond between practitioner and patient.

In signaling not just a reluctant willingness but an actual explicit desire to hear more from the patient, a strong nonverbal cue is being sent: "I'm here to help you, not just to get you out of my office fast." Reflective responses are strong and help build relationships, but they are even less widely used than paraphrasing statements. Health care professionals worry that patients will talk their ears off, or that patients will somehow breach professional boundaries because the invitation to talk more and the signal that "I care" might be misinterpreted for other things. Although this is always a possibility and every health care professional must always be vigilant about maintaining appropriate professional boundaries, reflective statements rarely produce this kind of problem. Instead, when used appropriately, they provide an invitation to actually build a stronger patient–practitioner relationship focused on the patient's needs and problems, not the time available to the practitioner.

In some cases, some health care professionals will quite naturally and effortlessly gravitate toward using reflective statements; this is how they are in their personal lives as well. In other cases, a deliberate conscious effort and repeat rehearsals will be necessary to use such responses appropriately and confidently. Importantly, not every response can be reflective. At a certain point, the health care professional will have to shift gears, ask more closed-ended questions, and use more focused summarizing and paraphrasing responses to achieve some kind of resolution or closure to the discussion. For now, however, and in response to what the patient has said, a reflective statement is an appropriate and reasonable response that will help strengthen the patient–practitioner relationship and help both of them get closer to the bottom of what the real problem is and what the patient is meaning by the words he is using.

The term *empathy* is sometimes defined as the ability to understand and share the feelings of others. It is a term that is widely used in health care and is sometimes framed as the ideal form of communication. Why is empathy so important? It is sometimes said that patients won't care about what you say unless they feel you care about them as people. The power of the empathizing statement is the connection it can help build between patient and practitioner.

This is an essential point to consider. Recall from Chapters 5 and 6 that health care professionals spend a lot of time trying to convince people to change their behavior by telling, lecturing, or warning. We want people to quit smoking, lose weight, accurately follow a complex medication regimen, complete a regular exercise regime to strengthen muscles, or floss teeth after every meal—complicated requests that are irritating to follow even if they are good for you. Most studies suggest health care professionals are shockingly ineffective at communicating with patients; much of what we say or suggest gets either forgotten or is actively ignored. Why? Because patients don't care about what we say unless they feel we care about them as people. If we are truly interested in helping people, truly motivated to positively influence their health outcomes, we cannot do this by simply being smart know-it-alls and telling them what they should do because, well, we know what's best. We first need to establish an empathetic relationship that truly demonstrates we care for them, so they in turn will care about what we say and pay attention.

The first step in this process is an appropriate and authentic empathetic response. For our patient who has said, "I don't know if I should even bother taking these pills. I mean, the last time I came here, you people gave me something just like this, I got a huge rash all over my body, had to call an ambulance to take me to the emergency department. Do you know how expensive that was? And nobody even cared afterward," what might be an example of an empathetic response? "I'm so sorry to hear about what happened the last time. I can't imagine how frightening that must have been for you. And then to feel like no one cared about it afterward, that just shouldn't happen. If you have a few minutes right now, I'd like to hear more about what happened, and we can try to make sure we're covering all the bases for you."

What's different about this empathetic response as compared with the summarizing and paraphrasing responses? First, it begins with an apology. Not an apology in the sense of taking personal responsibility, but in the sense of apologizing on behalf of an impersonal and cold system that left the patient feeling vulnerable. This kind of apology sends a strong signal to the patient that he has been listened to, heard, understood, and most importantly from the perspective of empathy, actually acknowledged. He is a real flesh-and-blood person, something terrible happened to him, and someone—the health care professional who happens to be in this clinic—is actually saying "I'm sorry." In this context, the apology is not an admission of guilt, but rather it is an expression of solidarity for what the patient has experienced. With this one small, two-word phrase, an empathetic relationship is building. Second, similar to the reflective statement, a strong emotional word has been used to summarize the nonverbal and emotional content of the patient's comment. In this case, the word was "frightening." It is a stronger emotional word than "upsetting" or "worried" and seems somewhat more in-line with the nonverbal cues being sent by the patient (defeated tone of voice, downward gaze, stooped shoulders). Is "frightening" the most accurate emotional label to use in this case? It's hard to know if the patient is frightened, or actually angry but feeling powerless. What if the practitioner uses the wrong emotional label, might not that make the situation worse? This is one reason why many practitioners shy away from making empathetic statements and responses for fear they will actually make things worse, not better.

Although this is always a possibility in interpersonal communication, in this situation it seems highly unlikely that a genuine attempt such as this would be rebuffed by the patient. The key here is that the attempt is genuine. Empathy must not and cannot be faked; it must be authentic. It is sometimes fashionable to believe it is possible to fake it till you make it. This is absolutely not the case with empathy. Empathy is not the words or deliberate nonverbal cues you choose to send to others, it is the genuine expression of interest in another person that is easily discerned by others as real or fake. Indeed, simply repeating the words of the empathetic response suggested previously, reading them out loud with no true feeling or emotion beneath it, would be profoundly insulting to the patient. When genuine emotion and nonverbal cues are being transmitted, the patient will be enormously forgiving if the exact right word in this case is not "frightening." The patient will understand and appreciate your intentions rather than focus on precision in language.

The empathetic statement also includes a clear statement that "this shouldn't have happened to you." This is another form of acknowledgment that this patient was not to blame for the situation. Recall the phrasing used for both the summarizing and paraphrasing responses, in which quick solutions were offered for complex problems. The suggestion that there is an easy answer to a problem may imply to a patient that they in fact were part of or at least contributed to the problem in the first place. Finally, the empathetic statement concludes with an invitation to continue the discussion in a genuine and committed way, through words and, hopefully, nonverbal cues such as body language, tone of voice, and eye contact. In this way, the health professional is signaling true interest in learning more about what happened.

Let's review this scenario now.

Patient: "I don't know if I should even bother taking these pills. I mean, the last time I came here, you people gave me something just like this, I got a huge rash all over my body, had to call an ambulance to take me to the emergency department. Do you know how expensive that was? And nobody even cared afterward."

Summarizing response: "Are you thinking you might have an allergic response to this medication? If that's the case, we can certainly arrange for you to have some allergy testing done."

Paraphrasing response: "You're worried something like this may happen again, and if it does, it will cost you a lot of money for another ambulance trip? Okay, if you have any problems with this medication, call our 24-hour service at this number and they will make sure you get to the hospital at no cost to you."

Reflecting response: "I can see the idea of all this is upsetting you, especially based on what you've experienced in the past. Can you tell me a little bit more about what happened that last time and let's see if we can find a way to make sure it won't happen again."

Empathizing response: "I'm so sorry to hear about what happened the last time. I can't imagine how frightening that must have been for you. And then to feel like no one cared about it afterward, that just shouldn't happen. If you have a few minutes right now, I'd like to hear more about what happened, and we can try to make sure we're covering all the bases for you."

If you were this patient, or if a beloved relative or friend were this patient, which response would you hope they would receive in this situation?

7.2 This Just Doesn't Come Naturally to Me

In the context of a written textbook, it may seem straightforward enough to learn the principles for composing a reflective or empathizing response to a single comment from an imaginary patient. But in the real world, there are hundreds of comments from dozens of patients each day, and in busy, time-pressured, interruption-driven health care environments, what can be done if this doesn't come naturally to you and you feel you've accomplished a lot if you simply avoid saying "uh-huh" and nothing else?

The reality of course is that much of what you've read in this chapter is aspirational and idealistic. No health care professional, including the author of this book, would ever claim they can always or even frequently or normally produce empathetic responses at a moment's notice delivered with true sincerity and authenticity. There are not enough hours in a day to be fully empathetic to every patient who needs our care, and even if there were, no human being has the emotional or intellectual capacity to be truly empathetic all the time. The key is not to set an unrealistic target of all empathy all the time but instead to realize that there will be circumstances—few and far between perhaps, but real circumstances nonetheless—where you will need to be empathetic and failure to be empathetic may have severe unfortunate conse-quences. The objective, therefore, is to ensure you have an understanding of how empathetic responses are structured and the skill and some confidence to do so when it is absolutely essential. In an ideal world, of course, all health professionals would be empathetic more often than not; however, in the real world, we must do the best we can with the resources we have available.

7.3   If You Can't Be Empathetic, at Least Avoid Being This!

For some talented, dedicated, smart, and well-intentioned health care professionals, even constructing and delivering a summarizing statement in real time in a complex situation will be too much and feel beyond their ability or control. This does not mean these people must abandon dreams of becoming practitioners immediately; it does, however, suggest there will be additional work in the years ahead to identify alter-native strategies that, although imperfect, are at least somewhat better than simply ignoring what the patient says.

If summarizing, paraphrasing, reflecting, and empathizing are simply too much too soon at the present time for you, it may be helpful to consider alternative com-munication techniques. One such technique is to not concentrate at first on what you should say, but instead, gain confidence in what NOT to say in a specific situation. Avoiding saying the wrong thing can sometimes be just as important (or at least a fair enough attempt) as saying the right thing.

Let's return to our previous example of a patient who says to you: "I don't know if I should even bother taking these pills. I mean, the last time I came here, you people gave me something just like this, I got a huge rash all over my body, had to call an ambulance to take me to the emergency department. Do you know how expensive that was? And nobody even cared afterward." What are the responses to avoid say-ing in such a situation?

Judging: A judging response is one in which an emotionally intensive evaluation of what another person has said is delivered from a position of authority and pow-er. An example of a judging response in this case might be, "There's no reason for you to feel that way." Imagine for a moment how the patient might feel if this is what was said. The practitioner uttering this response would likely not for a moment want to appear intimidating or judgmental, and perhaps selected those words thinking they would be comforting or reassuring. More likely, this response emerged from the practitioner without any specific or deliberate thought or plan. As you can see, a judging response sounds judgmental. It sounds harsh and dismissive, as though the patient's feelings do no matter and in fact there is something wrong with the patient if they actually feel that way. This is clearly not the way to build empathy or nurture a practitioner–patient relationship, and it will in all likelihood shut the door to future interactions. A patient hearing a response like this from a practitioner may actually get angry or perhaps simply find a new health care team or provider rather than put up with this kind of nonsense.

Advising: An example of an advising response in this situation might be, "Well, you should just take the pills you've been given; that's not going to happen this time." Once again, the practitioner speaking an advising response may think they are being firm and clear, and inspiring confidence in clinical decision making. In fact, an advising response such as this can be profoundly irritating to a patient. First, the response suggests nothing the patient said has even been listened to, let alone heard. Second of all, it sounds and feels dismissive, as though the patient's concerns don't matter. Third, from the patient's perspective, what's different this time around? At least with the summarizing response, the practitioner offered to send him for allergy testing, but with this advising response, there's no attempt to actually address any of the concerns raised by the patient's statement. When people offer unsolicited advice in a difficult situation, it can feel enormously frustrating or upsetting because it feels like you are being fobbed off and dismissed. The advising response should be avoided in recognition of the toxic effects it might have on relationship building and the counterproductive value it has in generating positive responses from patients.

Placating: A placating response involves use of empty platitudes in an attempt to soothe and reassure a person, all without actually addressing any of the underlying concerns. In this situation, an example of a placating response might be, "I'm sure it'll all be fine this time and you'll be okay, just you wait and see!" This kind of false cheerfulness and the rah-rah cheerleading quality of the statement itself can seem highly dismissive. How exactly do you know this time will be different and it will all be okay? Are you going to guarantee this in writing? Placating responses can appear to be an attempt to simply cut short a conversation, redirect attention away from the problem, and in this way can sometimes feel like infantilizing (or treating a patient like a child). The practitioner's intention in making a placating response might be to provide reassurance, but it can easily come across poorly and sabotage any future relationship with the patient. Therefore, empty platitudes and placating statements are best avoided if your objective is to build a strong and impactful relationship with a patient.

Generalizing: A generalizing statement is one in which an individual's unique needs, concerns, and circumstances are mistakenly compared with a larger group for the purpose of suggesting (or implying) that the individual needs to be like everyone else rather than being themselves. An example of a generalizing response in this situation might be "Yeah, everyone feels like that sometimes, but it all works out fine in the end." By reducing this patient's unique fears into a general statement, then adding on to the placating comment that it all works out fine in the end, this statement manages to alienate a patient in two different ways. Generalizing diminishes an individual's unique circumstances and implies there is something wrong with them because they have disclosed their feelings and thoughts. When generalized in this way, patients frequently feel diminished, and it will likely inhibit any future attempt at honest conversation with a practitioner.

In some cases, a variation of generalization called normalizing can, however, be a helpful and positive communication strategy to continue. Normalizing is the process of letting patients know that their specific feelings and experiences are in fact not only normal, but also perfectly reasonable and to be expected. Although generalizing is a diminishing or demeaning experience, normalizing can be an empowering one. In this situation, a more positive normalizing response might be, "I've heard lots of patients say the same thing you just said in similar situations. Here's what some of them have said worked for them." Note the subtle but important differences in tone associated with a normalizing versus a generalizing response in this case. In particular, note how the normalizing statement lacks the placating quality of the generalizing statement, and instead attempts to offer options and alternatives to the patient to consider, which in turn implies further conversation is possible. The generalizing response actually cuts off conversation, whereas the normalizing response encourages further dialogue and discussion.

Quizzing or Distracting: Arguably the most widely used communication by health care professionals in difficult situations, quizzing or distracting involves the asking of more questions (typically closed ended in their nature) or feeble attempts to change the subject as a way of simply avoiding dealing with an uncomfortable moment in a conversation. An example of a quizzing response in this situation might be asking rapid-fire series of questions such as, "I see. Were you in the hospital overnight? Did they do allergy testing? Was there a definitive allergy diagnosis? Do you have a medical alert bracelet?" The fatigue of answering a series of rapid-fire questions from a practitioner may simply exhaust the patient, who then loses interest in saying anything more, and the practitioner erroneously then believes "Great, problem solved!" An example of a distracting response in this situation might be, "Isn't it great we have such good ambulance services in town so they got you to the hospital in good time?" The absurdity of this response may be obvious when you read it; sadly, in reality, there are many unfortunate situations where stressed or overwhelmed health care professionals, in a momentary lapse, will say something like this, provoking a strong and negative response from a patient, and rightly so.

Just ignore it and maybe the patient will go away: Another favored response by some overwhelmed health care professionals, but one that should be avoided, is to simply pretend you didn't hear what the patient said and ignore the comment. Although such a technique can provide short-term relief from having to deal with a difficult problem, it will almost always result in longer term problems between the practitioner and patient. When you consciously ignore something important that is said by the patient, it sends a very strong signal that you literally do not care about the patient, and if that is the case, why should they bother to care about what you are saying?

This list of strategies to avoid is only illustrative; your common sense and good judgment should help you to identify other communication strategies to avoid that are not on this list. If the more positive and proactive communication strategies such as learning to deliver empathetic responses just seems to overwhelming for you, start by consciously choosing to NOT use some of the strategies listed previously. This may in fact open up space for you to take baby steps and try to develop your own strengths further.

7.4   There Is No One-Size-Fits-All Communication Strategy

Throughout this book, the point has been made that individual differences are real and matter, and that as a result, there are no simple one-size-fits-all communication strategies or psychological theories that will always and/or even usually apply. In Chapter 2, we discussed the importance of emotional intelligence and the idea that every health care professional and every patient possesses their own unique emotional intelligence, and as a result, effective communication involves a kind of unique chemistry that is built on the foundation of these two highly personalized emotional intelligences. Knowing your own emotional intelligence and understanding what it means for your strengths and preferences regarding communication is a first important step. Although it would be helpful to confidently know the emotional intelligence style of every patient and team member you will work with, it's simply not realistic or possible. As a result, finding ways of doing your detective work and assessing emotional intelligence strengths and preferences of others in real time, then responding appropriately, is as important a communication skill as anything else covered in this chapter. Avoiding the temptation or trap of believing there is a perfect solution to every communication problem is also essential. There are clearly better and worse alternatives, but there are no perfect options in the field of human interaction and communication.

This chapter has focused on communication strategies within a patient–practitioner context. While of course this is important, it is not the only kind of communication you will be engaged in as a practitioner. Equally important and sometimes equally difficult will be communication with colleagues, such as other health care professionals on your team and those who are outside your team. The same principles discussed throughout this chapter will apply to team relationships and interprofessional communication. The power of reflective and empathizing statements, and adequacy and unavoidability of summarizing and paraphrasing statements, and the statements to avoid apply equally to these important relationships as well. As with patient relationships, collegial relationships need to be nurtured carefully and cannot be faked. Taking baby steps toward learning some of these strategies is a great first step in building your confidence and skills for the time when it will matter the most for you to get it right.

7.5   Every Conversation Is a Series of Choices

The interpersonal communication model described in Chapter 4 highlights the notion that reciprocal interactions and exchanges of verbal and nonverbal information and cues represent a series of conscious and subconscious choices we must make in real time and under less than ideal conditions for self-reflection or trial-and-error decision making. When we ignore verbal or nonverbal cues sent by a patient or a colleague, or when we invest the time and cognitive energy required to carefully craft and deliver an empathetic response, we are demonstrating our choices. We are also propelling relationships with others down entirely different pathways and along new trajectories. It is sometimes said that you don't have a second chance to make a first impression, highlighting the reality that, in life, a few misplaced words or words never spoken can actually have an enormous steering effect on the future direction of any relationship.

Each of your conversations with other people will present these sorts of choices on a continuous basis. If, because you are too busy, too lazy, or burned out by the stress of your job, you are unable or unwilling to engage in reflective or empathetic conversations with others when the opportunity presents itself, a certain kind of relationship will evolve. It is one that in all likelihood will be highly transactional and focused on efficiency, but perhaps ultimately suboptimal from a health outcomes perspective and decidedly unfulfilling from a job satisfaction perspective. If, instead, you invest time and cognitive energy to learn new communication strategies, unlearn old ones, and recognize the potential transformational power of incorporating reflective and empathetic statements into your repertoire of behaviors (both professionally and personally), new possibilities for stronger and better relationships may emerge. This is difficult and can take a lifetime to achieve. Ultimately, it is a decision, and you will be the one who will need to live with the consequences that flow from it.

7.6 Mind Map Chapter 7

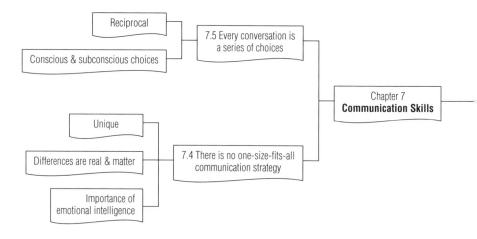

Mind Map for Communication Skills

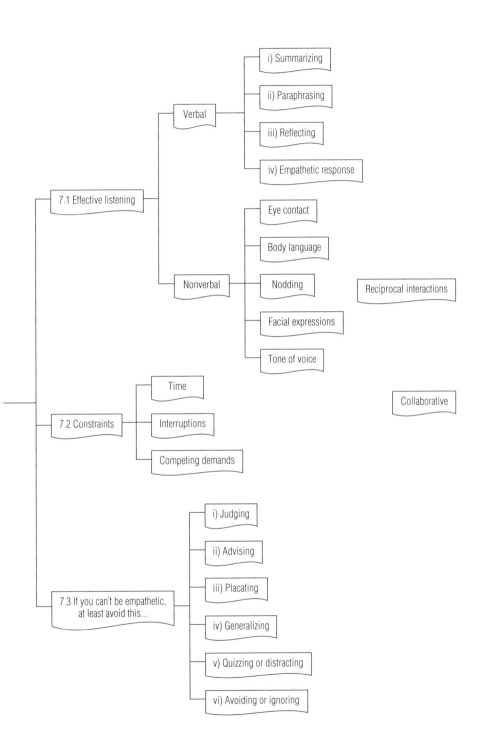

For Further Reading:

Chichirez C, Purcarea V. Interpersonal communication in healthcare. *J Med Life.* 2018;11(2): 119–122.

Christensen M. The consultative process used in outreach: a narrative account. *Nurs Crit Care.* 2009;14(1):17–25.

Irving P, Dickson D. Empathy: towards a conceptual framework for health professionals. *Int J Health Care Qual Assur Inc Leadersh Health Serv.* 2004;17(4):212–220.

Kaelber D, Bates D. Health information exchange and patient safety. *J Biomed Inform.* 2007;40:240–245.

King A, Hoppe R. "Best practice" for patient-centered communication: a narrative review. *J Grad Med Educ.* 2013;5(3):385–393.

Levinson W, Lesser C, Epstein R. Developing physician communication skills for patient-centered care. *Health Aff.* 2010;29(7):1310–1319.

Van Servellen G. *Communication Skills for the Health Care Professional: Context, Concepts, Practice, and Evidence.* Sudbury, MA: Jones and Bartlett; 2018.

Vermeir P, Vandijck D, Degroote S, et al. Communication in healthcare: a narrative review of the literature and practical recommendations. *Int J Clin Pract.* 2015;69(11):1257–1267.

Webb L. Exploring the characteristics of effective communicators in healthcare. *Nurs Stand.* 2018; 33(9):47–51.

8 Diversity in Interprofessional Collaborative Person-Centered Care

Health professionals have ethical responsibilities to provide the best possible care to all people, regardless of their background, economic situation, beliefs, or demographics. Although in our personal lives we may have some opportunities to choose those we wish to spend time with, as a health professional we must care for each person as they are, without favoritism or prejudice.

The importance of this ideal may be self-evident; however, the reality is that health care professionals sometimes have difficulty living up to it. In some cases, health care professional may have conscious or unconscious biases toward or against certain people or groups of people. In other cases, for nonprofessional reasons such as religious beliefs, health care professionals may experience psychological conflict while trying to balance ethical responsibilities. In many cases, health professionals may have good intentions and want to do what's best, but simply feel awkward or uncertain as to how to act or what to say with different individuals or groups of individuals. Despite political rhetoric and showmanship, the reality is that our societies and local communities are growing increasingly diverse. Learning to embrace, rather than simply tolerate or accept, this diversity and understanding how we as health professionals can better communicate with and care for our increasingly diverse patients and clients is essential. Importantly, the health care team itself is also composed of increasingly diverse individuals. Learning to work collaboratively within a highly diverse team of committed health care professionals is equally important.

8.1 What Is Diversity?

Diversity is a term that is frequently used in health care to describe differences between individuals. Importantly, the word itself is meant to reinforce the notion that difference does not mean better or worse. Diversity acknowledges the astonishing variation that is possible among human beings, which exists in every society in every place. There are many different kinds of diversities to consider. For example, consider the unique issues faced by adherent Muslims who must fast (i.e., abstain from eating anything) during the period of Ramadan. How can health care professionals support and respect this important duty of their patient's faith? What are the implications of fasting on, for example, taking certain antibiotics with food to prevent nausea? How can health care professionals integrate an understanding of religious needs into treatment plans and education they provide patients? Alternatively, consider the historical experiences of African Americans or the colonization experienced by indigenous peoples, and how this may influence their interactions with health care team members. How should we respect and acknowledge these historical realities that have shaped current beliefs and behaviors with respect to professional authority, perceptions of wellness and illness, and trust in institutions (like hospitals, which for some may represent a tool for oppression or submission, a place of hurt rather than a place of healing)? Further, consider the importance of intersectionality. All individuals simultaneously self-identify with different groups, and some of those groups may have encountered different kinds of systemic discrimination in the past or in the present. For example, consider the intersecting histories and realities of a recent immigrant, a person of color, who uses a wheelchair for mobility and who lives in poverty. The influence of each of these realities intersects in unique ways to produce a rich tapestry of a personality. Historically, health care professionals may have felt uncomfortable categorizing individuals or overtly noticing and responding to differences, for fears of appearing to stereotype or pigeonhole their clients. In some cases, practitioners studiously avoided even mentioning (let alone documenting in a chart) any of these differences to avoid the appearance or accusations of bias. This well-intentioned attempt to treat everyone the same, which ignores the impact and reality of diversity, results in suboptimal communication and care being provided. Recognizing, supporting, embracing, and responding appropriately and openly to the diversities we encounter is essential to providing person-centered care, and to ensuring our practices and our system can continue to improve to address the evolving needs of society.

8.1.1   Why Is "Difference" Even a Problem?

The differences that are at the core of human diversity make up the story of human history. Despite understanding that difference should not and does not mean better or worse, human beings will frequently act in ways that suggest they feel or believe otherwise. Why should it matter to us what the color of another person's skin happens to be? Why would anyone care if a man wants to love another man? What business is it of anyone's if a person who is born female chooses to self-identify as male? Why are we so interested in the clothes and headscarves worn by some people and not others?

Psychologists have struggled with understanding how the reality of differences—in appearance, behavior, choices, or preferences—translates into an array of negative emotional and behavioral responses in some cases. Understanding how the human ability to categorize tips into stereotyping and bias, and how the human tendency to cluster in groups or tribes manifests as racism and prejudice, is complex but essential. Although each individual's development will be different and subject to a variety of influences, it appears that there are some commonalities among human beings everywhere that perhaps predispose us to thinking about diversity and difference in troubling and unhelpful ways.

We are hardwired to feel before we think. As has been discussed previously in Chapters 5 and 6, our central nervous systems appear to be hardwired to route sensory information in a specific way, initially through the amygdala and emotional processing centers prior to higher level cognitive processing centers. In the past, there may have been significant evolutionary advantage to this hardwiring; in the time it takes to consider whether someone is friend or foe, we could easily be harmed or killed. Instead, by using a rapid emotional filtering system first, we can have virtually instantaneous feelings related to safety, security, and danger. The risk, of course, is that in some cases these instantaneous feelings may simply be wrong, and if we respond too rapidly and too emotionally without having the time and opportunity to engage our cognitive, logical selves, we risk making bad decisions based on feelings rather than logic. Our hardwiring may, therefore, predispose us toward sharp, strong, and sudden responses to anything we perceive as new, different, or unusual, and without conscious effort and will, we may succumb to interpreting our world emotionally rather than rationally.

Do we all have strong negative emotional responses to something new or different? Although our hardwiring may predispose us to respond emotionally rather than logically to diversity and difference, must this always mean this response is negative? Interestingly, the answer to this question may be broadly connected to our emotional intelligence (see Chapter 2). Recall that one of the important Big Five personality dimensions is openness, a baseline psychological state that describes our interactions with our environment. Those who are more open value novelty, change, and variety, whereas those who are less open prefer consistency, predictability, and stability. Recall as well that the Big Five personality dimensions are relatively fixed as we age, and somewhat resistant to conscious change or evolution beyond a certain age (around age 20–30 years). This suggests that, in addition to our hardwiring, we each have an individual psychological tendency toward either a more negative (i.e., less open) or a more positive (i.e., more open) emotional response to difference and diversity. Importantly, this does not mean that those who are more open are thinking or using their logical selves to process differences and diversity; they are responding just as quickly and just as emotionally as the less open individuals, but simply in a different direction. As a result, it becomes difficult to predict who will respond in what way to diversity, because these Big Five personality dimensions are highly individualized and do not necessarily have any kind of external manifestation.

Other Big Five traits may also be important in understanding our psychological response to diversity and difference. For example, those who score more highly on agreeableness may have a greater psychological need for harmony and to be liked and consequently may feel psychological discomfort in a strong negative emotional response. Those who score more highly as extroverts as opposed to introverts may find the external stimulation and novelty that may be a component of diversity and difference is of positive psychological value and consequently seek out or even crave to be with those who are different from them.

Beyond our emotional and logical processing systems, our underlying personal psychology (as described by the Big Five personality dimensions and emotional intelligence) may also influence whether a person is alarmed and frightened by diversity and difference or is intrigued and actively seeks it out.

The emergence of stereotypes. When our logical selves engage with difference and diversity, there are important additional issues that may arise. According to the psychologist Gordon Allport, stereotyping is part of normal human thinking and frequently influences our behavior. Our logical, cognitive selves appear to be hardwired to interpret the world by placing items into categories. Consider the complexity in our environment. From the time we are children, we learn to make sense of the world by creating categories into which similar things can be placed, to facilitate organization of our world and understanding of interrelationships between things, and to help us better predict future events. Some of our strongest initial categories relate to sex and gender—the biological differences between boys and girls, but also the socially acceptable (and unacceptable) things that are unique to either boys or girls. Categorization is a powerful cognitive tool that facilitates learning and human development. The human mind cannot function without categories. Unfortunately, this can produce an important cognitive trap: stereotyping.

A stereotype is an oversimplified assumption about a group (or category) most often based on some previous experience. As a child, we might see Daddy going to work and Mommy making dinner and therefore assume that all boys (and men) go to work and all girls (and women) make dinner. This is a type of mental shortcut to understanding our world: extending a single or a few experiences to a generalization we believe should or does apply to everyone. Stereotypes can have a veneer of being positive (e.g., "Women are caring and nurturing") or negative (e.g., "Men are violent and selfish"). Importantly, and an often overlooked power of stereotypes, is that even the seemingly positive ones can cause problems. What if a woman wants to run a business or be a leader? Does the seemingly positive stereotype cause a problem? Similarly, the negative stereotype about men may mask or cloud the truth of a situation. What if a man is acting in self-defense or in defense of another and strikes out. Might he be unfairly judged because of the stereotype?

Although categorization is an important cognitive tool to manage environmental complexity, it can often produce mental mistakes in the form of stereotyping. Worse, when stereotypes form, they can be stubbornly resistant to not only being changed but also to being questioned due to the twin problems of cognitive load and cognitive dissonance. Psychologists note that most human beings tend to minimize differences and overlook diversity within their own groups, yet maximize differences and be hypervigilant toward diversity when considering those outside their self-defined group. In part, this is because of cognitive load. The active and engaged thinking required to reflect on and change your mind requires psychological energy, and in some cases, individuals simply cannot or choose not to invest that energy in this way. In part, this is also because of cognitive dissonance. In order to change one's mind, one must first acknowledge that the original categorization and stereotyping was wrong or flawed, and this can provoke both a strong emotional and cognitive backlash. It is uncomfortable admitting we are wrong, and most of us would prefer not to do this. As a result, rather than truthfully acknowledging our own errors, we may double down and work even harder to find reasons to reinforce our originally erroneous categorization and stereotyping rather than experience this dissonance.

The power of socialization. Human beings do not exist in isolation, and human children are almost always raised and develop within some kind of group or community, whether that is a family, a religious belief system, or a patriotic national culture. The process of being raised and the psychological development that occurs during this time is generally referred to as *socialization*, the way in which the rules, norms, traditions, and values of a culture are transmitted from older to younger members of the group or community. Socialization exerts a powerful influence on both our thinking and feeling about different categories or groups. In some cases, a group's beliefs about a different category of people can become so unquestioned and matter-of-fact that the stereotype takes on the quality of unchanging, universal fact even though it is simply an oversimplified assumption not related to truth. Consider, for example, the strong negative response that has historically characterized homosexuality. Today we recognize homosexuality is simply a form of difference or diversity, but until the 1970s, even medical authorities used to categorize it as an illness.

Beliefs about different out-groups are transmitted from elders to children through school, religious education, and cultural artifacts (such as books and TV shows). Children, as they develop and engage in their own personal categorization, may absorb these beliefs and integrate them into their own categories. As a result, what was once simply categorized as different starts to take on the quality of bad, worse, or evil.

In addition to transmitting a moral connotation to the categorization of difference through stereotyping, socialization can also powerfully reinforce stereotypes and inhibit individuals from ever changing their minds. In our increasingly polarized times, we see this frequently erupt in the context of polarizing social issues (e.g., abortion, same-sex marriage, intercultural or interracial marriages, political affiliations). Polarization is frequently a cause and consequence of the echo chamber, the tendency for individuals to interact only with other individuals who share the same moral views on their stereotyped categorizations.

8.2 What Can Break the Vicious Cycle of Stereotype and Prejudice?

Although psychologists have attempted to explain why stereotypes and prejudice exist and why they are so tenacious, it is also heartening to note that there are ideas for how to transcend the logical and emotional mistakes that are at the heart of such behaviors. Our everyday experience showcases for us that, in fact, a variety of -isms (e.g., sexism, racism) and phobias (e.g., homophobia, xenophobia) are in decline, particularly among younger people, and that there is greater openness and embracing of diversity than ever before (despite the impression we may get from watching the nightly news). How does this happen, and how can we support this advancement?

The contact hypothesis: One of the most powerful theories of social psychology, the contact hypothesis suggests that despite categorization and stereotyping, and despite socialization and the power of the echo chamber, one of the most common and powerful counterweights to stereotypes and prejudice is simple, everyday contact with other people who are not exactly like you. When we come into contact with diverse others who demonstrate differences that are the subject of our stereotypes, this may initially provoke cognitive dissonance. For example, as women have become more visible in the workplace and have been promoted on the basis of competence, it is more commonplace to see women as managers, administrators, leaders, and executives. This challenges historical prejudices regarding the traditional role of women as caregivers and subservient to men, and in turn, this supports women to assume leadership roles outside of workplaces (e.g., as mayors, parliamentarians, senators, presidents). Coming into regular and routine contact with diverse others who do not conform to our stereotypes forces us to manage the cognitive dissonance that arises. Importantly one-off contact or a single instance of interaction will not have the same powerful effect as everyday, commonplace contact. As we interact with others on a daily basis, we begin to realize and feel more comfortable, and see them as fully rounded human beings, not simply stereotypes based on our categorization. Such contact also helps shatter the echo chamber and our tendency to want to only interact with those who remind us of ourselves. Coming into contact and interacting regularly with a diverse array of individuals highlights for us the commonalities we all share, not the superficial differences that we may unfairly dwell on.

Conscious and unconscious biases are important factors that shape our perceptions of others. Much of what was discussed in Sections 8.1 and 8.2 focused on unconscious bias, the ways in which categorization leads to stereotyping and eventually results in prejudice, which occurs without necessarily involving specific malice involved or intended. Conscious bias occurs when we are fully aware of our prejudices yet choose to continue to hold them and act on them, all the while finding ways of justifying these to ourselves (and to others) so we do not appear mean-spirited or small-minded. Both forms of bias are important, and both are difficult to manage, for different reasons. Unconscious bias is challenging to address because an individual is not necessarily aware of the implications of the bias and may not recognize the harm that is being caused. For example, a group of young men in a locker room making jokes about staring at each other in a shower may not be overtly or consciously homophobic. They are simply making jokes, trying to make an uncomfortable situation more comfortable through humor, and well, everyone makes these kinds of jokes, right, so what's the harm?

Of course, the harm with such an unconscious bias is that it establishes a tone and a pattern as to what is acceptable and unacceptable and who is "in" and who is "out." In challenging an unconscious bias, there is a risk of triggering both cognitive load and cognitive dissonance. Those young men in the locker room may not think of themselves as prejudiced or mean-spirited, they are just "boys being boys" in their mind. By calling them out on their behavior, it risks causing them to have to feel bad about themselves, and this is a choice few of us choose to make. Rather than feel bad about our own behavior, cognitive dissonance will sometimes cause us to turn around and actually blame the person who is calling attention to our negative actions. These young men may say, "Oh stop being so sensitive," or "Sheesh, I was just making a joke, I wasn't actually going out and beating anyone up!" When cognitive dissonance is triggered as a self-protection mechanism, it can make it even harder to reach the unconscious bias because now a protective overcoat has been constructed that allows the individual to shelter his initial perception of himself by denigrating those who dare criticize or comment on his behavior. Cognitive load may also be an issue with unconscious bias. If these young men have been socialized in a community where homosexuality is an unquestioned bad thing, asking them to reflect on their behavior in a locker room is asking them to do too much. Their mothers, fathers, relatives, friends, religious leaders, coaches, etc. have always said these things and behaved this way, so why should they change? Dealing with an unconscious bias is extraordinarily challenging and most frequently requires a light touch, effective communication strategies, and a realistic sense of what can be accomplished in the present situation. With conscious bias, there may be other issues to contend with. In conscious bias, a person is already aware of their prejudices and stereotypes yet will have likely constructed a well-reasoned argument as to why they are justified. Paradoxically, in many ways, conscious bias may be easier to manage than unconscious bias because the act of actually coming up with justifications for biases and prejudices indicates awareness and some defensiveness about one's beliefs and behaviors. Conscious bias may exist when, for example, we simply assume that older people are not capable of managing computers or technologies, and as a result, employers do not hire them. Rather than think about each person as an individual and allow each person to prove him or herself in action, conscious biases may direct us to make sweeping generalizations about categories of individuals simply based on our experience with our own parents, who may not be comfortable navigating technology.

Increasingly, workplaces have begun to explicitly tackle issues of conscious and unconscious biases through formal training and human resource interventions. To address either, tactics such as those discussed in Chapter 7 in the Transtheoretical Model for Change (Prochaska) can be helpful. Unconscious bias is analogous to precontemplation; the individual is not even aware there is a problem either in her beliefs or in her behaviors. Labeling these as wrong or mean does not help her to gain this awareness; instead, all it will do is trigger a powerful emotional response, shut down conversation, and further harden attitudes. Similarly, a conscious bias is analogous to contemplation; the act of articulating a justification for one's biases indicates there is self-awareness of prejudice, and this can be a useful starting point for respectful discussion and exploration of alternatives. In both cases, the focus needs to be on building self-awareness rather than castigating or insulting, and on providing individuals with a face-saving way to change their minds, attitudes, and behaviors. Effective communication and civil discourse are essential in facilitating this change.

Cultural and media influences: The influence of popular media (e.g., television, Web-based programs, movies, books, YouTube influencers) in shaping our beliefs is crucial. Unfortunately, politicians of all persuasions have increasingly tried to weaponize the media as a tool to shape public opinion and thinking. Traditionally, media such as television and movies have been an important tool for socialization because they allow us to see how other people live. Even though these depictions have historically been fictionalized, the power of theatre (whether on stage, on TV, or in movies) is undeniable. We connect powerfully with characters, and our perceptions of entire categories of people will change because of a character we have seen on a TV show. For example, the actor Sidney Poitier is often credited with advancing the cause of civil rights in the United States in the 1960s and 1970s through his sensitive portrayals of the effects of racism, not only on African Americans but on the white American perpetrators. His quiet dignity and grace stood in sharp contrast to the bigoted and racially charged language of other characters in the movies in which he starred (e.g., *Guess Who's Coming to Dinner*, *A Raisin in the Sun*, and *They Call Me Mr. Tibbs!*). Films and TV provide a useful mirror on society and can provoke considerable discomfort, which in turn must be managed as cognitive dissonance and can, in the longer run, promote widespread social change. The fact that hundreds of millions of people will see the same movie or watch the same TV show means that the socialization effects of media can be far reaching and long lasting; in the 1960s, the movie characters played by Sidney Poitier were, for some Americans, among the first times they had ever seen an educated, articulate African American man on screen, and these portrayals changed the hearts and minds of a nation. Of course today, as our awareness of the power of media to shape public opinion has increased, media itself has succumbed to the echo chamber problem. We no longer have television or movies that will be seen by the entire or even a substantial proportion of a population. Instead, people self-segregate and tend to watch media that conforms to their preexisting worldviews, rather than something that stretches their thinking and imagination in new or different ways.

The importance of political change: Among the most important accomplishments of most Western democracies, and many other countries too, is the way in which the political system and rule of law have been used to protect minorities and legally manage prejudice and discrimination. For example, the use of tribunals and other judicial mechanisms to ensure people are not discriminated against with respect to housing means that there are legal solutions to complex interpersonal conflicts. Recently, many countries have passed legislation making same-sex marriage legal, and in the case of South Africa, this is enshrined in that country's constitution. Legal and political change such as this may never change some people's minds and hearts, but legal protection and political influence can help shape what is considered acceptable and unacceptable in society as a whole. Using the legal and political systems as a way to counter unconscious and conscious bias, and to manage the messy reality that human beings are hardwired to stereotype and thus potentially to be prejudiced is never easy, but it is an important tool to ensure fairness and justice.

8.3   Civil Discourse

As this chapter has highlighted, managing diversity at the individual, workplace, community, and societal levels is complicated and difficult. Understanding the psychological factors and influences that lead to stereotype, bias, and prejudice is important because it helps us to identify potential alternatives and solutions. Perhaps the most important personal and societal tool we have available to support diversity in our homes, our communities, and in the broader society is effective communication.

Civil discourse is a term that is frequently used to describe a type of communication that demonstrates respect for all. Rather than think about individual sources of discrimination or oppression (e.g., sexism, racism, homophobia, ageism, ableism, xenophobia) and try to identify a specific strategy for each -ism or phobia, civil discourse is a pattern of communication that builds on the psychological understanding of categorization, stereotyping, and bias, and uses communication as a tool to diffuse conflict, build relationships, and enhance trust between individuals.

Civil discourse begins with the understanding that our human hardwiring around emotions versus cognition, and around categorization of others, has evolutionary roots. In a hostile environment where everyone is at war with everyone else, there is a need to establish safety and security. In such an environment, sameness evolved as an indirect marker or proxy for such safety. Those who look, sound, act, think, and behave like us were more likely to be of our kind or of our tribe, and consequently were more trustworthy than those who were different in any way. Although we no longer live in such environments, and such tribalism no longer is a feature of most human societies, these patterns of thinking and behavior have been enduring. To this day, the signal that sameness sends with respect to safety continues to be strong for many people.

Increasing disregard for civil discourse, even the belief that somehow civil discourse signifies weakness, is corrosive and an epidemic infecting relationships within families, communities, and across society. If a community cannot communicate effectively within itself, it cannot advance or sustain itself. Civil discourse encourages productivity and respect, not necessarily agreement. When practiced properly, it actually builds relationships even when people disagree in substance. Civil discourse is as much about psychology as it is about communication techniques. It requires understanding of another person's motivations, beliefs, and ideas and an acceptance of their legitimacy, even if you strenuously agree with the substance of these motivations, beliefs, or ideas.

8.3.1   Find Common Ground

The starting point for civil discourse is common ground. In any disagreement, including disagreement related to bias, prejudice, or stereotyping, two people oppose one another. Finding common ground means identifying as early as possible the things you actually agree on. For example, although people who belong to different political parties may have very negative views of one another, if they can both accept that everyone who takes the time and trouble to join a political party actually loves their country, this is the foundation for common ground. What might the common ground be around difficult issues associated with difference and diversity? Simple human truths around safety, security, parents loving children, and fairness are common grounds. Corny though it may sound, diversity is facilitated and supported when individuals discover they have something in common.

8.3.2   Avoid Us-Versus-Them Language

As we have seen in this chapter, the human tendency toward in-group favoritism and out-group derogation (i.e., us versus them) is a fundamental challenge to diversity and embracing differences. Civil discourse demands we very carefully consider and use words that minimize the us-versus-them combat. Simply paying attention to and avoiding unnecessary or inflammatory use of collective nouns such as "us," "them," "most people," "most of us," "everyone," or "no one" will go a long way toward establishing a tone of respect between individuals. Further, in difficult situations, there may be a tendency for individuals to circle the wagons and try to protect the reputation and integrity of others they self-identify as "us." Use of words such as these can send inflammatory verbal signals to others, suggesting they do not belong or are outsiders, and therefore, are either inferior or less deserving than us. In some cases, there may be backhanded compliments that reflect stereotyped beliefs that also use us-versus-them language. For example, saying, "Those people work very hard," or "My goodness, they all have such talent!" with respect to individuals from particular ethnocultural groups might sound like a compliment, but in fact are just as biased and offensive as other more obvious insults. Civil discourse recognizes that individuals are first and foremost individuals, not representatives of a group. The difference between saying, "Wow, you're really talented" versus "Wow, you people are all so talented!" should be clear. It can be very challenging, and often will require conscious effort, to monitor and minimize the use of us-versus-them language in day-to-day conversation, but it is essential for civil discourse.

8.3.3   Discuss Ideas, Not People

When a person feels attacked, minimized, or disrespected, they will stop listening, and frequently, they may feel compelled to respond in kind. Civil discourse that embraces diversity requires conscious effort to not focus on individuals or groups of individuals but instead on ideas. For example, when discussing leadership qualities such as decisiveness, assertiveness, or forceful communication, it is not helpful to use one set of words to apply to male leaders (e.g., strong, powerful) and another to apply to female leaders (e.g., nasty, pushy).

In some cases, it may not be possible to discuss ideas without directly involving people. For example, as same-sex marriage has become legal and more commonplace in the last decade, those who are opposed and/or who are homophobic may carefully choose words and say, "I am opposed to same-sex marriage" as a way of not denigrating or directly insulting the lesbian and gay people who, by definition, are those involved in same-sex marriage. Conversely, there are those who object to the label "same-sex marriage" to describe a marriage between loving adults, as though somehow it is different or lesser than opposite-sex marriages that have no label or clarifier attached. This can produce significant strife and hurt feelings on both sides and accusations that opponents and proponents of same-sex marriage are opposed to diversity and are stifling free speech. The reality is, of course, in an issue such as same-sex marriage, that it is difficult logically to accept that one can be opposed to same-sex marriage and still be embracing (or at least accepting) of gay and lesbian people, because love and marriage are so foundational to the human condition. How then can civil discourse be used to express disagreement without triggering polarizing arguments? There is no easy answer. At the very least, it is essential to publicly affirm and support existing legislation and evolving positive social norms, and recognize that what was once the majority opinion (opposition to same sex marriage) is no longer the case. Establishing this common ground prior to articulating one's own opinion and belief may (or may not) make a difference in how the message is received, but at the very least this will help everyone recognize a person's attempt to discuss a concept or ideas, rather than to demonize or vilify a whole category of people.

8.3.4 Listen Before You Speak

Central to civil discourse is respect for others and the notion of reciprocity: If you listen to what I have to say, I will listen to what you have to say. When individuals remember this important rule and actually listen before speaking, civil discourse is facilitated. Listening does not mean simply standing and looking forward as someone else speaks; it implies an active and honest attempt to hear and understand what the other person is saying, regardless of your preconceptions about that person or the topic being discussed. Listening requires good faith and the sincere intention to try to communicate as respectfully and honorably as possible. This of course can be challenging, particularly if the other person is not listening, is not demonstrating good faith, and is behaving dishonorably. Still, it is always important to maintain your own self-respect and dignity by behaving appropriately, even in inappropriate circumstances.

Importantly, listening before speaking also provides opportunities to send important nonverbal messages rather than having to use strong and adversarial language. Listening before speaking provides opportunities for tactical, but clear, use of silence as a way of expressing disagreement and an opportunity to refocus the other person's attention on your facial responses and body language, and can transmit enormous amounts of information without using words that may potentially be inflammatory.

8.3.5 Acknowledge Your Own Stereotypes and Biases

Regardless of one's beliefs and political orientation, we all have conscious and unconscious biases that influence our interactions with others. Verbally acknowledging these conscious biases is an important first step in civil discourse. Simply being aware of one's biases without verbalizing them publicly is less impactful and frankly unfair to others. Learning to express your conscious biases may be challenging and may feel awkward, but it can help establish a more trusting interpersonal relationship with others.

More challenging is the process of becoming aware of your unconscious biases, which by definition, are those predispositions of which you are not aware. Uncivil discourse is rarely if ever helpful in triggering awareness of unconscious bias; instead, it is more likely to harden attitudes and produce toxic interpersonal relationships. Civil discourse, founded on common ground, respect, and a listening rather than speaking stance, can be extraordinarily helpful in surfacing unconscious bias. When this happens, it is important to remember the lessons of precontemplation from the Transtheoretical Model; that is, moving from unconsciousness to awareness of a bias will take time for both cognitive and emotional processing. Do not expect individuals to immediately apologize, change behaviors, or even acknowledge this new awareness. The shift from unconsciousness to awareness is more likely to be communicated nonverbally through, for example, a facial expression of surprise or worry. Attentiveness to this kind of communication is essential to civil discourse.

8.3.6 Nonverbal Cues and Messaging

A major challenge in managing diversity and difference is the strong emotional responses that may be provoked, especially in situations involving disagreement or conflict. Recall from Chapter 5 that close to 80% of all communication is nonverbal in nature, and this can go even higher in situations that are at their foundation more emotionally rather than logically focused. Civil communication involves active attention to the nonverbal cues and messaging that are transmitted; for example, avoiding rolling your eyes or making exasperated sighing noises in response to someone's comments or statements. Although such nonverbal slips may be difficult to control, they transmit enormous amounts of information and can be quite inflammatory. Maintaining composure—your ability to control and monitor the nonverbal messaging you are transmitting to others—is essential, particularly if you are highly and emotionally charged by a discussion or debate. Similarly, observing and responding appropriately to the other person's nonverbal cues and messages will be equally important. Recognizing that the other person may have difficulty maintaining composure and controlling their nonverbal messaging may reduce the risk of you reacting strongly to a cue they are sending. Important elements of nonverbal cues include tone of voice (e.g., sarcasm, superiority, dismissiveness), eye-rolling, dismissive hand gestures, and a closed body language stance; controlling these for yourself, and not overreacting to these when transmitted by others, will support respectful, civil discourse.

8.3.7 Know When to Walk Away

Intense emotional and unconscious responses to diversity and difference are an unfortunate reality, and in some cases, there will be no easy option or right answer to manage individual responses. Regrettably, but realistically, in some cases, issues of personal safety and security will be of primary importance, rather than attempting to engage individuals in discussion or debate. Civil discourse will have limits, and there will be circumstances where outright hatred toward others will pose a risk to personal safety. In less dramatic circumstances where personal safety is not an issue, there may simply be an impasse. In some cases, it may be possible to disagree without being disagreeable; in other situations, this is not possible.

Recognizing the limits of civil discourse means it may be necessary to politely and safely remove yourself from certain conversations, situations, or people when it is clear that there is no possibility of common ground *at the present time.* Walking away today may allow you to get back together tomorrow.

It is impossible to generate a list of "correct" communication strategies for civil discourse in the context of all possible diversities and differences. Further, it would be inadvisable; simply following a list of prescribed behaviors in a textbook is neither genuine nor authentic and would be immediately detected and dismissed as offensive by some people. Instead, understanding the psychology behind how human beings interpret diversity and difference, and considering the principles of what constitutes civil discourse, it should become possible to construct your own, genuine, personal, and authentic communication strategies and techniques to enable better interactions with diverse audiences. One area of increasing importance of course is cultural diversity, as our societies and workplaces become ever more ethnoculturally diverse and enriched by the presence and contributions of people from all over the world.

8.4 Cultural Diversity and Difference

We use the word *culture* a lot and, in recent times, the term itself has been used both positively and sometimes negatively to label individuals and groups. No single definition of culture can quite capture what it means to us in our day-to-day lives, largely because culture is like the air we breathe. Without culture we cannot function and we cannot thrive, but it is often invisible to us and something we take for granted. One way of thinking about culture is a series of rules, or a computer operating system, that dictates how we respond and interact with everything in our world. These rules are almost never written down, and we almost never spend time to think critically or reflect upon them. We simply follow them, respond to them, and use them as a filter to interpret and judge the actions, behaviors, and words of others to see whether they are part of the in group or outside of it. In this way, culture is one of the most powerful, important, and overlooked nonverbal cues that we transmit and receive on a regular basis. Culture is the lens through which we observe and draw inferences about others–whether we like them, trust them, can rely on them, want them to be our friends, want to work with them, or simply feel safe and comfortable spending time with them. Given its central importance to day-to-day life, it behooves us to think more about our own unquestioned cultural rules and how we use them in our interactions with others.

8.4.1   Ethnicity and Race Are Not Culture

Ethnicity describes an individual's membership or association with a distinct group of individuals, usually based on some form of common national tradition. It is most frequently connected to race and visible racial characteristics, although not always. As all reasonable people recognize, race is an extraordinarily imprecise and unreliable way of categorizing anyone, yet unfortunately, it persists as one of the most commonly used ways human beings have of sorting individuals. Ethnicity may be somewhat broader than simple racial categorization. For example, someone who self-identifies as having Spanish ethnicity may (or may not) have dark hair, eyes, and skin tone, but beyond that they have absorbed elements of Spanish national cultural factors and norms, which may be different from his neighbor who self-identifies as having Portuguese ethnicity but who may visibly look quite similar.

The problem of ethnicity and race as the basis for categorizing people is further exacerbated by the reality of widespread immigration. For example, there are millions of individuals who may "look" like they are from a different country (due to the color of their hair, skin, or eyes) and who may have absorbed cultural norms of a different nation, yet who were born and bred in your community and who have no nationality other than yours. The absorption and integration of generations of immigrants from around the world is what has made immigrant-receiving nations such as Canada, the United States, Australia, New Zealand, and the United Kingdom the great countries they are today and the greater countries they will be tomorrow.

Unfortunately, human prejudice and stereotyping are enduring, and visible racial and ethnic differences can sometimes trigger problems. Many second-, third-, or fourth-generation immigrants—those whose grandparents or great-grandparents moved here from another country—may occasionally still be asked where they're from simply because ethnically or racially they appear different from those around them. Ethnic and racial differences may produce subconscious bias that, in turn, results in unfair treatment or behavior, which is both fundamentally unfair and eventually toxic to the general health of an individual, a community, and a society.

8.4.2   Culture and Diversity

We live in increasingly complex societies. Regardless of where you live, a big city or a small town, or where you practice—whether a suburban strip small, a big box store, an ambulatory care clinic, or an institutional setting—the patients we see, the colleagues with whom we collaborate, and the interprofessional team that delivers care are becoming more diverse in terms of culture and background. Building relationships with different people means embracing the cultural differences that are becoming more commonplace in our day-to-day lives. Thinking about the cultural dimensions of our interpersonal communication is an important element in building better relationships and involves more than the application of effective communication techniques we have previously discussed in this book. Let's look now at culture: What it is, why it matters, and how embracing cultural differences can help us to build and nurture relationships to support providing the best possible patient care.

In daily life, we tend to use the word and the concept of culture to label obvious visible things that are different or unusual to us. For example, the way people dress, the kinds of head coverings they may choose to wear, or the food they eat are some of the more visible or obvious facets or factors of culture and the way we use to describe it to others. Sometimes, we may make judgments about these visible factors without reflecting on how our own cultures may appear to others. Think about the issue of head coverings. In some cultures, men and/or women are expected to wear certain articles of clothing to cover part of their head. It is easy to dismiss this kind of cultural expectation; however, one need only enter any college classroom to see an explosion of head coverings (we call them baseball caps) that are a common part of that culture. The time, attention, and energy that some people place on selecting and wearing the right baseball cap in the right way may seem extraordinary to many of us, but good luck trying to get someone to remove a baseball cap when they do not see the need or value of doing so. The meaning and significance to the individual of that part of their culture can be an important part of the way they present themselves to the world. In today's somewhat polarized world, there is a lot of attention placed on the visible factors of culture, and there are many who would like to change the way others eat, dress, carry themselves, etc. This focus on the visible factors of culture may be understood as feelings of discomfort, perhaps fear, about what these visible cultural symbols mean about a rapidly changing world. However, it is focusing literally on only the tip of the iceberg.

The nonvisible indicators of culture run far deeper than what we wear and eat. Our cultures shape us as human beings throughout our lives, and the cultural rules we were raised and grew up with form indelible imprints in our adult personalities. These may rarely manifest in any outward or visible way, but they are a form of culture as important and real as the holidays we celebrate. Examples of invisible cultural factors include our understanding and response to authority. In some cultures, there is an expectation that all people—men and women, adults and children—are equal and deserve equal treatment. In other cultures, there is a hierarchy in which some individuals, generally older men, may have specific roles, responsibilities, duties, and opportunities that others do not. Growing up and being socialized in such cultural norms influences many of our interactions and responses as adults, and learning this culture makes unlearning it very challenging. Is one cultural norm inherently better or worse than another? This is of course an important but very challenging philosophical question. Although culture can explain certain differences, using culture as an excuse for certain behaviors can be problematic. Ultimately, as pharmacists and as human beings, we are constantly juggling the need to be respectful and polite with the need to also protect certain nonnegotiable cultural values of our own in a way that is practical and meaningful. There are sometimes no easy and right answers with respect to this balancing act; as a start, however, understanding the distinction between visible and invisible factors of culture and recognizing that at least some of the cultural biases and assumptions we may hold about our own culture influence our interpretation of others is important.

An understandable response to the increasing diversity in all societies today is to wish we could go back to a seemingly simpler, uncomplicated time where everyone knew and followed the same rules. There may be more than simple wishful thinking and a misremembering of the past in this sentiment. The reality is, of course, that multiculturalism has been part of our communities and countries as long as communities and countries have existed. Although the specific newcomer group may change with each generation, the general principles of cultural difference have remained similar. When we reminisce about simpler times and fail to recognize the challenges inherent in those times, it may make nostalgia sweeter, but may not be an accurate representation of the numerous parallel subcultures that have always coexisted in all communities. Culture matters because it is integral and inherent to who we are as human beings. Disagreement about culture can quickly escalate to disrespect for individuals; disliking an important cultural factor or expressing tacit or overt disregard for a cultural norm cannot help but be interpreted personally. If you reject an important part of my culture, you reject me, and this will often escalate quickly and unfortunately into conflict. Thinking in cultural terms and being careful in the way we understand others' behaviors is essential to prevent and avoid inadvertently hurting others' feelings, offending them, harming them, or provoking unnecessary escalation for both individuals and entire communities. Although thinking in cultural terms cannot prevent all these problems, it can help us to establish a more respectful tone with which we can discuss differences.

We know from our own day-to-day experiences how challenging intercultural communications can be, but also how rewarding it can be as we learn more about our world. A central challenge to navigating intercultural communications is to be mindful of our own biases and assumptions, both about cultures and individuals. As we know from our own experiences, although we are members of different cultural groups and subgroups, we as individuals do not necessarily accept, support, or demonstrate every single facet of any culture. We are shaped and formed by our culture, but that does not mean we completely abandon individuality and personal choices to those cultures. As individuals we can benefit and grow from our own cultural affiliations, but we also need not be entirely subsumed by them. As we reflect on our own personal development within a culture, we need to afford that same generosity of spirit to individuals from other different cultural backgrounds. Simply because someone looks a certain way, dresses a certain way, eats certain foods, or self-identifies as a member of a specific cultural group or subgroup does not mean we can immediately attribute all characteristics of that entire group to a specific individual. Assuming we understand and know everything or even most things about an individual because we have one label to describe them means we reduce the complexity of that individual to nothing more than a list of preformed, stereotyped attributes, and this is fundamentally unfair. Just as we can be proud of our culture, and respectful of our heritage, we also know that there are some aspects of that background that we may not entirely embrace ourselves. We feel we have the latitude to cherry pick in this way and so we need to provide that same latitude to everyone else and try to check our assumptions regarding how a label shapes our interpretation of others. It is entirely possible, of course, that we may have personal objections to or dislike individuals because of individual characteristics they demonstrate. Extending one individual's characteristics to an entire group and judging an entire group by the characteristics of one individual is simply unfair. Within any group, even a group bound together by a common cultural label or beliefs, there will always be significant variation. Treating each individual as an individual, not as the representative of their entire group, is essential.

8.5 **Summary**

Diversity and differences enrich our societies and communities, and our personal lives. It is erroneous to believe that just because someone looks like you, dresses like you, speaks like you, and eats like you that they will actually think, act, or be-have like you. Diversity is everywhere, perhaps nowhere more obvious than in one's own family. Societies have made progress toward greater inclusion. Those who have historically been marginalized and excluded can now contribute more freely and fully than ever before. Communication with diverse individuals and communities is built on civil discourse and an understanding of the psychology of how human beings perceive difference. Learning to develop your own authentic and personal communication style will be rewarded by better and more fulfilling personal and professional relationships.

8.6 **Mind Map Chapter 8**

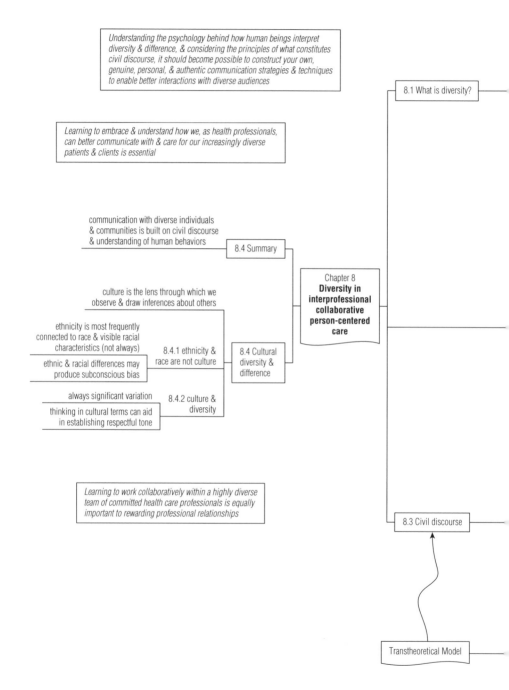

Understanding the psychology behind how human beings interpret diversity & difference, & considering the principles of what constitutes civil discourse, it should become possible to construct your own, genuine, personal, & authentic communication strategies & techniques to enable better interactions with diverse audiences

Learning to embrace & understand how we, as health professionals, can better communicate with & care for our increasingly diverse patients & clients is essential

communication with diverse individuals & communities is built on civil discourse & understanding of human behaviors

8.4 Summary

culture is the lens through which we observe & draw inferences about others

ethnicity is most frequently connected to race & visible racial characteristics (not always)

8.4.1 ethnicity & race are not culture

ethnic & racial differences may produce subconscious bias

always significant variation

8.4.2 culture & diversity

thinking in cultural terms can aid in establishing respectful tone

8.4 Cultural diversity & difference

Chapter 8 **Diversity in interprofessional collaborative person-centered care**

8.1 What is diversity?

Learning to work collaboratively within a highly diverse team of committed health care professionals is equally important to rewarding professional relationships

8.3 Civil discourse

Transtheoretical Model

describes differences between individuals

categorizing vs. stereotyping & bias

sometimes the reality of differences translates into negative emotional & behavioral responses

are we predisposed to thinking about diversity & difference in troubling & unhelpful ways?

i) we are hardwired to feel before we think

8.1.1 Why is "difference" a problem?

ii) do we all have strong negative emotional responses to something new or different? | Big Five personality dimensions useful to predict responses to diversity

iii) the emergence of stereotypes
- part of normal human thinking - Gordon Allport
- categorizing - cognitive tool to manage environmental complexity
- changing opinions requires owning mistaken assumptions, coping with cognitive dissonance, & truthfully acknowledging our own errors

iv) the power of socialization
- process of being raised & the psychological development that occurs
- beliefs are transmitted from elders to children, school, religious education, & cultural artifacts
- can reinforce stereotypes & inhibit change

8.2 What can break the vicious cycle of stereotype & prejudice?
- i) The Contact Hypothesis
- ii) conscious & unconscious biases
- iii) cultural & media influences
- iv) the importance of political change

understanding influences that stereotype, bias, & prejudice helps to identify potential alternatives & solutions

demonstrates respect for all

builds on psychological understanding of categorization, stereotyping, & bias

increasing disregard is corrosive

requires understanding & acceptance of another person's motivations, beliefs, & ideas

8.3.1 find common ground | identify things agreed upon/commonalities

8.3.2 avoid us-vs-them language | essential to civil discourse

8.3.3 discuss ideas, not people | try to establish common ground & then discuss concepts

8.3.4 listen before you speak
- reciprocity
- nonverbal (e.g., eye contact, nodding)

8.3.5 acknowledge your own stereotypes & biases
- expressing conscious bias is a key to establishing trust
- surfacing unconscious bias via listening rather than speaking, respect, common ground | 80% of all communication is nonverbal

8.3.6 nonverbal cues & messaging
- maintaining composure
- controlling your nonverbal messaging

8.3.7 know when to walk away
- recognizing an impasse
- leaving the door open

For Further Reading:

Barak M. *Managing Diversity: Toward a Globally Inclusive Workplace*. 4th ed. Thousand Oaks, CA: Sage Publishing; 2017.

Betancourt J, Green A, Carrillo J. Defining cultural competence: a practical framework for addressing racial/ethnic disparities in health and health care. *Public Health Rep*. 2003; 118(4):293–302.

Ko M, Sanders C, de Guia S, Shimkhada R, Ponce N. Managing diversity to eliminate disparities: a framework for health. *Health Aff (Millwood)*. 2018;37(9):1383–1393.

Ontario Regulators for Access Consortium. Managing cultural differences. Available at: regulatorsforaccess.ca/wp-content/uploads/2017/03/ManagingCulturalDifferencesEnglish.pdf.

Roberson Q, ed. *The Oxford Handbook of Diversity and Work*. Oxford: Oxford University Press; 2013.

Seeleman C, Essink-Bot M, Stronks K, Ingleby D. How should health service organizations respond to diversity? A content analysis of six approaches. *BMC Health Serv Res*. 2015;15:510.

Whelan A, Weech-Maldonado R, Dreachslin J. Diversity management in health: cross national organizational study. *Int J Divers Organ Communities Nations*. 2008;8(3):125–137.

9 | Applying Communication Theory: Feedback

You have a colleague on your interprofessional team who is clever and technically skilled but displays some peculiar and disturbing interpersonal mannerisms from time to time. Frankly, you're concerned that he simply doesn't respect women's opinions despite appearing to be polite and attentive. He has never said or done anything that reaches the threshold of outright sexism or misogyny—yet. You are not sure if this is a behavior that can or should be excused culturally or for another reason, and you are concerned that this attitude will be problematic for you personally, the rest of the team, and most importantly, for the patients you serve.

Learning to communicate effectively with colleagues, particularly when managing difficult situations such as in this example, requires both cognitive flexibility and a high degree of skill and self-confidence. Relationships with colleagues are important. We typically spend more time at work than anywhere else, and the friendships and professional relationships we form there are very important to us. The term *work wife* or *work husband* highlights just how important our colleagues can be. We often spend more time with them and have more intense ups and downs than we may with our own family members. As a result, communication is essential. Our work relationships are not transient or temporary, and as a result, we have a strong investment and high stakes in nurturing and sustaining them, which means particular care must be taken in communicating with one another in difficult situations.

Feedback is one of the most important communication skills necessary for health care professionals. Feedback is a process by which we communicate information to one another about our performance and learn from one another about how we are perceived within our environment. Learning to deliver effective and constructive feedback is both an art and a skill. We must provide feedback to student learners in our environment and to peers with whom we work, and for those who have managerial or administrative responsibilities, we must learn to provide helpful feedback to enhance performance and functioning.

9.1   Feedback Versus Evaluation

A central challenge in delivering effective feedback is that it may be interpreted emotionally if focused on criticism rather than on quality improvement, and few of us gain emotional satisfaction from criticism even if we gain valuable information to perform better. Although effective feedback should provide reinforcement of the things we do well, most of us have become accustomed to the "gotcha" moment or the "everything is great BUT . . ." in which our deficiencies are pointed out by another person.

The emotional context for feedback may therefore bias many people, including well-trained health professionals, to anticipate the worst and expect problems. Recall from previous chapters that our emotional self provides the primary and initial filter through which we interpret the world. When we become aware or suspect that feedback is about to be provided to us, we may immediately adopt a negative or defensive emotional posture that will adversely influence the way we hear and interpret the other person's words and nonverbal cues.

In part, this problem may be due to definitions and understanding of words. Words such as *feedback*, *evaluation*, *assessment*, and *criticism* are sometimes used interchangeably, and even if they aren't used in this way, many people expect that feedback will involve an evaluation and that assessments are really criticisms. Increasingly, educators favor the use of the term *assessment*, understood as the description and estimation of the nature, quality, and ability of something or someone. From this perspective, feedback is sometimes defined as a formative assessment, that is, an assessment of performance that is meant to perform, guide, coach, and support quality improvement and personal development. In contrast, an evaluation is sometimes defined as a summative assessment; that is, a judgment that utilizes benchmarking, ranking, rating, and comparisons to evaluate performance.

Although these definitions may seem vague, you will have already personally experienced the difference between feedback and evaluation. Evaluation has a sorting function; it attempts to weed out and to rank individuals, and consequently the results of an evaluation have practical significance beyond simply quality improvement; a person's salary, job title, place in a line, or promotion prospects may be fundamentally changed because of an evaluation. In contrast, feedback is meant to be more personal and should not influence external standing, rank, or position. Although an evaluation can be risky but rewarding, feedback should feel safe and nurturing. A central challenge in any team, organization, or in any interpersonal relationship occurs when individuals are unclear or simply do not know whether they are receiving feedback or an evaluation. Am I being judged or am I being coached? Will what has been said be held against me or are you really just interested in nurturing and mentoring me? Because we rarely explicitly say to one another, "I am now providing you with summative assessment" or "that was just a formative assessment," the somewhat vague term *feedback* gets frequently used, which can provoke both confusion and, consequently, emotionally negative responses. As a person delivering or receiving feedback, ensuring you are clear as to what is going on and whether a summative or formative assessment is being utilized is essential. Worse, when a person tries to use both summative AND formative assessments at the same time in the same conversation (i.e., providing simultaneous feedback AND evaluation), this can further heighten confusion and emotional anxiety, and precipitate negative responses.

9.2   Why Is Feedback Important?

It may be tempting to believe that well-educated health professionals already know when they perform well and when they don't. The reality, of course, is that all individuals and workers must constantly adapt to their environments, and as result, all of us benefit from and need both summative and formative assessments to ensure we are aligned with a team's objectives and goals. We literally cannot see ourselves in action, and as a result, we must rely on others to be external eyes and ears on our performance and to use this information in a constructive way to support quality improvement and personal and professional development.

Feedback (a formative assessment) is particularly crucial because it is low stakes and not connected to external rewards such as salary, status, or position. When we trust the feedback we hear, we have an opportunity to reflect and adjust our behaviors with the hope of improving our performance. We need feedback because, for most of us, our own self-assessment and self-perception is notoriously unreliable, particularly when we are novice or new practitioners. The *Dunning–Kruger effect* is a term used to describe the consistent overestimation of one's skills and abilities that most of us will experience, including health care professionals. This effect is sometimes summarized in the expression: "We don't know what we don't know." When we are unable to truly see ourselves in 360° from multiple perspectives, there are crucial pieces of information we are missing. As a result, a self-assessment will be compromised; therefore, we need trusted others around us to fill in these gaps and allow us to more honestly and fully understand how we come across and are viewed by others.

9.3   Pendleton's Rules for Feedback

At its best, feedback helps us to fill in self-awareness gaps to allow us to see the big picture regarding our performance. Because it is not linked to external rewards but is focused on our personal development, it should be nonthreatening, supportive, and truly aimed at improvement rather than judgment. Unfortunately, because many of us will have already have had negative experiences with an evaluation disguised or mistakenly labeled as feedback, we may not be as open and trusting as we could be, and this in turn may inhibit our ability to truly benefit from it.

In medical education, Pendleton's Rules are a widely used model to provide a structured approach for the delivery of feedback. The importance of this structure is clear: It helps alert the recipient of feedback as to what is coming, involves them directly in a conversation (rather than a download of information), and provides both parties with an opportunity to share observations and thoughts. The following are seven steps in the adapted Pendleton's Rules model.

Rule 1: Check that the person actually wants and is ready right now to receive feedback. This first—and arguably, most important—rule is frequently overlooked in day-to-day life. It is easy to believe that everyone around us is so interested and so eagerly awaiting our thoughts and feedback that we can just dive in and start talking. The reality, of course, is that human beings need to be psychologically ready and primed to receive feedback. Delivering feedback to someone who has just finished having a fight with someone else, is in the middle of a complex task, or is in a rush is worse than pointless, it actually may heighten that person's aggravation. Remember that feedback will likely be initially experienced and filtered emotionally, not cognitively. As a result, it is essential that the environment and timing of feedback are well considered to optimize delivery and receipt. If a person says or behaves in a way that suggests now is not a good time for feedback, then wait. Feedback cannot be delivered on a rigid schedule and should be adapted to the unique needs and circumstances of the individual.

Rule 2: Let the other person speak first. Perhaps paradoxically, the second Pendleton rule states that the best way to offer feedback is to first listen, then speak. Encouraging the other person to self-reflect, self-assess, and speak first by giving general comments about their performance helps to establish a comfortable and respectful environment. It demonstrates that you are actually interested in what the other person has to say and that you are willing to take the time needed to discuss and share. Equally important, by inviting the other person to speak first, it will give you time to figure out how best to phrase and say things, and to get a sense of the challenges that await you in delivering feedback on certain topics. As noted in Chapter 7, this is a variation of the principle of effective listening and starts to approach the level of empathizing by letting the other person speak, reflect, share, and vent if necessary. Most importantly, letting that person actually hear themselves discussing their own performance can be a powerful form of feedback and an important first step in opening a dialogue or discussion.

Rule 3: What are you doing right? What are you doing well? If the first two Pendleton rules are followed in structuring a feedback discussion, you may frequently encounter the situation where the person you are speaking with becomes unnecessarily or unfairly self-critical. This is particularly true for health care professionals (and even more true for those who have an emotional intelligence style of assimilator). The perfectionist tendencies that are frequently noted among practitioners can sometimes make us our own worst critics. Although appropriate, accurate, and fair self-criticism is of course an essential part of self-awareness and self-assessment, it can easily go too far. Some practitioners can become so self-critical and so self-doubting that they fall into a negative spiral. The third Pendleton rule is aimed at preventing this downward spiral and reminds practitioners that no matter how badly you think you performed, there were still many good things that happened. Explicitly asking the other person to reflect on and articulate, "What are you doing right?" and "What are you doing well?" helps to reorient the discussion in a positive way, provides opportunities to pull out of any downward negative spiral, and again will signal that you are not evaluating and judging but instead are focused on personal development and quality improvement. Starting with the positive can help shift a negative emotional state and can make both parties more open and willing to engage in honest conversation. It also sends a strong signal to the person receiving feedback that you are letting them steer the direction of conversation and take primary responsibility for their own development. Finally, by using this Pendleton rule, it will create a more positive interaction and keeps both parties more open to continuing the discussion.

Rule 4: Here's what I saw you doing well . . . The first three Pendleton rules are all focused on having the other person speak and self-reflect; although this is valuable for a number of reasons, there is of course a point where you will need to start actually providing feedback of some sort. The fourth Pendleton rule suggests the way to do this is to focus on the positive by corroborating and reinforcing what was identified in the third Pendleton rule by the individual. The value of positive reinforcement is clear: It helps to engage the listener, it helps them to remember to keep doing certain things, and it establishes your role as being one of coaching and mentoring, not judging or evaluating.

There is, of course, an inherent challenge in this fourth Pendleton rule: What if the person says or thinks they are doing something well or correctly but you, in fact, disagree? Using this fourth Pendleton rule, it means you simply do not mention it at all. Instead, you only focus on the strengths and things done well or right that you both agree on. Do not explicitly state, "No, I think you're wrong" or "Actually, I didn't think you did this well." This will be emotionally provocative, sound evaluative and judgmental, and will diminish prospects that this conversation will be experienced as a formative assessment and feedback. Instead, by simply concentrating on the positive elements you both agree on, for now, you can strengthen your relationship and allow yourself a future opportunity to discuss areas of disagreement.

Rule 5: What do you think you could have improved on? Providing an opportunity to focus on the positive and to receive appropriate positive reinforcement can lay the foundation for the more demanding Pendleton's rules. The fifth rule highlights the need to eventually begin focusing on quality improvement and areas for personal and professional development. Asking the individual to answer the question, "What do you think you could have improved on" only AFTER they have described and reflected on the things they did well provides a psychological and emotional safety zone to discuss deficiencies. If this were the first question asked, defensiveness and negativity would likely interfere with feedback, and the entire exercise would devolve into an evaluation. Asking the individual this question can be highly illuminating. It will allow you to start to gauge the accuracy of self-assessment, the honesty with which disclosure occurs, and the person's comfort level with you in terms of a difficult conversation. A key element of Pendleton's Rules—and why they are framed as rules—is the sequence of questioning. Prematurely focusing on improvement (Rule 5) before first moving through Rules 1 through 4 fundamentally changes and negatively impacts the relationship between teacher and student, manager and employee, or colleagues sharing feedback.

Rule 6: How can we fix what YOU (not I) want fixed? The sixth rule focuses on action, specifically helping the individual figure out how to fix or address deficiencies and areas for improvement identified in Rule 5. This is crucial. As a teacher, parent, manager, or colleague, you may have your own thoughts, ideas, or priorities in terms of feedback and what you would like to see the other person do. Using the Pendleton's Rule model, however, it is important to take cues and priorities from the person himself and his reflections and observations, not yours. In the sixth rule, you simply help that person identify and formulate strategies to address what he wants to fix regardless of whether it is your priority.

This can be challenging for many of us, but it is an essential aspect of what makes this a process feedback (a formative assessment) rather than an evaluation (a summative assessment). In some cases, this might mean that you will simply have to bite your tongue and not actually say everything you want to say or believe to be important to preserve the relationship and reinforce the formative nature of the feedback being presented. Failure to do so will change how the other person perceives you and receives this entire conversation. This means you must honestly assess HOW important your suggestions for improvement for the other person really are. In some cases—for example in situations involving legal issues, patient safety or risk, or where timeliness of behavioral change is essential—you simply may not be able to abide by Pendleton's sixth rule and in fact, will need to switch to an evaluative (a summative assessment) delivery style. If this is the case, avoid tricking or giving the appearance of double-crossing the individual by abandoning feedback only at this stage. It will make it difficult for the other person to ever trust you again to deliver nonjudgmental feedback. If the corrective suggestions you feel are essential must be made in a timely fashion and it is not possible, in your opinion, to do so while adhering to Rule 6, then feedback may simply not be the appropriate mode for communication. Best in this case to be honest and clear about this up front and indicate you are providing an evaluation rather than try to sugar coat at first, only to confuse and disappoint later.

Rule 7: Now, let's make the change we've discussed. The final rule focuses on the implementation of whatever plan was discussed in Rule 6, and providing the other person with the opportunity to continue to ask for and receive your feedback as needed. This invitation to continue the conversation in the future and maintain the relationship as change is being implemented indicates you are in this for the long haul and that you have a strong interest in nurturing and sustaining the interpersonal relationship you have built. It also helps the other person feel more accountable to implement the ideas and strategies discussed.

The value of Pendleton's Rules in providing a systematic structure to follow in delivering feedback has been demonstrated in many different situations. By emphasizing speaking and by allowing the other person to speak, reflect, and prioritize for problem solving first, and by valuing maintenance and nurturing of the interpersonal relationship over downloading of suggestions for improvement, this approach defines what effective feedback—rather than evaluation—can be. However, this model does not explicitly address many of the other communication issues described in previous chapters. Pendleton's Rules focuses on WHAT is said, not HOW it is said. As a result, conscious effort to ensure you use appropriate and supportive body language, tone, nonverbal gestures, facial expressions, among others is essential. As was discussed in Chapters 5, 6, and 7, attentiveness to these important aspects of interpersonal communication are essential when discussing feedback.

Pendleton's Rules can, in some cases, appear ham-fisted and somewhat belabored. In particular, for those whose emotional intelligence tends toward a stronger accommodator or converger type, the methodical structure demonstrated previously may appear forced, unnecessarily time consuming, and somewhat infantilizing. As you may recall from Chapter 2, accommodators and convergers tend to favor efficiency and directness in communication and feedback, so they may be less oriented toward the approach described previously. It may take them longer to learn and apply with finesse. In other cases, you may still want to adopt a feedback orientation but feel you simply do not have time to go through the seven rules. An abbreviated feedback model has been developed that captures many of the elements of the rules but in a more efficient and direct manner. This abbreviated model consists of three feedback questions that are asked in sequence as a vehicle for opening a discussion and dialogue:

1. What did you do well?

2. What could you have done better?

3. What did you learn about this experience for the next time this situation comes up?

As can be seen, these questions bear similarity to the Pendleton's Rules, and adopt a similar philosophy of asking questions, listening attentively, and engaging in dialogue rather than a download of suggestions for improvement. By being more focused, this approach may save time and may simply be more appealing to direct communicators such as accommodators and convergers, while still emphasizing a formative assessment and a feedback rather than an evaluation orientation.

9.4 What If My Feedback Isn't Getting Through?

Pendleton's Rules may at times simply not appear to work, and there may be a temptation to shift into an evaluation (or a summative assessment) mode to fix the problem quickly, even if this may compromise or adversely impact the interpersonal relationship among colleagues. By definition, processing feedback will take time. Remember that feedback works to support professional and personal development because:

*   it is built on a model of reflective practice—sustainable quality improvement can only occur through honest self-appraisal;

*   it utilizes a nonjudgmental inquiry model—instead of telling or lecturing, you are asking and listening, and this interpersonal strategy builds rapport and a relationship; and

*   it keeps the other person thinking, talking, and actively engaged in the process rather than simply passively listening and agreeing to what you're saying.

When this is not working as hoped or planned, there may be alternative approaches to consider that can still utilize a feedback orientation.

What if the other person has inaccurately self-assessed? If, in listening to responses to Pendleton's Rules 2 and 3, you believe the other person "doesn't know what they don't know" and is demonstrating inaccurate or incomplete self-assessment, it may be tempting to immediately switch to an evaluation because feedback cannot work if self-assessment is flawed. Prior to making this decision, there are alternatives that could be tried first. You could ask the other person to provide some more clarification or more detailed evidence to support their self-assessment. This can sometimes cause the house of cards of a flawed self-assessment to collapse as the other person struggles to find and articulate evidence, then realizes there is none to support their initial statements. Alternatively, asking a question that forces the other person to look at a situation from another stakeholder's perspective (e.g., "How do you think the patient felt about this?" or "What was the team's response when you said this?") can also have a similar effect.

What if the other person just doesn't want to self-assess or reflect and isn't interested? At worst, this may mean that feedback is not possible and an evaluation is now needed. However, before reaching that stage, it may be useful to consider an alternative approach. For example, demonstrating how self-assessment or reflection works can sometimes trigger a positive response. Give a personal example from your own experience of how feedback helped you, how you learned to self-assess, and how you improved your ability to reflect. Demonstrating the process using yourself as the subject might, in some cases, loosen blockages and open opportunities for feedback.

What if the other person is just really good at faking feedback? Sometimes, you will detect that an individual really isn't interested in engaging in feedback with you but feels for political, social, or other reasons they have to play the game. They may look and sound like they are engaged, but subconsciously you register that this is not authentic. In such a circumstance, you may simply want to be honest and say what you are thinking, and give the person a chance to reconsider their response to Pendleton's Rule 1: Are they truly ready, interested, and open to feedback? If not, let's save this for another time. Do not disregard or overlook cues that suggest the other person is faking interest. Responding to these cues genuinely may enhance the quality of future interactions by signaling to the other person that you respect their time and their opinions and are not there to foist yourself on anyone.

There's so much to fix here … where do I even start? In some cases, your genuine desire to be helpful and supportive may run contrary to your perception that there are so many issues to contend with that there is no time for feedback. All you have time to do is provide a summative assessment and hope for the best. Mindful of the potential impact of an evaluation on an interpersonal relationship, it is frequently beneficial to try to make feedback work first. Where there are many different but important issues that you'd like to discuss, finding a way of prioritizing the low-hanging fruit (i.e., those problems or issues that have the highest likelihood of being successfully addressed in the shortest time) can build confidence and success, and open opportunities for future discussion and feedback. Additionally, limiting your problem-solving discussion to no more than two or three specific issues or problems will ensure this does not become overwhelming or daunting for the other person, increasing the likelihood that they will at least try something rather than thinking this is hopeless and giving up entirely. In essence, this means knowing that everything cannot be fixed all at once, and doing the easiest things first can be a good starting point.

9.5 General Principles for Making Feedback More Effective

Pendleton's Rules provide a useful structure for organizing a feedback dialogue, but of course other issues are also important if feedback is to be helpful, acceptable, and meaningful. Important principles to consider include the following.

For every statement, suggestion, or comment you make, be prepared to provide specific evidence or a specific example from what you have observed, not just what other people have told you or what you assume to be true. Using specific, personally observed behaviors is impactful and indicates that you are interested enough in the person to be connected with them in practice. Referencing what others say or think gives the impression of a bureaucratic or impersonal process. It also opens up the possibility that these others are wrong, biased, or misunderstood.

Use "I" statements more frequently than "you" statements. As discussed in previous chapters, the word "you" can be profoundly impactful for some people, particularly divergers and assimilators. The word can trigger a strong emotional and defensive response in some cases, which can completely shut down a feedback dialogue. Paying careful attention to your own verbal language and the extent to which the word "you" is used is essential. For example, saying, "You shouldn't use the word 'you' so much in conversation" sounds very different than, "When I hear the word 'you' in conversation, I become quite defensive." The first sentence is an order or a directive and implies what the other person has been doing all along is wrong or deficient. The second sentence is simply you sharing your experiences and feelings and inviting the other person to reflect on it. The second sentence conveys an important thought but may be less likely to provoke a negative or defensive response.

Do not give negative feedback without also being able to provide a concrete alternative option. Simply pointing out someone else's deficiency without offering any kind of alternative, solution, or improvement will be interpreted as an insult and will trigger a defensive response. Carefully considering which issues are your priorities for discussion in feedback means ensuring you have concrete, viable, and helpful ideas for addressing these priorities that will be feasible and acceptable to the other person. If you don't have these alternatives, don't bring up the issue or problem as this becomes a discussion point that will go nowhere and do nothing other than create bad feelings between the two of you.

Ensure alignment between your verbal and nonverbal messaging. Recall from Chapters 5, 6, and 7 the importance of alignment between WHAT you say and HOW you say it. Myriad nonverbal tells (such as eye contact, sighs, gestures, body language, etc.) all transmit large amounts of information about what you are really thinking and feeling in a situation. For example, if you say you are interested in feedback and a dialogue, do not be distracted by your cellphone, other people, or your own notes. Maintaining eye contact, responding appropriately with "uh-huh," and an open body language are all essential to demonstrating your interest in the other person, rather than simply SAYING you're interested. Feedback should not be a chore and should not feel onerous to you. Although it may be challenging, it should also feel like an opportunity to help solidify and nurture a relationship with someone who is important to you.

9.6 Conscious and Unconscious Competence and Incompetence

One of the most important but difficult elements of effective feedback is the extent to which it helps drive new learning and awareness of issues that another person may simply have not ever considered. One model for understanding is built on the notion of conscious and unconscious awareness.

Unconscious Competence: Many practitioners are perfectly competent but perform their day-to-day work in an almost unconscious way, as though they are simply following a formula or a routine approach to a problem. Unconscious competence can allow us to appear as though we know what we are doing, but unfortunately it can lead to errors, compromise patient safety, and leave us unequipped to deal with any situation where the formula or routine may not completely apply. When a person cannot quite explain what they are doing or why it is appropriate, this can be an important signal of unconscious competence. What they are doing might be perfectly fine and reasonable, but it should be worrisome if they cannot explain it. One feedback strategy to help address this and prevent small problems from becoming bigger ones may be to use a talk aloud approach. Asking someone to use words to explain their behaviors can focus attention on unconscious behaviors, and in the process, can help to surface them and make them less automatic and therefore more amendable to conscious control and quality improvement.

Conscious Competence: In some cases, practitioners can demonstrate their competence but only in situations that are unnatural, contrived, or somehow simulated. This may be the case when someone is book smart or able to perform well in a clinical simulation, but somehow cannot translate this into real-world behavior. It suggests they KNOW what they're supposed to say and do but become overwhelmed by real-world context and environmental constraints, which may result in a failure to perform. A useful strategy in this case can be an incremental building of responsibilities and a gradual introduction of real-world complexities into the environment, if this is possible. Giving people, especially young practitioners, an opportunity for an incremental and gradual transition to the real world can build confidence and enhance performance, allowing them to shift away from conscious competence to effective performance.

Conscious Incompetence: Some practitioners are perfectly aware of their shortcomings but have no ideas or skills for actually doing anything about these deficiencies. These individuals, in particular, may be very interested and open to supportive feedback, and may be desperate for nonjudgmental support, guidance, and mentorship. Awareness that self-improvement is needed does not automatically translate into actual self-improvement; in some cases, people need a coach and supportive feedback to make this transition successful. Individuals in this category may be particularly helped by the approach discussed previously in Pendleton's Rules.

Unconscious Incompetence: This category is probably the most challenging and the most resistant to traditional feedback. In unconscious incompetence, individuals are not aware there is a problem and may not even know they have shortcomings. Similar to the precontemplation stage of the Transtheoretical Change Model discussed in Chapter 5, unconscious incompetence is difficult to manage within either a feedback or evaluation orientation. It requires first and foremost a shift in thinking and a recognition that there is a problem; leaping prematurely to a solution or answer before the person even realizes there's a problem to solve can be insulting and counterproductive. Where unconscious incompetence is an issue, the focus should be on simply raising awareness that there may be an issue to reflect on, rather than telling someone to change their behavior.

Let's consider these various models using the case presented at the opening of the chapter. You may have defined this issue as one of unconscious incompetence. For whatever reason, your colleague may not be aware that he is sending signals or demonstrating behaviors that are being interpreted by others as vaguely or potentially offensive and dismissive toward women. Although some may try to excuse this as cultural, it is not something that can be simply ignored, especially as it is interfering with team functioning and patient care. Can you simply tell a person like this to shape up and change their behavior? Of course not. If they perceive they are being evaluated and judged in this way, this will naturally provoke defensiveness and shut down the relationship you have. An evaluation orientation is, therefore, not likely to be helpful or successful in managing this situation; instead, a feedback orientation, one focused on unconscious incompetence and first raising awareness (rather than solving the problem) may be most helpful.

If we follow Pendleton's Rules (or the abbreviated version, depending on context and time available), we begin by first ensuring our colleague is ready, interested, and open to feedback. Assuming he is, we need to hear from him first. It is essential to focus on managing your own nonverbal communication and cues you are sending during this conversation. His behavior may offend you, but if you display or demonstrate that you are offended, this will register as judgmental and, again, will shut down the conversation. Managing your own emotional response to this difficult situation is important if your objective is to support your colleague in his personal and professional development. The reality, of course, is that not everyone is going to be able to manage their emotional response in this situation. Understandably, some individuals may take personal affront to this or other kinds of behavior and cannot help but feel defensive, which turn may prompt a somewhat offensive communication interaction that could lead to argument rather than resolution. Closely and honestly monitoring your own emotional involvement and entanglement in such situations is essential to prevent an escalation of the problem. Not everyone is going to be well equipped to adopt a feedback orientation in this situation. If you simply cannot reconcile your personal emotional responses in this case, it may be necessary to have another colleague engage in the discussion with this person, rather than risk inflaming the situation through inadvertent demonstration of your emotions, feelings, and judgments about his behavior.

In unconscious incompetence, people do not know what they do not know. The traditional sequence of questions using Pendleton's Rules may be frustratingly ineffective the first time around; you should probably expect this in this situation. As a result, it may be necessary to use redirecting statements (e.g., "That's an interesting point, and makes me wonder if there might be different ways of handling this situation") and questions (e.g., "How do you think other people respond when you say that?") to prompt further reflection and discussion, all delivered in a nonjudgmental tone with supportive nonverbals consistent with a feedback orientation.

9.7 Summary

Feedback is one of the most important tools available to individuals in teams to nurture and enhance team functioning. The communication skills necessary for effective feedback are similar to those required in any other interpersonal situation. Important issues to keep in mind include clear differentiation between a feedback orientation (focused on a formative assessment) and an evaluation orientation (focused on a summative assessment); careful attention to your own emotional state and your ability to truly adopt the coaching, mentoring, and nonjudgmental stance required for feedback; effective use of nonverbal cues to complement verbal communication; and attentiveness and appropriate responsiveness to nonverbal and emotional communications being sent. Delivering effective feedback is both an art and a science, one that is supported by an understanding of the psychology of human interaction and the careful application of communication theory.

9.8 Mind Map Chapter 9

You have a colleague on your interprofessional team who is clever and technically skilled but displays some peculiar and disturbing interpersonal mannerisms from time to time. Frankly, you're concerned that he simply doesn't respect women's opinions despite appearing to be polite and attentive. He has never said or done anything that reaches the threshold of outright sexism or misogyny - yet. You are not sure if this is a behavior that can or should be excused culturally or for another reason, and you are concerned that this attitude wil be problematic for you personally, the rest of the team, and most importantly, for the patients you serve.

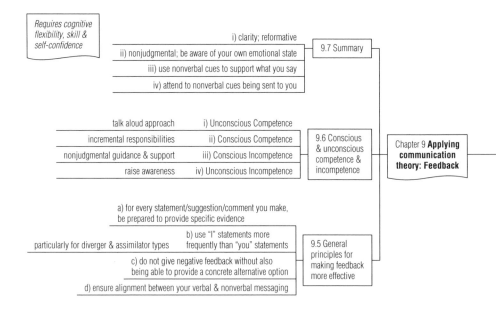

Requires cognitive flexibility, skill & self-confidence

i) clarity; reformative
ii) nonjudgmental; be aware of your own emotional state
iii) use nonverbal cues to support what you say
iv) attend to nonverbal cues being sent to you

9.7 Summary

talk aloud approach   i) Unconscious Competence
incremental responsibilities   ii) Conscious Competence
nonjudgmental guidance & support   iii) Conscious Incompetence
raise awareness   iv) Unconscious Incompetence

9.6 Conscious & unconscious competence & incompetence

Chapter 9 **Applying communication theory: Feedback**

a) for every statement/suggestion/comment you make, be prepared to provide specific evidence
b) use "I" statements more frequently than "you" statements
particularly for diverger & assimilator types
c) do not give negative feedback without also being able to provide a concrete alternative option
d) ensure alignment between your verbal & nonverbal messaging

9.5 General principles for making feedback more effective

Process to communicate information about performance & learn from each other how we are perceived

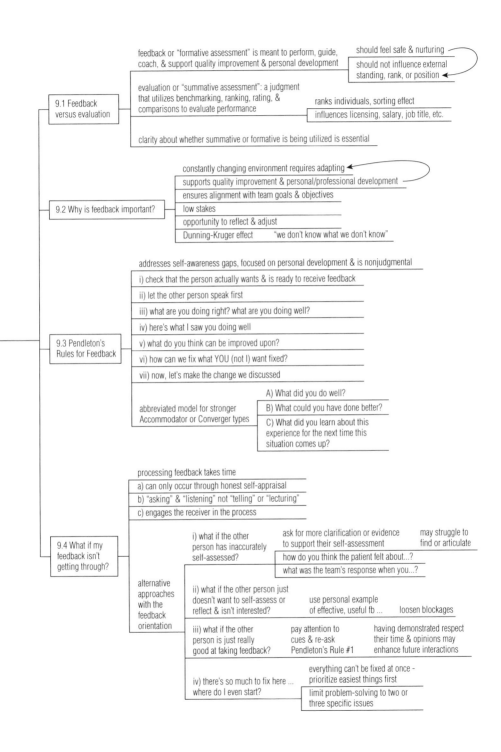

9.1 Feedback versus evaluation

feedback or "formative assessment" is meant to perform, guide, coach, & support quality improvement & personal development

should feel safe & nurturing

should not influence external standing, rank, or position

evaluation or "summative assessment": a judgment that utilizes benchmarking, ranking, rating, & comparisons to evaluate performance

ranks individuals, sorting effect

influences licensing, salary, job title, etc.

clarity about whether summative or formative is being utilized is essential

9.2 Why is feedback important?

constantly changing environment requires adapting

supports quality improvement & personal/professional development

ensures alignment with team goals & objectives

low stakes

opportunity to reflect & adjust

Dunning-Kruger effect   "we don't know what we don't know"

9.3 Pendleton's Rules for Feedback

addresses self-awareness gaps, focused on personal development & is nonjudgmental

i) check that the person actually wants & is ready to receive feedback

ii) let the other person speak first

iii) what are you doing right? what are you doing well?

iv) here's what I saw you doing well

v) what do you think can be improved upon?

vi) how can we fix what YOU (not I) want fixed?

vii) now, let's make the change we discussed

abbreviated model for stronger Accommodator or Converger types

A) What did you do well?

B) What could you have done better?

C) What did you learn about this experience for the next time this situation comes up?

9.4 What if my feedback isn't getting through?

processing feedback takes time

a) can only occur through honest self-appraisal

b) "asking" & "listening" not "telling" or "lecturing"

c) engages the receiver in the process

alternative approaches with the feedback orientation

i) what if the other person has inaccurately self-assessed?

ask for more clarification or evidence to support their self-assessment

may struggle to find or articulate

how do you think the patient felt about...?

what was the team's response when you...?

ii) what if the other person just doesn't want to self-assess or reflect & isn't interested?

use personal example of effective, useful fb ...

loosen blockages

iii) what if the other person is just really good at faking feedback?

pay attention to cues & re-ask Pendleton's Rule #1

having demonstrated respect their time & opinions may enhance future interactions

iv) there's so much to fix here ... where do I even start?

everything can't be fixed at once - prioritize easiest things first

limit problem-solving to two or three specific issues

For Further Reading:

Aguinis H, Gottfredson R, Joo H. Delivering effective performance feedback: the strengths-based approach. *Bus Horiz.* 2012;55:105–111.

Algiraigri A. Ten tips for receiving feedback effectively in clinical practice. *Med Educ Online.* 2014;19:10.3402/meo.v19.25141.

Chaowdhury R, Kalu G. Learning to give feedback in medical education. *Obstet Gynaecol.* 2004;6:243–247.

Hamid Y, Mahmood S. Understanding constructive feedback: a commitment between teachers and students for academic and professional development. *J Pak Med Assoc.* 2010;60(3): 224–227.

Jug R, Jiang X, Bean S. Giving and receiving effective feedback: a review article and how-to guide. *Arch Pathol Lab Med.* 2019;143:244–250.

Ramani S, Krackov S. Twelve tips for giving feedback effectively in the clinical environment. *Med Teach.* 2012;34(10):787–791.

Richardson B. Feedback. *Acad Emerg Med.* 2004;11(12):e1–5.

van der Leeuw RM, Slootweg IA. Twelve tips for making the best use of feedback. *Med Teach.* 2013;35(5):348–351.

10 Resilience and Preventing Burnout: How to Communicate When You Need Help

The work that health care professionals do is extraordinarily important. We are there with and for patients and their families during some of the most difficult times and transitions in any human being's life. Although some events can be extremely joyful (for example, the birth of a child), others can be extremely painful. In some cases, events that might be considered joyful may become tragic because of unexpected circumstances, or be filled with sadness due to context-specific reasons. The nature of health care work means that we engage with people during particularly emotionally intensive periods of time.

This emotional intensity can sometimes become overwhelming and can produce unanticipated knock-on effects or consequences for the health care professionals themselves. Professional work is always intellectually challenging and exhausting; learning new skills, performing delicate procedures, maintaining your competency in a field that is always changing due to new scientific and clinical innovations is part of what stimulates and drives people to choose health care work in the first place. What many young practitioners may underestimate or not really consider is the extent to which professional work is emotionally draining and exhausting, especially for those whose emotional intelligence is of the assimilator type. The constant interactions with others, the day-to-day realities of conflict and disagreement, and the high level of emotion that characterizes many conversations can be daunting. Having the intellectual capacity to become a health care professional is one thing; having the emotional stamina to sustain a career over 30 or 40 years is entirely different.

There is very little that can be done to truly prepare someone for the real-world emotional and interpersonal demands of professional practice. Because most people who choose health care as a career are smart, nice, and well-intentioned, it is sometimes simply assumed that such people will just handle it, as though somehow their inherent niceness and intelligence will help them to navigate interpersonally complex and emotionally intensive situations. Unfortunately, and increasingly, we are beginning to recognize the long-term negative impact of such situations on the morale of the workforce and the mental health of individual practitioners if individuals do not have the ability to actually communicate with colleagues when they need help to manage the difficult realities of their jobs.

10.1 The Health Care Workforce

Health care work can be the best of times and the worst of times. On the one hand, the opportunity to help other people during some of the most difficult times in their lives is extraordinarily personally rewarding. On the other hand, these difficult times can produce strong and negative emotional responses, and as a result, health care professionals can sometimes end up becoming embroiled in family arguments or being at the receiving end of someone simply venting or complaining. Although intellectually it may be easy to say to yourself, "I know the patient is not mad at me personally. The patient is mad at the situation they are in, and they just need someone to shout at right now," most of us cannot help but have some strong and negative personal emotional response when a patient is shouting at us even though we are doing the best we can.

Occupational surveys suggest the morale of the health care workforce is a problem. Across all health professions, there are concerns regarding the emotional state of health care workers themselves. What are some of the issues they face? On the one hand, opportunities for health care professionals have never been better. With new technologies, new scopes of practice, and greater opportunities for interprofessional collaboration, the positive impact health care professionals can have on patient care has never been greater.

Simultaneously, health care providers have never experienced more pressure. Caring for another person, at the very best of times, is difficult. It consumes both emotional and cognitive space, and can leave you with very little in reserve to take care of yourself and your own day-to-day responsibilities. Such caregiver exhaustion can be worsened by other factors. Patient expectations have never been higher, with more and more individuals viewing themselves as clients or customers. Historically, health care professionals enjoyed a high level of deference, and people listened to and respected what they said. Increasingly, some members of the public have grown suspicious of professional privilege and are more demanding than ever. Health care professionals may not be accustomed to being questioned or to the increasingly assertive (sometimes aggressive) style of communication they encounter. On a day-to-day basis this kind of communication starts to become grinding and wearisome; it starts to produce a negativity or dread of patient interaction, because few health care professionals particularly enjoy arguments or emotionally intense discussions. As patients, clients, customers, and consumers demand and expect more and more from us, our capacity (and frankly our desire) to deliver on these expectations may diminish. Accountability requirements have never been more strenuous, particularly for health care professionals who work in large organizations like hospitals. External scrutiny and auditing of clinical decisions is a constant feature of daily professional work, and such scrutiny may produce a kind of hypervigilance in decision making that is exhausting. Knowing that everything you say and do will be subject to review and criticism may help improve clinical performance, but it also produces a kind of emotional exhaustion over time. Further, the sense of professional autonomy and independence that used to characterize the work of practitioners has eroded considerably; in many cases, professionals today feel like they have jobs rather than vocations, which may in turn diminish pleasure and enthusiasm in the work itself. The technical and continuing learning demands of the professions have never been higher. In every profession, scientific advances that translate into clinical practice are occurring at a breathtaking pace. By one estimate, within the first 7 years of clinical practice, virtually everything that was learned in school will be obsolete. The notion that you go to school, you get a degree, and then you work is completely out of date; instead, there is an absolute requirement to constantly learn and update knowledge and skills continuously for fear of becoming obsolete. This takes time, intellectual energy, and dedication precisely at the same time as other life demands (such as relationships, children, parent care, and other personal commitments) are also increasing. Are there even enough hours in a day for a health care professional to do all of this? In addition, economic conditions for many health care professionals are less reliable than ever before. Traditionally, health care professionals were paid well, in recognition of the importance of the work they do, but also in order to ensure that, as they were performing this important and sensitive work, they were not simultaneously burdened worrying about day-to-day issues like paying for groceries or school fees. Today, health care professionals will frequently graduate from school with an enormous student debt load even before they've earned a single dollar of income. The cost of housing and living in many urban centers makes everyday expectations (such as home ownership, marriage and children, and summer vacations) seem out of reach or unrealistic. Although most health care professionals make good incomes, the reality of course is that it is possible to make the same or better money doing other jobs that are less stressful, less demanding, and simply easier. The intersection of these issues becomes fertile ground for the emergence of one of the most important, and corrosive, features of the health care system today: occupational stress.

10.2 Occupational Stress

Occupational stress develops when day-to-day pressures become a constant, unavoidable, and unmanageable part of the work environment. Where stress can sometimes be positive and productive, and cause us to surpass ourselves and find better and more creative solutions to problems, occupational stress is problematic because it is not a sometimes event but a chronic, consistent feature of the workforce. When we feel occupational stress is unavoidable and insurmountable, as many health care professionals feel today, it can trigger a cascade of emotional responses and symptoms ultimately leading to negative behavioral changes.

Classic emotional symptoms of occupational stress include irritability, anger, anxiety, and apathy. Most health care professionals are kind and caring people, that's why they selected this line of work in the first place. They are generally understanding and patient. The ability to be understanding and patient is very closely associated with one's emotional capacity to manage and process negative environmental cues. Over time, occupational stress grinds down one's capacity to do this, and as result, patience and kindness toward others may evaporate. When formerly caring and sympathetic individuals become abrupt and harsh, it may be a sign of irritability caused by occupational stress. Anger, as discussed in Chapter 5, is one of the six core emotions that characterize all human beings. Anger is an essential emotion because it allows us to convey enormous amounts of information in a highly condensed manner, thereby triggering others in our environment to respond. The ability to productively channel and communicate anger is, however, equally essential to our ability to get along with others and to work effectively in organization. When irritability tips into anger, it may be an indication that occupational stress has hijacked our normal control mechanisms that allow us to manage anger impulses and convey them in a more productive and socially appropriate manner. Anxiety is a natural outcome of uncontrolled occupational stress. Anxiety describes the experience associated with hypervigilance, catastrophizing, and ultimately, a lack of self-confidence that can produce negative behavioral changes. When anxious, individuals are excessively sensitive to environmental and nonverbal cues and triggers and expend enormous emotional and cognitive energy attempting to decipher and manage these cues. As a result there is diminished capacity to do anything else, such as being caring or sympathetic. Anxiety tends to rob individuals of their ability to be empathetic and altruistically concerned about others, and will often manifest as a desire to withdraw from social and interpersonal interactions. Apathy describes an emotional response to interpersonal situations characterized by numbness, lack of interest, and a general lack of concern or care. Apathetic individuals may intellectually understand a problem, but are incapable of finding an emotional connection or investment in the situation. Because emotional engagement is often the psychological fuel that allows us to demonstrate empathy or to care for others, apathy can be a catastrophic problem for health care professionals. When we approach our patient's health needs as logical problems to be solved rather than situations that require us to care for them as people, we are not able to truly fulfill our potential or to meet these patient's needs.

These emotional symptoms of occupational stress will often, in turn, lead to a variety of behavioral symptoms which can further worsen the initial emotional symptoms. Behavioral symptoms of occupational stress include sleeping problems, alternations in diet and appetite, diminished interest in our own lives, and avoidance of personal and present realities. Sleeping problems, one of the most common early warning indicators of occupational stress, include alterations in normal sleeping and sleep–wake patterns. As we know, healthy and restorative sleep is essential for both cognitive and emotional functioning. Missing a few nights of good sleep can cause immense problems in attitude and behavior, and if this persists for months or years, it can fundamentally change one's personality. Because health care must be provided 24 hours a day, some professionals must work midnight shifts or long hours. Beyond the already high occupational stress demands of such work, the structural requirement for night shifts can make health care professionals uniquely vulnerable to this behavioral change.

Alterations in diet and appetite can also be a result of occupational stress. It can begin simply enough. A long and busy shift as a health care professional might mean you do not eat a proper lunch, you skip a meal, or you grab a coffee and donut for breakfast just to save time. If this behavior only happened occasionally, it would not be a problem; unfortunately, workplace demands make such events commonplace, and finding time and space for a healthy diet can sometimes take a backseat to simply getting through a day in the clinic. On top of this issue, many of the emotional symptoms of occupational stress, such as anger, anxiety, and irritability, can frequently trigger their own kinds of eating-related problems. Many of us eat our emotions. When feeling emotionally depleted, vulnerable, or amplified, we may find comfort in unhealthy foods such as carbohydrates, ice cream, or chocolate. Over time, a negative pattern of eating associated with both workplace conditions and occupational stress can begin to feel normal and comforting, and in the longer run, this can deprive us of the necessary healthy nutrition we need in order to combat occupational stress in the first place. Alterations in diet may not happen suddenly or noticeably; instead, over a period of months or years, we may find ourselves slipping into unhealthy eating habits and then experience consequences in terms of unnecessary weight gain, bloating, constipation or diarrhea, lethargy, lack of energy, and sugar crashes.

Diminished interest in our own personal lives is also an important indicator of occupational stress. Many health care professionals will know that, after a busy and chaotic day at work, sometimes there is nothing left over to give to family, friends, and relationships. At times this may seem unavoidable; however, in some cases, this becomes a pattern that amplifies over months and years, adversely diminishing our personal relationships and distancing us from our loved ones. As we start to withdraw and avoid personal contact and intimacy, sexual problems or lack of sexual interest might become more prominent, and this again may serve to distance us even further from those we are supposed to be closest with. Sacrificing personal relationships for professional work is not sustainable. Ultimately, it will lead to larger problems for everyone. What many of these behavioral symptoms of occupational stress have in common is the notion of avoidance of personal and present realities. Avoidance behaviors—not attending family dinners, missing children's music recitals because of a work commitment, forgetting dear friends' birthdays because you are simply too busy, excessive screen time playing video games or online—all serve to further isolate us from our support networks and relationships precisely at the time when we actually need these relationships and support the most.

10.2.2 Communicating Your Needs in Times of Occupational Stress

Emotional and behavioral symptoms of occupational stress such as those described previously can sometimes serve as early warning indicators that corrective action is needed to prevent larger problems from occurring. Health professionals sometimes disregard these early warning indicators, believing it to be a sign of weakness or "something I can just deal with." This is fundamentally flawed thinking. Learning to recognize you are experiencing occupational stress begins by honest self-appraisal of your emotional and behavioral symptoms. If you see yourself reflected in these descriptions, do something about it.

What can be done? In some cases, you may still have sufficient residual energy and cognitive or emotional space to take action on your own. For example, take a vacation. Most health professionals work in environments where vacation time is part of the condition of employment, so use it. It is surprising that close to 60% of health professionals do not use their entire vacation allotment each year. They may claim, "I'm too busy" or "I'm too important, there's no one to cover for me." Although it can be difficult to plan a vacation, it can be done with advanced notice and thought. Taking a break from your job is essential to maintaining your emotional and cognitive balance.

Limit your work to work. With smart phones and ubiquitous Internet access, many health care professionals find they can seamlessly shift from work to home and continue to stay connected to the clinic or office. At times, this flexibility may be great if it allows you to control the location of your work. However, in many cases, we can overdo and allow work to invade personal time to the point where we are never disconnected. Learning to turn off your phone or choosing not to check your email before sleep and first thing on awakening can be challenging, but it is absolutely necessary to manage occupational stress and provide you with the cognitive and emotional space necessary to rebalance.

Learn to say no. Most health professionals, particularly younger ones, are eager, helpful, and want to do the best job possible. In some cases, this can lead to a tendency to always agree to take on more and more work, regardless of the personal consequences. Hoarding of opportunities creates occupational stress and personal problems, but it is also sometimes fundamentally unfair to others in your workplace who may also want to do interesting things. Honest self-appraisal of your capacity and learning to simply but firmly say, "Thanks for thinking of me for this, but I think I'm at my limit right now. I'm going to have to say no" takes practice but is essential to prevent occupational stress from becoming burdensome.

Let someone know you are experiencing signs and symptoms of occupational stress. This can be one of the most humbling and difficult things to do, because for many health care professionals, it can feel like failure to admit that, in fact, you need help. It is not failure, and it is absolutely essential if you are going to continue to be able to work in this field. Reaching out to a friend, a family member, a boss, or a colleague and sharing your experiences—the emotional and behavioral symptoms you are experiencing—requires courage. You may fear that by admitting you need help now you may never, ever get a promotion or be thought of in the same way as in the past. Despite what you may think, such catastrophic predictions rarely are the case. Virtually everyone in health care recognizes and understands the importance of early management of occupational stress, and you may simply be telling yourself a story about how others will respond. Simply saying, "I think I need some help to manage something right now" is perhaps the hardest but most important words you can say to prevent small problems from escalating and getting beyond your control. Remember that one of the classic emotional symptoms of occupational stress is anxiety. Your sense of dread or fear of repercussions for asking for help may in fact be anxiety rather than the truth of a situation. If you are working in a large organization such as a hospital or clinic, you may have access to an important resource, an EAP, or employee assistance program. EAPs are widely available but regrettably underutilized resources for health care professionals. They provide confidential referral to a trained therapist, social worker, or psychologist and allow you to begin to have important conversations with trained professionals who can help you to strategize, prioritize, and rehearse what you are going to say to whom and what remedies you are going to seek. The EAP service does not solve the problem of occupational stress; instead, it can give you some breathing room to begin to figure out how you are going to manage occupational stress rather than allow it to control you. EAPs are anonymous services; you will not be reported to your boss or colleagues. In some cases, EAP consultations can be arranged by telephone rather than in person if that is your preference. Even if your employer does not offer an EAP service, many licensing bodies and professional associations do, and this can be accessed by any licensed or regulated member of that profession. Learning about what EAP services you have access to before you actually need to use them can be helpful. Simply by virtue of the fact that you are employed or are a member of a union, a professional association, or a profession, you will likely somewhere have access to the EAP service. If you need it, use it.

We ignore the signs and symptoms of occupational stress at our own peril. Failure to recognize (or simply ignoring) and not proactively managing occupational stress is problematic because, ultimately, without intervention, it can lead to burnout.

10.3 **Burnout**

Burnout is a form of extreme professional exhaustion, sometimes referred to as occupational stress on steroids. It is a condition in which professional and personal demands chronically outpace a person's ability to manage, complete, and control them. Worse, burnout is not contained to the workplace; it spreads like a disease into one's personal and daily life, diminishing capacity for self-regulation of emotions. Over time, it literally can rewire our cognitive and perceptual systems, and become a vicious cycle, ultimately leading to full blown psychiatric illness including depression. Burnout is unfortunately all too common in the health care professions.

Many of the emotional and behavioral symptoms of burnout are similar to those of occupational stress; the difference is in the magnitude of these symptoms, their unrelenting quality, and the seemingly endless suffering it causes. Many psychologists believe the true tipping point between occupational stress and burnout occurs when individuals begin to feel diminished self-worth and a sense that they are useless. At this point, the crisis that is burnout is potentially in full control. Beyond "just" anxiety, burnout produces feelings of pessimism, activates behaviors related to social isolation and detachment (including lying to family members), and a corrosive sense that there is simply no hope.

Importantly, burnout is NOT something that you as an individual can actually manage on your own. It cannot be dealt with in isolation, any more than one can perform self-surgery on a knee joint. Although occupational stress may still present opportunities to reach out and ask for help, those in burnout may simply be incapable of even asking for help. Burnout itself fundamentally distorts the cognitive and emotional lenses through which we interpret the world and makes it very difficult to actually see reality as it truly exists.

Anyone who has spent any time in a health care setting will, no doubt, have seen colleagues in burnout. Burnout can lead to significant and sometimes life-threatening errors in judgment and behavior that fundamentally compromise patient care. Burnout can poison a team atmosphere and act as an infectious disease, causing others in a team to experience similar negativity. As a result, although the focus in occupational stress may be to learn how to ask for help from others, in burnout it is sometimes necessary for these others to let you know that you actually need help now, before something terrible happens to you, your patients, or to the team.

Burnout is everyone's problem and everyone's responsibility. If you fear a colleague or a friend is experiencing more than occupational stress, ask them about it. A simple open-ended question like, "How are you doing?" might be a start. If you get a diversionary response such as, "Fine, fine, everything's good," and you still worry or suspect there is a problem, consider a redirecting statement, one that honestly displays both your concern and your willingness to listen and help: "I need to let you know that I'm concerned for you. You're not behaving like your normal self and I hope you know that I'm here if you ever want to talk."

Effective management of burnout requires coordinated support, and honest disclosure, from colleagues, family, friends, and employers. It will frequently require additional support from other trained health care professionals, particularly mental health professionals. Those at highest risk of burnout in the health care system tend to be female (particularly with family care responsibilities), those with an administrative role in addition to clinical responsibilities, and those in the first 15 years of professional practice. It is essential for these people to realize they are not alone. It is, therefore, imperative that every health care professional knows how to recognize signs and symptoms of occupational stress and burnout, and acquires communication skills necessary to provide empathetic support to those who need your help.

10.4   Resilience, Grit, and Perseverance

How can we manage occupational stress more effectively? How can burnout be prevented? Beyond the clinical knowledge and technical skills you will acquire during your educational program, there are additional competencies that are essential for every health care professional: resilience, grit, and perseverance.

10.4.1   Perseverance

Perseverance is defined as the ability to maintain attention, focus, and commitment in the face of environmental challenges or obstacles. It is a type of steadfastness that allows us to overcome impediments to our goals, objectives, and dreams.

Most health care professionals have learned perseverance simply by completing academic and licensing requirements required to practice their profession. In most cases, perseverance means taking small steps in order to make small achievements. By subdividing a seemingly huge and impossible objective (e.g., become a health care professional) into smaller, manageable steps (e.g., apply for my program, get good enough grades to get into my program, show up to class, pass first year exams), we ultimately achieve the larger objective. Human cognitive and emotional capacity is limited and can easily become overwhelmed in the face of an unrealistically daunting goal. Those who have learned perseverance have generally mastered the art of subdividing into manageable steps. Start with the easy things first, master those, then move forward to the more complicated things with the wind at your back.

10.4.2 Grit

Grit is sometimes described as a kind of self-control, and although this is certainly part of what makes grit an important competency for health care professionals, it is more than simply that. Grit is related to the ability to defer immediate gratification and maintain a sense of hope and optimism that the future will be better. Although perseverance is about actions (subdividing complex tasks into smaller manageable steps), grit is essentially a psychological characteristic that allows us to believe and understand that today's sacrifices will be more than rewarded by tomorrow's rewards. Those demonstrating grit learn to accentuate the positive without completely ignoring the negative. Instead, they learn that there may be only 10% of factors that they can control. No matter the number, 10% is still a large enough number to matter, so focus energy, enthusiasm, and attention on what can be controlled first. Once that is controlled, some of the remaining 90% will suddenly become available for control, and in this way success and accomplishments are built incrementally. Those without grit would simply focus on the 90% that is beyond control in the first place and give up hope immediately. Grit is sometimes referred to as a growth mindset and is very closely connected to the psychology of positive thinking. If we believe failure is inevitable, it will be. If, instead, through our grit we move beyond simply talking about success or failure but now focus on one small step, or this next job, we incrementally and gradually conquer challenges, build confidence, enhance self-esteem, and in the process, generate positive energy that can allow us to continue to grow and advance.

10.4.3 Resilience

Resilience is defined as the ability to bounce back after adversity or disappointment, or the ability to manage and adapt when things do not go as expected. Interestingly, many health care professionals may have little experience with resilience in their academic lives. In some cases, health care profession students have had relatively untroubled academic trajectories, getting the marks they needed to get into the program they wanted. Never having experienced academic adversity or disappointment may mean that some practitioners have simply never had their resilience truly tested.

No matter how successful an individual is—academically, professionally, or personally—all human beings will at some point experience adversity and disappointment. Within a health care profession, this disappointment is sometimes completely beyond your control. Despite every possible and heroic intervention, sometimes a patient will die. Despite all the time and effort you take to educate and support a patient, sometimes they will not listen to you. Despite all your best intentions and efforts, sometimes you will make a mistake. In such situations, demonstrating resilience is essential.

Resilience is possible if we have the capacity to think realistically and act in accordance with realistic plans. When we engage in magical or fantastical thinking disconnected from reality and probability, we are not being resilient. Resilience is enhanced when we can manage our immediate emotional response to a situation (e.g., sadness, anger, fear) and instead cognitively examine it and attempt to subdivide a realistic plan into specific, concrete, and actionable steps. It is crucial that we maintain a positive self-impression and positive self-image; if we succumb to negative thoughts or beliefs about ourselves and our characters and blame ourselves emotionally, resilience may not be possible. A positive self-image, however, does not mean that we excuse our own deficiencies or errors. We need to be honest and realistic in appraising both our strengths and our weakness in order to move forward. Resiliency is all about moving forward in a way that allows us to accept what has happened in the past but not become emotionally overwhelmed by it.

10.4.4   Learning Perseverance, Grit, and Resilience

Although the definitions of each term are somewhat different, the connections between these concepts should hopefully be clear. One commonality shared across all three concepts is the central importance of networks and relationships: Without social and human interactions, perseverance, grit, and resilience become difficult to manage.

Although there is no step-by-step guide to learning perseverance, grit, and resilience, there are several important characteristics of each that are important to consider.

Other people are crucial. Social networks appear to provide the psychological fuel necessary to sustain our interest and our energy in managing adverse and difficult circumstances. These social networks are most typically characterized as warm, filled with humor, familiarity, inside jokes, and mutual care and concern. When what we do matters to other people, and when other people matter to us, the reciprocal social energy that is produced is essential to sustaining perseverance, grit, and resilience. Sustaining and nurturing your personal and professional relationships with others is not simply a feel-good exercise. It is absolutely essential for your success as a professional.

Managing emotional responses. Recall from Chapter 5 the unique human hard-wiring that means we are built to feel before we think. The fact that our emotional selves are engaged before our logical selves sometimes can mean that strong emotions (such as fear, sadness, or anger) can easily overwhelm us. This is not only natural, it is our default hardwiring. This is, however, something we can learn to manage and control. Each person will learn their own best method for doing so. For some, it will mean taking a deep breath before talking. For others, it will mean repeating back a question or statement to someone before responding. For others, it will mean taking a sip of water or writing down a few notes to buy the time necessary to allow our cognitive, logical selves to engage and manage our initial emotional response. Whatever technique works for you, learn it and use it.

Be grounded in reality. One of the most difficult aspects of managing occupational stress and burnout can be the ways and extent to which they can distort our perception of reality. Catastrophizing refers to the tendency of amplifying negative outcomes or consequences beyond what is real and probable. In part this relates to being able to manage emotional responses, but is also related to the ability to honestly self-assess one's strengths and weaknesses as well as environmental opportunities and threats. Although it is tempting to frame our thinking around re-mote possibilities, learning instead to focus on realistic probabilities is essential. Of course, virtually anything is possible (theoretically), but estimating the likelihood or mathematical probability of a specific outcome can be a better way of guiding behavior and helping support resilience, grit, and perseverance.

Stay positive. As noted, grit is the ability to maintain a growth mindset and positive outlook, and it is an essential attribute in effectively managing adversity. At first glance, it may be tempting to cynically note, "How can I be positive AND grounded in reality, don't you see what's going on?" This time of ironic attachment may be mildly amusing, but it is ultimately unhelpful. Remember that positivity is not about mind-less enthusiasm or ignoring realities around you; instead, it is identifying the 10% that you have some control over, successfully managing that 10% and taking plea-sure and building self-worth through this accomplishment as a springboard to the next 10%. Mindless positivity is neither necessary nor actually helpful, particularly if it somehow blinds you to reality. Instead, the positivity that comes from successful completion of small steps on the way to a larger objective is both sustainable and necessary to build resilience.

Take care of yourself. Occupational stress and burnout are corrosive, and begin to affect us not only psychologically but physiologically. Learning to detect early warning signals, such as sleep disturbances, lack of interest in relationships, or alterations in diet, is essential. Equally essential is doing something about it once the early warning signal is detected. Making a conscious effort to eat better, sleep longer, and truly engage with others in social interactions may be exhausting in their own ways, but are necessary to prevent these small problems from becoming larger ones. Successfully managing one's own sleeping, eating, and pleasure also builds a sense of mastery and self-confidence that can contribute to positivity.

It goes without saying that taking care of oneself also means being cautious and prudent with respect to use of alcohol, cannabis, vaping, and other licit or illicit substances, and with overreliance on social media or screen time as a distraction. It is all too easy to succumb to the temptation of self-medicating with these sorts of substances when one is emotionally vulnerable. Every health professional already knows the dangers associated with reliance on substances as a coping mechanism for psychological or occupational stress; it will not work and is not sustainable. The short-term buzz, escape, or relief that may be achieved is illusory, and relatively quickly, things can spiral out of control. Taking care of yourself may, in some cases, mean being extra vigilant in these areas. In some cases, other kinds of substances—for example, gambling, unsafe and risky sexual behaviors, or simply driving too fast—may also be relied on to provide short-term psychological relief. In all these cases, recognizing that emotional needs and short-term relief may actually be harmful to long-term goals and objectives is important.

Ask for help, and offer your help to others. Possibly the most important element of perseverance, grit, and resilience is the ability to communicate effectively within our social and professional networks, and to find the vocabulary we need to ask for help when we need it. In many ways, this is less of a communication challenge and more of a psychological barrier to overcome. We all know the words "I need help," but there are so many intermediate psychological decisions that can interfere with us being able to say this aloud in the right place and the right time. In part, we can help ourselves by maintaining and nurturing a broad array of personal and professional relationships with others. When we feel like we are part of a connected network, it is simply easier for us to find the courage to say these words out loud. In some cases, this might not be possible, or it is too late; due to occupational stress or other factors, we may have allowed our networks to fray or disappear. In such cases, remember there are ALWAYS other resources available, including your personal physician and health care professional, your EAP, and even anonymous phone-in lines in virtually every community. Although these may not be as helpful or effective as a close friend or relationship, it will still be helpful and is an important first step. Do not succumb to the catastrophizing thinking that you are all alone. You are not alone, no matter how negatively you happen to feel at any given time.

Equally challenging can be offering your help to a colleague (or friend) who needs it. Sometimes we may feel shy or awkward doing so, fearing we are invading their privacy or making assumptions. This is rarely the case; instead, an honest attempt at clear communication coupled with transmission of empathetic nonverbal cues will send a strong message to the other person that you are there and you want to help, if not right now, then when that person is ready to accept your offer.

10.5 Connecting to Others

Throughout this chapter, a common theme has emerged: the protective and therapeutic benefits associated with social connection with other people. We know that in today's world, loneliness is of epidemic proportions. Loneliness is sometimes likened to an epidemiologic risk factor in terms of physical and mental health; like smoking or obesity, loneliness has real health consequences and mortality and morbidity associated with it. Social connection and communication serve as inoculations to loneliness and are as important for your success as a health care professional as any clinical skill you have acquired in your education.

You may feel you are an introvert and therefore do not require such connections. This is simply not the case. Creating social networks takes energy and commitment—it takes perseverance—but is absolutely essential to support your professional life as a practitioner. Sustaining these networks and relationships requires grit. The reward in all of this is an infrastructure that will support your resilience in challenging circumstances. Sociologists tell us that middle-aged men may have the most difficult time finding connections, creating these relationships, and consequently building this infrastructure for resilience. Other groups that may have challenges include those who have historically or traditionally experienced discrimination or marginalization (e.g., racialized minorities, LGBTQ+ people, those with physical disabilities). Those with family care responsibilities (particularly, young mothers) may have additional logistical issues to contend with that make it difficult to nurture and sustain personal networks.

Across all these different groups, an important common thread is effective and honest communication. Although everyone experiences time pressures associated with day-to-day life as a busy practitioner, communication is the way we keep our social relationships alive and vigorous. It need not be an hour-long conversation each day, but focused attempts to maintain connection and to honestly share and authentically engage with friends, family, and colleagues are essential for all human beings.

10.6 Summary

At some point, every health professional—and human being—will likely experience the crushing symptoms associated with occupational stress. It is essential to not ignore the early warning symptoms and instead develop proactive communication strategies to learn how to ask for help from others before it becomes a crisis or turns into burnout. Developing the attributes of perseverance, grit, and resilience can play an important role in supporting your professional development and helping you to more effectively manage the risks associated with occupational stress. To do so will require careful attention to both your personal and professional relationships and conscious effort to sustain and nurture these relationships to provide you with the shock absorbers necessary to help better manage occupational stress. Although communication is an essential aspect of nurturing these relationships, there may be psychological and emotional barriers that interfere with your intentions and desires to maintain friendships and family connections. Learning to identify your own risk factors, and your own preferred techniques and communication strategies to manage these, is as important a clinical skill as any other learned in your profession.

For Further Reading:

Bridgeman P, Bridgeman M, Barone J. Burnout syndrome among healthcare professionals. *Am J Health Syst Pharm.* 2018;75(3):147–152.

Brindley P, Olusanya S, Wong A, Crowe L, Hawryluk L. Psychological 'burnout' in healthcare professionals: updating our understanding and not making it worse. *J Intensive Care Soc.* 2019;20(4):358–362.

Dyrbye L, Shanafelt T, Sinsky C, et al. Burnout among healthcare professionals: a call to explore and address this underrecognized threat to safe, high-quality care. *National Academy of Medicine Perspectives.* Washington, DC: Discussion Paper, National Academy of Medicine; 2017. Available at: https://www.ama-assn.org/sites/ama-assn.org/files/corp/media-browser/public/ipp/i17-ipps-lotte-dyrbye-burnout-among-health-care-professionals.pdf.

Nordang K, Hall-Lord ML, Farup P. Burnout in health-care professionals during reorganizations and downsizing. A cohort study in nurses. *BMC Nurs.* 2010;9:8.

Ray S, Wong CD, White D, Heaslip K. Compassion satisfaction, compassion fatigue, work life conditions, and burnout among frontline mental health care professionals. *Traumatol.* 2013;19(4):255–267.

Reith T. Burnout in United States healthcare professionals: a narrative review. *Cureus.* 2018;10(12):e3681.

Robertson H, Elliott A, Burton C, et al. Resilience of primary healthcare professionals: a systematic review. *Br J Gen Pract.* 2016;66(647):423–433.

11 Communication in Leadership, Management, and Administration

Sam is an award-winning clinician in your practice in a small town with a great reputation among colleagues and your patients. Recently, Sam wrote an article in the local town newspaper complaining about same-sex marriage, claiming homosexuality was "an illness," that it was "ruining society," and that Sam sympathized with those who "felt the need to get violent about the current situation." No patients have complained about this article, and you have personally overheard some of them congratulating Sam on this article. You have not observed any patient-specific or patient-related performance issues with Sam in the clinic, although some of your colleagues have expressed disgust and anger to you (but not Sam) about this article.

Life in organizations, including health care teams, can be fraught with difficult and challenging interpersonal situations. Even when smart, well-intentioned, and generally nice people (clinicians) work with one another, there will be disagreements and issues that need to be sorted out. The scenario presented represents one such situation. This case will provoke a wide array of different responses from different readers based on their own beliefs, values, and expectations for what it means to be a professional and a health care provider. Some readers may view this as nothing more than the legitimate expression of free speech; although such readers may not necessarily agree with Sam's point of view, they do not view it as problematic because Sam has a right to his opinions. Other readers will view this as seriously problematic. Sam is making outright false claims (no reputable health care professional or organization today considers homosexuality an illness) and is inciting others to commit acts of violence. Most readers may wonder at how professional it is to make such claims in a public forum such as a small-town newspaper, and virtually all readers will concede that simply because no one has complained about Sam (and even though some patients have actually congratulated him), this popularity does not mean Sam is right.

In such situations, there is often a temptation to ask, "Who's in charge around here anyway?" The belief that there is a leader, a manager, or an administrator who is supervising or in charge of someone like Sam, and who consequently has both the responsibility and the ability to discipline if that is necessary, may mean everyone else in the practice simply shrugs shoulders and says "not my job." Complex situations like this require significant and nuanced communication skills, not simply from those who have a title or job description related to leadership, but from every-one in the practice who is interested in ensuring the workplace maintains a positive and diversity-embracing role in the community.

11.1   "Who's in Charge?" and "It's Not My Job!"

Health care workplaces are unique insofar as the health care workforce is composed of professionals with a high degree of education, a high level of skill, significant re-sponsibility, and a great deal of autonomy. Health care work deals with some of the most important and personal and intimate parts of a human being's life; it is not the same as working in a factory or any other office setting. Health care professionals must exercise both clinical skill and compassionate wisdom and judgment in their day-to-day work with patients, including the central importance of maintaining con-fidentiality and privacy for patients. As a result, traditional top-down management structures in which a boss tells a worker what to do and the worker does it is not well suited for health care settings. Health care professionals must be independent critical thinkers who can question authority and the traditional chain of command to ensure errors are not made. If every health professional simply did as they were told, the system would be much less safe and much less humane. This is not to say health care settings are leaderless or filled with autonomous professionals who do as they see fit, it simply means that leadership, management, and administration in health care settings are experienced quite differently than in other organizations without the same sensitivities associated with patient care.

As a result, it is important to carefully distinguish what kinds of different roles and responsibilities exist within a health care team or organization, and in particular, differentiate between terms that are sometimes used interchangeably, such as man-agers, administrators, and leaders.

Managers typically have formal responsibilities and specific tools available to them to help direct or control some of the day-to-day activities of people in an orga-nization, including clinicians, technicians, and support staff. In health care settings, managers are most frequently clinicians themselves, and have been frontline patient care providers before they assume a management role. In many health care set-tings, managers must work within unionized settings, in which workers (e.g., nurses) have self-organized and work collectively to advance their own interests and agenda. These interests and agendas are usually focused on ensuring the highest possible care for patients while maintaining the best possible working conditions for staff. Managers usually have specific roles and responsibilities that will be carefully ne-gotiated and agreed upon by unions and/or other clinicians (e.g., scheduling, hiring, promotions, annual performance reviews, vacation planning). Importantly, manag-ers tend to focus their attention on people-related issues and problems, and work within a system of policies and procedures to ensure fairness, transparency, and accountability. This emphasis on people-related issues means managers need to have a well-developed set of communication tools. They rarely can simply tell people to do things or punish them if they do not comply. Instead, in a health care context, management requires the ability to communicate, motivate, explain, and support others in doing difficult tasks in complex environments.

Administrators most frequently have responsibility for a diverse portfolio of non–people-related issues, including budgets, physical space, equipment, and materials, all of which are essential to allow the people in the organization to do their job safely, efficiently, and effectively. Administrators frequently focus on the quantitative (i.e., numbers-intensive) aspect of an organization (e.g., how many dollars do we have to spend on a particular intervention, how much space will we need if we try to hire new staff, are we in compliance with federal requirements with respect to narcotics audits). It is easy to dismiss administrators as bean counters who are more interested in the bottom line than in patients, staff, or other human concerns. Of course, this is simply wrong. Without the care and oversight provided by well-qualified administrators, no health care organization can be sustainable. Although administrators may sometimes be seen as people behind the scenes, they still have important responsibilities for day-to-day activities, and must have strong communication skills in order to implement their work and make difficult decisions. Similar to managers, administrators rarely have the ability to force their views or opinions on others; instead, they must use effective communication strategies to help others understand important details regarding budgets, space, and logistical constraints that means difficult choices must be made.

Leaders are crucial to the success of every organization, particularly in health care. Although managers and administrators will often have a formal title and role in an organization, leadership may not be this clear-cut. In some cases, leaders will have a formal title, but in many cases they will not. Some people argue that every health care professional needs to think, behave, and communicate like a leader because every health care professional needs to be a leader for a practice to work effectively. Unlike managers and administrators, the role of a leader is not necessarily clear or defined. It sometimes is described as the ability to drag others kicking and screaming into a future they don't necessarily embrace but ultimately will recognize is for the best. From this perspective, leadership is not necessarily about day-to-day details but instead about big-picture thinking regarding a collective future that is better than the present. It requires vision, commitment, and the ability to recognize that we must always be improving and advancing or else we will fall behind. The communication requirements for leaders are significant, especially in health care. They cannot bully or shout their way to success, but must inspire, persuade, and stimulate others to buy into a vision of the future and the hard work necessary to get there. Every health care professional has this responsibility and opportunity, because every health care professional should be invested in making their practice better than it is today. Whether you have an official title or job description or not, you will be a leader and need to think and act as a leader within your practice and your profession. This means learning to communicate effectively as a leader.

Beyond these roles of manager, administrator, and leader, in some cases there may be an *executive*, a person or a group of people with ultimate responsibility and accountability for the activities of everyone within an organization. These individuals are rarely involved in day-to-day operational decisions, and instead provide general oversight to an organization. Their most important role, it can be argued, is to ensure selecting and nurturing the best managers, administrators, and named leaders within the organization, and the cultivation and support of unnamed leaders who will ultimately lead change and progress.

11.2   Roles, Responsibilities, and Sometimes Confusion Too

Health care organizations and teams are complex, and as a result, there may be confusion or ambiguity about who does what and who is in charge, particularly when difficult or sensitive cases arise. The clear distinction described in Section 11.1 between managers and administrators may not always be so clear-cut in real life. Often, especially in small organizations or teams, one individual will be both a manager of people and an administrator of resources. One disadvantage to this approach can be that the skills required of a manager may not necessarily be the same as those required of an administrator; conversely, sometimes administrative responsibilities and goals can be at odds with managerial responsibilities and goals. This can produce a difficult burden for the one individual who must reconcile them and find a way to act.

As noted, not all leaders have formal titles or job descriptions. This too can lead to confusion because those with formal titles may sometimes overlook the potential contributions of those without. Conversely, those without titles may sometimes forget that they have leadership responsibilities too. Importantly, in some cases, leaders without titles can be more impactful and carry greater weight than those with formal job descriptions. Leaders without titles sometimes speak from a position of greater objectivity or moral authority and can be more effective at persuading peers than someone who is viewed generally as the boss. Leaders without titles can sometimes be closer to a problem and closer to the people involved, and so may actually have deeper insights than those who are in a different location in an organizational chart. A central challenge in most organizations is finding a way to recognize and nurture leaders without titles without devaluing or diminishing leaders with titles.

Part of the confusion in many organizations arises because, at times, the goals of managers, administrators, leaders, and executives can actually be in conflict with one another. Consider the case described at the beginning of this chapter. Who is responsible for Sam's behavior? A manager might note that what Sam does on his own time and out of the clinic is no one else's business. If Sam walked around with signs in the practice or said overtly hateful things directly to patients, then the manager must intervene, but an article in a town's paper is outside the scope of the workplace and consequently is not about management. An administrator may say Sam's behavior is a human resources problem, and nothing to do with finances, operations, physical facilities, equipment, or budgets, and consequently, not the administrator's responsibility.

Most health care professionals (but not all) will consider the case of Sam and experience some (or great) discomfort at this colleague's behavior and choice of words. Few, however, are likely to challenge Sam directly because they may feel uncomfortable provoking conflict, feel "it's not my job," or believe "well, you can't change what people believe, so why bother opening that can of worms?" To a certain extent, both the manager and administrator are correct. Dealing with Sam's behavior is not their job. But if Sam's behavior is not addressed and explicitly called out, there may be people in the community who read what he has written as a respected health care professional and actually believe homosexuality is an illness because, well, Sam said it is. They may be motivated by Sam's sympathy toward "those who get violent" and think it is socially acceptable to verbally or physically attack other people. Or perhaps some members of the community will simply not seek out health care, believing other professionals think like Sam. If everyone believes "it's not my job," what are the consequences for the community?

11.3 Your Role as a Leader

Every health care professional must think, behave, and communicate as a leader because every health care professional is a leader. As well-educated and respected professionals, you have a standing in the broader community and a unique set of privileges and responsibilities that must be upheld. Although you may not be Sam's boss, you are his colleague and his peer, and the need for peers to lead in a situation like this is critical. Leaving Sam's comments unchallenged will imply to the general community that other health care professionals agree. Indeed, Sam may actually believe everyone else agrees with him because, well, no one has said anything negative and patients have actually been congratulatory!

Remember the central role of leadership is to drag organizations (or people) kicking and screaming into the future, and it appears as though Sam actually requires some dragging into the present day reality. Failure of other professionals around Sam to take a leadership role in this issue could be seen as both unethical and ultimately damaging to the overall public reputation of professions in general.

At this point some readers may wonder, "But what about free speech?" or "But he was acting in his capacity as a private citizen, not as a health care professional!" These are of course important and reasonable points; however, these must be balanced against the reality of the potential and actual harm Sam's words may cause for some individuals and the medical inaccuracies of some of his statements. If Sam is known in the community as a health care professional, when he says "homosexuality is an illness," it does not matter if he feels he is speaking as a private citizen or not. His words will be interpreted by others as having the weight and significance of medical accuracy. As a result, others in his professional community have a responsibility and an opportunity to lead and address this issue directly.

11.3.1 What Does It Take to Lead?

As can be seen in this discussion, effective leadership sometimes requires moral and ethical clarity. It is all well and good to debate philosophical issues related to free speech and citizen versus professional rights, but at the end of the day effective leadership means being able to take a clear and unambiguous stand on an issue that is informed by professional ethics and personal morals and is not influenced by fear of conflict or a desire to simply avoid responsibility. Leaders need to actually know and believe what they think and feel about an issue before they can find a way to communicate it to others.

11.3.1.1   Understanding What You Think and Feel When You Are a Leader

Effective leadership requires tremendous self-insight and self-awareness. Leadership is as much a psychological state as it is a series of behaviors. In reflecting on a challenging case such as this in order to acquire self-insight and self-awareness, there are several important concepts to consider.

Dissonance: Cognitive and emotional dissonance are important issues to manage for any difficult situation, and for leadership in general. Dissonance refers to a psychological state of discomfort that is produced when contradictory ideas collide, producing both confusion and uneasiness. For example, you may have a long relationship with Sam and have always seen him as a nice and thoughtful person, and suddenly this article he has written has exposed a different, unpleasant side you never knew existed. This can produce dissonance. You may be inclined to think, "Well, it's not that serious because, after all, Sam's a great guy normally, right?" It may produce another form of dissonance in which you find it challenging to recognize what you KNOW you should do (i.e., address the issue with Sam) versus what you FEEL might happen (i.e., what if Sam gets mad at me and doesn't want to work with me anymore?). Dissonance is an important psychological issue for leaders to manage internally. If you do not resolve whatever dissonance you are experiencing, it will be impossible for you to be authentic and effective in the leadership role because you will be constantly conflicted about what is the right thing to do.

Load: Another important issue for leadership is the concept of cognitive and emotional load. Load presumes there is a finite and fixed capacity for human beings to effectively process cognitive and emotional tasks. When we exceed this capacity we become overloaded, which compromises our ability to think effectively and to respond appropriately to different situations. Load theory suggests that leaders need to be attuned to their ability to focus and concentrate on important issues rather than to become overwhelmed by administrative or managerial details. Keeping the big picture perspective, rather than getting lost in the weeds or details, is essential to preserving cognitive and emotional capacity to be a leader. In a difficult situation such as this case with Sam, it will require significant cognitive and emotional resources to be able to act as a leader and do what is right. In some cases, an individual may simply lack the capacity to do this right now; for example, you may be experiencing significant personal challenges due to an illness of a loved one or other personal problems and do not have the ability to focus and concentrate on this problem adequately. At times, of course, people may use load as an excuse to avoid difficult conversations or leadership responsibilities. Although the issue of load is real and important to consider and manage, its use as a tool for avoidance is also real and must be managed honestly.

Risk balancing: The concepts of load and dissonance speak to the complex psychology of leadership, and in particular, the issue of balancing emotional and cognitive needs and risks. Risk balancing represents a cognitive process, informed by controlled emotional responses, in which risks and benefits associated with different options and interventions are assessed and compared against one another. Leaders must consider both cognitive and emotional factors while risk balancing; for example, the emotional cost of losing Sam's collegiality versus knowing the harm that may be inflicted on others by not challenging his behavior. Risk balancing requires cognitive and emotional capacity as well as the ability to manage dissonance. It is sometimes described as the process of actually making a decision as to what to do in a complex case by looking at all sides carefully.

Looking for least worst alternatives rather than perfect answers: One of the most challenging aspects of leadership is the reality that, in many cases, there is no perfect answer but only a series of imperfect options that must be selected from. For example, in this case, there is no perfect response to Sam; this is a messy problem that you likely wished never occurred and for which there is no easy answer. In risk balancing, we seek to find the least worst alternative, in other words, the best approach among a series of less-than-desirable options. This can trigger its own kind of dissonance. Recall that leaders need to know what they believe and feel the strength of their convictions. It is difficult to feel positive toward a least worst alternative. At best we can feel reconciled or resigned to it, but to actually feel any conviction to a least worst alternative can be difficult. Yet, without conviction and positivity, it is difficult for leaders to communicate effectively and clearly. Managing this reality and this dissonance is essential. It usually requires us to abandon the naïve notion of perfect answers to complex problems and instead recognize that, no matter how imperfect, a least worst alternative is still better and will produce a better outcome than doing nothing at all.

Being aware of and learning to manage the psychological dimensions of leadership are essential in helping you to do the difficult work of communicating effectively in challenging situations such as this. If you are internally conflicted, unconvinced, or simply resentful that you've been put into this situation, this emotional subtext will seep into conversations and become confusing nonverbal cues to others that will undermine your message, sabotage your communication, and ultimately lead to more confusion. Failure to manage issues of dissonance, load, and risk balancing prior to communicating will most likely result in failed communication and this risks actually amplifying, rather than dealing with, a problem.

11.4 Your Emotional Intelligence and Your Leadership

In Chapter 2, we discussed the concept of emotional intelligence and its important role in shaping our thinking and behavior. Arguably, self-awareness regarding personal emotional intelligence is one of the most important psychological underpinnings of successful leadership. The real and important differences between emotional intelligences means that each of us needs to have an accurate and grounded sense of ourselves prior to attempting to lead or communicate with others. It also provides us an opportunity to consider the complex intersections that exist when individuals with different emotional intelligences sometimes collide.

Ongoing reflection regarding personal emotional intelligence can—for some emotional intelligence styles, such as divergers and assimilators—be helpful in managing issues of load, dissonance, and risk balancing. For others, such as accommodators, such reflection will be neither natural nor easy, and as a result, they may require a trial-and-error approach to trying different least worst alternatives. Convergers, with their general high level of confidence, may be at risk of overestimating the influence they have on others, and may be at some risk of being subverted by assimilators in particular. It is simply impossible to list every possible combination and permutation of emotional intelligences and provide a neat answer as to how to manage these intersectional difficulties. As a result, it is most important that each of us is able to understand ourselves, our emotional responses to challenging situations such as this, and have an accurate self-appraisal of what strengths we have in managing or leading change in such circumstances, based on emotional intelligence theory.

For divergers, with their high need for interpersonal harmony, it may be personally difficult to deal with high stress and potentially confrontational situations. They may find themselves relying more on charm and humor rather than forcefulness to try to exert managerial control or leadership. At their best, divergers can demonstrate a great deal of empathy, which can help them navigate difficult situations. For example, in this case, a strong diverger may be able to temporarily suspend his or her own sense of outrage toward Sam's statements and words, and instead approach Sam collegially, asking him to reflect on the article and its impact and using effective listening and empathy try to get him to see alternative perspectives. A strong diverger may not want to actually call out Sam on unprofessional behavior for fear of poisoning any future relationship or to simply avoid a potential conflict, but instead may rely on the strength of their relationship to provide a gentle nudge, rather than a forceful push, toward a constructive solution. At their worst, divergers' fear of conflict may lead them to become paralyzed in such a situation and unable to actually manage or demonstrate leadership effectively. However, if the diverger is able to harness her empathetic communication and listening skills to their fullest, it may be possible to help Sam see the impact of his statements in a different light. Although this will likely not result in Sam changing his mind or opinions, it may at least lead to Sam reconsidering his actions in the future.

Assimilators, with their high need for structure, organization, and planning, may feel quite uncomfortable simply jumping into this kind of situation without first reflecting, preparing, developing a series of what-if scenarios, and then rehearsing different approaches. As managers and leaders, this focus on preparation and rehearsal can be the assimilator's greatest asset or their greatest weakness. In some circumstances, of course, there is simply not enough time to prepare for every what-if scenario that may occur in a delicate conversation; the strongest assimilators may struggle to think on their feet or roll with the punches as a conversation evolves rapidly. At their best, however, assimilators are able to harness the power of logic and preparation constructively to create strong and persuasive arguments and provide clear instructions and directions for how to proceed. In general, assimilators do not have the same need to be liked as divergers and may view Sam's situation in a more straightforward manner as unprofessional behavior that needs to be managed or addressed, rather than as a challenge to a friendship or professional relationship. This view of the situation can help provide a layer of emotional insulation for the assimilator, who may be better able to focus on the issue itself rather than the person involved. At their worst, strong assimilators may be so consumed with planning and preparation for difficult conversations as managers and leaders that they lose momentum or overload these conversations with so much detail that the actual point may be lost.

Convergers, with their natural sense of self-confidence and ability to think on their feet, may have no hesitation or difficulty in assuming a managerial or leadership role in a situation such as this. Strong convergers rarely feel inhibited in sharing their opinions and beliefs, which can be both an advantage and a disadvantage. At their best, convergers can clearly convey their feelings in a forceful and direct manner, and this force of personality can be quite a powerful tool for changing other people's thinking and behaviors. At their worst, however, convergers can appear somewhat bullying, which can build resentment and encourage subversion from others. The strongest convergers may, at times, have difficulty with effective listening and demonstrating empathy; they may simply miss nonverbal cues from others that are either negative or contrary to their preconceived notions of how a conversation should evolve. Although the converger's strength of conviction can be a powerful tool for management and leadership, if it is not mellowed with effective listening skills and authentic empathy, it can actually escalate conflict and problems rather than diminish them. A converger will rarely back down from a strongly held belief simply because he is afraid of conflict or fears the rupture of a relationship. At their best, convergers learn to be more attuned to nonverbal cues transmitted by others and to demonstrate effective listening and empathy more frequently in order to more effectively manage and lead.

Accommodators in general like to get to the point. They are not naturally inclined toward reflection, self-assessment, or discussion, but instead prefer to simply give or receive directions and act accordingly. As a result, for the strongest accommodators, management and leadership roles can be somewhat challenging, and in many cases, strong accommodators simply do not perceive such roles to fit them very well. This is unfortunate; at their best, accommodators bring a direct and somewhat unemotional style of communication to challenging situations such as this, which can be productive without appearing to be as intimidating or bullying as strong convergers. At their worst, however, accommodators can sometimes be less interested in monitoring and follow-up, erroneously believing that once they've said something, that should be enough. Accommodators can be particularly blindsided by subversion because they rarely subvert others and, consequently, do not necessarily understand either the psychology behind subversion or the mechanics of how someone subverts another person. At their worst, accommodators can sometimes appear unfeeling or dispassionate and will rarely think of a situation such as this in terms of the impact on others. At their best, however, accommodators will keep a cool head, not allow their personal emotions to interfere with discussion, and be able to communicate in a clear, direct, and succinct manner.

Although your personal emotional intelligence style will of course greatly influence how you interpret and deal with a situation such as this, there are some general communication skills and tactics that are applicable in all cases.

Manage your personal emotional response to this situation before engaging in any kind of conversation with Sam. For some, Sam's letter will be absolutely infuriating. The frank disregard he has shown for others may be interpreted as homophobic and discriminatory and may provoke a strong emotional response before any kind of logical response emerges. As has been discussed previously, conversations that start with an emotional response may not be the most productive. This is particularly important where you are a manager or a leader. Maintaining your emotional control and being able to engage productively and calmly will be important. For others, they may personally agree with what Sam has said, even if they don't necessarily agree with the words he selected or the tone he has used. Philosophical agreement with Sam's perspective should not, however, cloud thinking and evaluation that Sam has behaved in a fundamentally unprofessional manner. Agreeing in any way with Sam's beliefs and statements must also be reconciled with the inaccuracies in Sam's article, labeling homosexuality "an illness." In this case, managing one's positive response to Sam's general thinking, while simultaneously addressing the professionalism deficits he has demonstrated, can be a challenge but must be done in order to communicate effectively.

Management and leadership in this case will involve feedback. In Chapter 9, we reviewed principles of effective feedback. Regardless of your role as a manager or a leader, this is a situation that requires you provide feedback to Sam based on the principles discussed in Chapter 9. As noted in that chapter, it is important to be realistic in terms of what you hope to accomplish with feedback and what you can reasonably expect Sam to do as a result of this feedback. It seems somewhat unlikely that any kind of feedback or conversation will actually change Sam's opinions or mind with respect to the issue of same-sex marriage, and arguably, that is not your job or role anyway. A central principle of feedback is that you are focused on behavior, not thinking or philosophy. As a manager or a leader, it may be more important to identify a concrete behavior (e.g., an apology letter, a meeting with local LGBTQ+ community members) that may have a greater likelihood of success than asking him to change his fundamental beliefs. It may also be important to recall the important lessons from Chapter 6 regarding the Transtheoretical Model for Change (Prochaska). If Sam is in precontemplation regarding his behavior, he may not even be aware that he has behaved unprofessionally, and as a result, a different strategy for feedback may be required.

What's the least worst alternative? In this situation, there is no right answer. If Sam's article was prompted by discriminatory beliefs or by a deeply felt kind of religious or other conviction, he is going to be extremely resistant to any reasonable alternative you propose. Having a clear and practical understanding of your bottom line, rather than a naïve belief that you will be able to change him after one or two conversations, is important. In some cases, the least worst alternative may be nothing more than you simply telling Sam your opinions, expressing your disappointment in his behavior, and agreeing to disagree. For others, the least worst alternative (in the event that Sam is entirely resistant to an apology or meeting with community members) may be that you feel compelled to report Sam to the regulatory body or professional association for conduct unbecoming of a professional. In writing such an inflammatory and medically false article, Sam has demonstrated not only unprofessional behavior, but he has also actually demonstrated he is not competent to continue to practice his profession. If he believes homosexuality is an illness—contrary to every reputable medical and health professional organization's statements—what else does he believe? For example, if a health professional actively encouraged patients to NOT receive vaccinations, would that be considered a form of gross incompetence? Or if a geography teacher believed the earth was flat, should that person be allowed to teach? There are foundational concepts in every profession that speak directly to competence to practice in the field, and Sam's article suggests there may be fitness to practice issues that must be investigated further to ensure that patient care is not compromised. As can be seen, there are an array of different least worst alternatives that must be considered and carefully weighed using risk-balancing approaches.

Find common ground. In order to be productive and as nonconfrontational as possible, any conversation with Sam needs to begin from a place of respect and commonality, regardless of the emotional response you may have initially had after reading his article. It may be easy to forget that Sam is your colleague and that, over the years, you have built up a collegial relationship with him based on mutual respect and trust. This collegial relationship can be an important starting point for any conversation with Sam, because it can allow you the opportunity to find and keep common ground with one another. Common ground refers to the things you agree on, and if Sam has been your colleague, you will have some or many things you see eye to eye on. Beginning your conversations acknowledging this common ground is important. Saying, "I know we both want to do the best job we can to help our patients," or "We both know how important it is to demonstrate respect and to show compassion to everyone we serve," strikes a positive and constructive tone, and acknowledges that despite your disagreement over the article, you know that you have many things in common with Sam. Failure to find common ground can set this conversation up for conflict and failure. Common ground can also be a neutral zone you can return to as the conversation becomes more dominated by things you disagree about. Reminding yourself and Sam of the values, beliefs, experiences, and professional standards you share demonstrates respect, builds rapport, and enhances communication.

Be conscious about "you" and "I." The topic of Sam's article may, in some places, be highly polarizing. The words that are chosen to discuss this situation can contribute or worsen such polarization. A conversation filled with, "When you wrote this . . . " or "I believe that . . . " highlights differences, eliminates common ground, and verbally establishes an us-versus-them polarization mentality that can be counterproductive to a collegial discussion. This is particularly important for strong convergers and accommodators to remember, because these individuals may more naturally gravitate to the direct communication style characterized by use of "you" and "I" than divergers or assimilators. Being careful, without being clumsy or awkward, in trying to construct sentences that minimize use of the words "you" and "I" may help to de-escalate potential conflict in this situation.

What you say is important, but how you say it will be even more important. Management and leadership situations are frequently highly emotional, dealing with difficult or sensitive issues about which people may have strong feelings and beliefs. This situation is no different; it is inherently an emotional situation that pits one person's strong beliefs against another's. Where emotion is at the core of an issue, nonverbal messaging and cues become even more important. As discussed in Chapters 5, 6, and 7, alignment between verbal messaging and nonverbal cues is essential. If you are subconsciously disgusted and appalled by Sam, there is a strong likelihood that this will creep into your body language, tone of voice, and gestures, which will send negative nonverbal cues that will provoke a strongly negative emotional response back from Sam. Managing how you say what you say in any conversation will be just as important (if not more important) than the specific words you use. To help you to manage this, it may be best to carefully plan a time and place for a conversation that provides privacy, that supports face-to-face conversation, and that minimizes distraction or interruption. Assimilators in particular may want to try to rehearse a conversation with someone else before going live with Sam, as a way of helping to manage diverse what-if scenarios. This is not a situation or a circumstance where it is safe to fake it till you make it or to simply wing it. There is much that could go wrong with a poorly conducted conversation, and you owe it to yourself and to Sam to be as prepared as possible.

11.5 Communicating as a Manager Versus Communicating as a Leader

This situation provides an interesting opportunity to compare and contrast communication as a manager and communication as a leader. As Sam's manager, you may have certain responsibilities and tools that allow you to work with Sam constructively and positively around the issue itself. As a manager, you will be focused on Sam's professional development and how he addresses the situation. As a leader, however, you may need to take a wider perspective than simply Sam's development.

Sam's article was very public and no doubt read by many in the community. This is not an internal health team or collegial issue; it is something that an entire community may be watching with some interest. A leader cannot manage this as simply an internal issue. Despite the facts of the case, which suggest that "no one has complained and some patients have actually congratulated Sam on his article," it should be obvious that there will of course be some or many people in the community who will be most upset by Sam's article but may not say so publicly. Leaders must recognize that situations such as this are not a popularity contest.

As a leader, it is important to recognize that, in some cases, a compromise may not be possible or desirable. It may not be possible to simply agree to disagree on some issues that are so fundamental to people's lives and beliefs. Leadership in this case will mean making a clear and unequivocal public statement that Sam's assertions are wrong, not medically defensible, and that you personally do not agree with or support what he has said. This may sound confrontational and provocative, and without good communication, it easily could become that way. However, good leaders recognize that clarity is not necessarily provocative, and that being principled does not mean you have to be confrontational.

Whether communicating in writing or verbally with others, it is important to remember that the tone with which you deliver your message will make all the difference. You can disagree with Sam respectfully and without being disagreeable, but also in a way that is clear and unequivocal. If communicating verbally, this will mean selecting words carefully and also ensuring that nonverbal cues such as gestures, eye contact, and tone of voice are steady, calm, and nonemotional. If communicating in writing, this will mean being direct, respectful, and concise and not trying to make everyone happy (which usually results in no one being happy).

As a leader, this means taking a clear and public stand in support of fully embracing diversity in your community and ensuring the public understands professional responsibilities to serve every patient with respect and compassion. No doubt, some people in the community may disagree with you, for example, those who publicly congratulated Sam on his article. Preparing yourself for this reality may be challenging, especially if you are a diverger, but having the strength of your convictions is essential for leadership. Even if a majority of the community disagrees with you, your professionalism and code of ethics should guide your behavior as a leader in this situation.

11.6 Summary

Communication as a manager, an administrator, or a leader is built on many of the same principles that have been previously discussed, including the need to demonstrate empathy, use effective listening, and be attentive to individuals' emotional intelligence styles. Although the mechanics of communication are important, the underlying psychology of management, administration, and leadership are also important to help provide support for effective conversations. The need for authenticity, clarity, and a forward-looking vision for improvement is particularly important for leaders. Not all health professionals will aspire to formal management or administrative roles; however, all health professionals, whether they have a named role within an organization or not, are leaders and will be called on to demonstrate leadership in difficult circumstances.

11.7 **Mind Map Chapter 11**

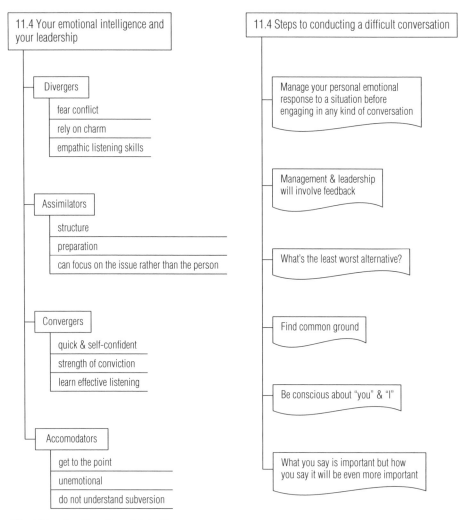

Mind Map for Emotional Intelligence

For Further Reading:

Booher D. *What More Can I Say? Why Communication Fails and What to Do About It.* New York: Penguin Group; 2015.

Collins S, McKinnies R, Collins K. Leadership characteristics for health care managers. *Health Care Manag.* 2015;34(4):293–296.

Delmatoff J, Lazarus I. The most effective leadership style for the new landscape of healthcare. *J Healthc Manag.* 2014;59(4):245–249.

Goleman D, Boyatzis R, McKee A. *Primal Leadership: Learning to Lead with Emotional Intelligence.* Boston: Harvard Business Review Press; 2002.

Hargett C, Doty J, Hauck J, et al. Developing a model for effective leadership in healthcare: a concept mapping approach. *J Healthc Leadersh.* 2017;9:69–78.

Lake D, Baerg K, Paslawski T. *Teamwork, Leadership, and Communication: Collaboration Basics for Health Professionals.* Edmonton, Canada: Brush Education; 2015.

Luxford K, Safran D, Delbanco T. Promoting patient-centered care: a qualitative study of facilitators and barriers in healthcare organizations with a reputation for improving the patient experience. *Int J Quality Health Care.* 2011;23(5):510–515.

Maccoby M. *The Leaders We Need and What Makes Us Follow.* Boston: Harvard Business School Press; 2007.

12 Conflict Management, Resolution, and De-escalation

It's happened again! Sarah, the young pharmacist working in the dispensary is approached by an angry physician. The physician, an older, experienced family doctor, had written a prescription for misoprostol two tablets per vaginal insertion for a patient who had just suffered a miscarriage. The medication was dispensed by the pharmacy as by mouth and the patient took it as instructed on the label and by the pharmacist. As a result, the medication did not work and now the patient has to undergo a surgical procedure instead. Worse, this is the third time this exact same situation has happened in this pharmacy. After the first incident, the doctor explained to the pharmacy the problem. After the second time, he wrote it down and emailed it. Now it has happened a third time and the doctor is very, very angry. The pharmacist on duty didn't dispense the medication, wasn't around for the first two incidents, and is now caught in the wrong place at the wrong time. The first thing the doctor says in anger is, "I can't believe you pharmacists. You're more interested in making money off prescriptions than actually helping my patients. How can you keep on making this same mistake over again?"

12.1 What Is a Conflict?

There are many different ways of describing or defining conflict. For this module, we are going to define it as an interpersonal struggle between two individuals. This struggle will typically have two components: intellectual or philosophical disagreement and some level of emotional involvement. Conflict rarely occurs when people simply and only disagree about something. Having different points of view or perspectives, by itself, can spark friendly and fun debates or dialogue. Where conflict occurs, it is generally because this intellectual disagreement is coupled with some level of emotional involvement or entanglement. When you actually CARE or have STRONG FEELINGS about the source of the disagreement, this emotional connection produces a sense of being threatened, disrespected, or feeling afraid, which is generally the spark that leads to open conflict. Without this emotional component, a disagreement is simply a different point of view. With the emotional overlay, disagreement rapidly escalates into conflict. Learning to recognize, manage, and mitigate this emotional component is a crucial part of conflict management.

Within health professions and teams of health professionals, there are unique reasons for conflict development and escalation. As we saw in the previous vignette, conflict can occur simply because we are doing our job. A major source of conflict in practice is our attempt to actually enforce or implement rules that other people may disagree with or may not like. When patients are not well, or preoccupied due to health concerns, our attempts to simply do our job can be misinterpreted as being aggressive, unhelpful, or disrespectful. Intellectual disagreement becomes connected with emotional involvement and conflict may erupt. Further, health care facilities are physically challenging places where there are lots of distractions, noises, and cramped working spaces, all of which heightens our emotional fragility and primes us for experiencing conflict. Perhaps most importantly, many practitioners report that the nature of the professions themselves mean we have responsibility to enforce rules without any real power, and this sense of powerlessness is a strong emotional foundation for conflict development and escalation.

An important principle of conflict management is to separate the intellectual disagreement from the emotional involvement we may be feeling. Of course, this is easier said than done, particularly in the heat of the moment! Root cause analysis is a technique that can help us to emphasize the cognitive rather than the emotional sources of conflict. If we can analyze a situation, it can help us to compartmentalize and contain our immediate emotional response to it in a way that is both productive and may help de-escalate conflict. Although this can be a challenge to apply, it is a technique that allows us to think through—rather than simply emotionally experience or feel—a conflict. One approach to root cause analysis involves categorization of conflict based on one or more reasons.

12.1.2 What Are the Root Causes of Conflict?

One model of root cause analysis suggests there are five major reasons why conflicts occur: personal differences, disagreements over methods (not outcomes), informational deficiencies, role incompatibility, and environmental stress. More detail about each of these follows.

Personal differences: Conflicts rooted in personal difference are frequent and can be very challenging to manage. Each of us as individuals has a unique and highly personalized worldview that forms over many years and decades. Our worldview is central to who we are as individuals and forms the foundation of our personalities, our psychologies, and our way of interacting with others. This worldview is shaped from childhood by our families, our communities, and our societies, religions, and cultures. No two people have the same worldview. When an intellectual disagreement is built on a personal worldview difference, it is generally and immediately viewed as an insult—a challenge not to our ideas, but to our personalities and selves, which can quickly lead to strong emotional involvement. We feel threatened, disrespected, or diminished when people do not agree with something as foundational as our worldview. Sadly, in such cases, emotional entanglement can occur swiftly and sometimes even violently. It also makes reaching a consensus or compromise challenging because few of us wish to compromise something as foundational as our worldview. As a result, when personal differences are truly the source of conflict, an impasse may occur quickly and a resolution may not be feasible or practical in the short term. In such cases, it may be best for one party to simply withdraw to allow time for emotions to subside and cooler heads to prevail before attempting to address the impasse. Examples of personal differences causing conflict in pharmacy practice might include individuals' differing views on sensitive issues such as emergency contraception, medical aid in dying, or medical cannabis. People may have strong personal beliefs that clash on such topics, and this can lead to an impasse. It is not generally possible to convince someone or change their mind on such topics; worldview is notoriously unchangeable at times, and the use of strong emotions in conflict situations is least likely to succeed in such situations of impasse. It is better to find ways of simply working around or withdrawing from such situations where possible.

Disagreements over methods, not outcomes: In many workplace settings, disagreements over methods are a root cause of conflict. It is easy to observe others and think, "I wouldn't do it that way!" Such observations may lead us then to actually tell others what we think about the way they are doing things. When such observations are unsolicited, they can provoke a strong and negative emotional response. We may feel lectured to, or feel like we are being treated as children in a disrespectful way. Interestingly, in debating methods or processes, we lose sight of the actual outcome. When we are busy telling other people HOW to do their job, we may forget that they are achieving what they are supposed to be achieving, so why are we so fixated on the process? In situations where the root cause of conflict is a disagreement over methods, focusing on outcomes rather than processes can provide us with COMMON GROUND, something that we can all agree on is more important. Discussing this common ground is a powerful way of stripping away the emotion from a situation and demonstrating respect for another person. Focusing on what we agree on (i.e., the outcome, the common ground) rather than what we disagree on (i.e., the process, the method) helps us to keep emotions in check and can be a powerful tool for conflict de-escalation. Examples of disagreements over methods in a pharmacy may focus on work style; for example, an individual may prefer to batch fill similar prescriptions for different patients to increase efficiency, whereas another person may feel this approach might lead to errors and instead prefers to fill prescriptions for one patient at a time even though it is more time consuming to do it this way. Neither method or process is inherently right or wrong; so long as all prescriptions are filled accurately and in a timely manner, does it really matter which process is used if the outcome is achieved?

Informational deficiencies: We live in a complex world, and it is impossible for any one person to know all the facts and rules that govern day-to-day life. When we don't know something, we may accidently behave or make statements that can be misinterpreted by others who assume we should know better. Information deficiencies are a common cause of conflict in practice as scientific knowledge, policies, procedures, and practices constantly evolve and change. Keeping up with this can be daunting. When we assume someone's statements or behaviors are based on them actually knowing EVERYTHING, we seriously underestimate how frequently lack of knowledge causes disagreements. If we assume they are knowledgeable, it leads us then to believe their statement or behavior reflects on their underlying feelings of disrespect for us. When a conflict's root cause is framed as informational deficiency, the most effective strategy is to teach and learn, rather than respond emotionally. Helping the other person learn what they currently do not know—in a respectful and constructive way—can move the conflict away from emotion and toward a more positive resolution. An example of information deficiency in this case may be a new staff member (e.g., a medical resident) who lacks awareness regarding the protocol for managing a miscarriage. It is easy to understand why someone might assume that misoprostol, which is an oral tablet formulation, should be swallowed like a regular tablet. No malice is intended when the medical resident, or the nurse before her, or the pharmacist before him provided a patient with the wrong instruction. This error—although unfortunate, preventable, and difficult for the patient—does not necessarily mean the professionals involved were incompetent or lazy. However, if other team members are now speaking to them in a tone that makes them feel disrespected or diminished, the emotional collision can lead to conflict.

Role incompatibility: As practitioners, we are all justifiably proud of our contributions to our communities regardless of our specific professional designation or degree. Our professional roles are an important part of who we are as individuals. Human beings frequently think of themselves in terms of the multiple roles they play in different circles. We are parents, children, students, teachers, friends, neighbors, etc. Our roles are central to our understanding of ourselves. When we feel someone questioning our role or diminishing the importance of that role, we cannot help but respond negatively and sometimes emotionally, which in turn can escalate into conflict. When our role is disrespected, overlooked, or ignored, we as individuals feel disrespected, overlooked, or ignored. It is important, however, to recognize that when someone disagrees with us about a specific problem, it does not necessarily mean they are disrespecting us or our role. For example, if a pharmacist questions a prescription from a physician and suggests an alternative, that pharmacist may expect the physician will defer to the pharmacist's professional expertise and agree. If the physician disagrees, the pharmacist may feel it is more than a simple intellectual disagreement; instead, it may be interpreted as "the doctor thinks he is better than me because I'm just a pharmacist," and a negative emotional spiral may result. Separating disagreement about a situation from disrespect for a role is an important way of helping to prevent conflict escalation. Clarity around roles and responsibilities and demonstrating ongoing respect for each other's roles are essential for harmonious workplace functioning.

Environmental stress: The connection between our work environment, the psychological stress it provokes, and the escalation of conflict is clear. Challenging environments and workplaces take a psychological toll. The noise, distraction, competition for scarce resources and space, and competing priorities for our time are both exhausting and stress inducing. In such situations, our emotional selves are constantly on edge and primed to experience conflict. Our capacity to coolly and rationally analyze root causes of a conflict are significantly diminished when we feel such environmentally linked stress, particularly day in and day out. As any harried commuter will tell you, the experience of having to drive on busy highways with other angry motorists every day just to get to work sets a negative foundation for all interpersonal experiences that day. Learning to recognize when environmental stress is making us more vulnerable to conflict and more emotionally fragile is essential. Sometimes, the trigger for a conflict—the intellectual disagreement at the root—can be the environment itself. If we feel suffocated, like we are drowning in our work and our environment, we will naturally respond emotionally and strongly, which can start the negative spiral of conflict with others. Sometimes we can address this issue; we can fix our physical environment, reduce our workload, better manage our emails, etc. Sometimes we can't really do anything about this issue other than recognize the impact it is having on us and our tendency to conflict and look for other coping mechanisms outside of the workplace, such as yoga, meditation, or running. The reality, of course, is that most health care settings are filled with interruptions, small pieces of paper that frequently get misplaced, phone calls that never end, noise, and congestion. These distractions produce a high level of cognitive and emotional load that literally block out the ability to coolly and rationally think through problems and situations, and instead prime us to respond to environmental triggers in an emotional, rather than logical way—a sure recipe for conflict escalation.

Root cause analysis is an important tool for helping us to manage conflicts as they occur and to prevent future conflicts from arising. It works by helping to engage us in cognitive rather than emotional problem solving and, in the process, helps us to separate factual issues from emotional ones and gain greater control over our own responses. Applying some form of structured or systematic approach to conflict management and de-escalation is a valuable tool to prevent small disagreements from spiraling into bigger conflicts. There are many different approaches that have been proposed and tested, some of which may work better for some people than others. It is important to simply pick some kind of an approach and try it, learn from the experience, and refine your own approach as time goes on. Let's turn now to one type of systematic approach that many people find helpful in managing conflict.

12.1.3   From Analysis to Action: Techniques for Conflict Resolution

This five-step process draws on many different ideas and techniques in the conflict management literature. The first step involves identifying and actually naming the issues involved in the conflict, then clarifying opposing viewpoints before finding common ground. Once common ground is identified, then it becomes possible to evaluate best possible outcomes and acceptable alternatives for consideration. Finally, implementing a plan or change and monitoring to see the impact follow. Let's now look at each step of this process more closely.

First, identify and accurately name the issue—what's the problem we are really trying to solve? The root cause analysis approach we have just discussed is an important first step in the process. It allows us to engage cognitively with a problem and then use the power of language to help contain and control it. Along with using root cause analysis to frame the reasons behind factual disagreements, we can also then start to understand and name the emotional responses that accompany it, both in ourselves and with the other party involved. Our emotional responses to factual disagreements provide a window into both our thinking and feeling processes, and as such, are important sources of data in understanding an issue. Correctly identifying an emotional response can be difficult, but is essential for helping to understand all dimensions of a conflict. Emotional responses such as fear, anger, sadness, and grief are strong and each is different; mislabeling anger for sadness or fear can lead us to misinterpret the signals being sent by the other party, which then risks escalating the conflict further. Anger is very often driven by fear and/or sadness. In many cases, if a person is given the space to vent their anger, the next wave may be tears. Learning to maintain your composure, keeping appropriate eye contact, and achieving emotional control and calmness in the face of strong emotion is important. Do not underestimate, however, how challenging it can be to identify and name others' emotional responses when we are ourselves are in a highly emotional state. Care must be taken to avoid assumptions in this case. If you're not sure, reflect on what you've heard and ask the person to confirm and continue. This demonstrates that you want to understand and can accept the emotion and anger.

Clarify opposing viewpoints: Focus on the facts while respecting the emotions. The power of root cause analysis and an assessment of the accompanying emotion should not be underestimated. When done properly, it provides the gateway to helping to de-escalate and manage conflict effectively. More importantly, it allows us as individuals to engage with a conflict situation cognitively rather than emotionally, which is the objective of this next step of the process. If we are able to transform our understanding of the root causes and emotional consequences of a conflict situation, we are in a better position to focus on the factual while respecting the emotional. We can use dialogue to start to clarify and better understand opposing viewpoints and, ultimately, help the other party engage with the issue cognitively rather than emotionally. An important part of this clarification may be determining whether the person is simply venting rather than actually blaming you. For example, in this case involving Sarah the pharmacist, the physician may not actually be angry with her personally, but is angry at the overall situation. Sarah just happens to be the one working in the pharmacy that day and so is on the receiving end of his venting.

Find (and protect!) common ground. Common ground is the term used to describe those things that we agree on in an effort to not only ensure they do not become affected or contaminated by the strong emotion of conflict, but also to provide us with an opportunity to hear ourselves agreeing and saying yes rather than no to one another. The objective of identifying and naming factual and emotional issues then clarifying opposing viewpoints is to help us to establish and confirm the common ground we will share with the other party during a conflict situation. Common ground is the basis on which conflict resolution can occur. Establishing and protecting this common ground is crucial and requires both acknowledgment of legitimate factual differences and respect for emotional responses, which may be difficult to accomplish unless we are in control of our own emotional responses. Once achieved, however, common ground becomes the foundation within which compromise can take root and meaningful conflict de-escalation and prevention can occur.

Identify the best reasonable outcomes and acceptable alternatives. Conflicts occur because there are no perfect solutions or right answers available; we must all concede the need to compromise in order to move ahead. As discussed in Chapter 11, the least worst alternatives, rather than perfect answers, are frequently the only option available to us. A discussion of options and alternatives should build on a foundation of common ground, the things we already all agree on. Focusing initially on the outcome that is desired before discussing specific actions and alternatives can frequently be helpful. With common ground achieved, it becomes possible to consider moving forward in a way that respects our emotional responses and factual disagreements but is not paralyzed by them. If common ground has been truly achieved, there will be recognition that both parties in a conflict have legitimate points of view that need to be respected and that compromise is not only possible but is in fact the only positive and constructive path forward. There are rarely perfect answers to conflicts. Instead, we search for the least worst alternative—options that are acceptable by both parties—imperfect though they may be. It is common in a conflict situation to try to leap quickly to an answer or a resolution. Such leaps may paradoxically slow down the conflict resolution process and may risk even worsening the conflict through further emotional entanglement. Rather than jump to a solution at the outset, it is often helpful to initially focus on what a desirable outcome would look like from both parties' perspectives. This outline of the characteristics of a successful resolution to a conflict situation can help to guide discussion of specific alternatives and options and can provide a framework for evaluating and prioritizing them.

Identify the plan or a step to be implemented, monitored, and recalibrated as necessary. As cooler heads prevail and alternatives are agreed on to de-escalate and manage conflict, it is important to be mindful that implementation of alternatives requires as much attention to detail as the initial negotiation of options. One of the best ways to both implement and monitor conflict resolution alternatives is through ongoing respectful communication and dialogue among the parties. The objective here is to learn from the past and ensure small disagreements do not escalate into major conflicts. Being mindful of root causes, such as personal differences, information deficiencies, role incompatibility, disagreement over methods and environmental stress, allows us to carefully observe ourselves in real time, and when small issues arise and flash points occur, try to diffuse them quickly before emotional entanglement occurs. Conflict resolution is not a linear process; it will ebb and flow and emotions will rise and fall during the process. At times it may feel like two steps forward, one step backward, which can be frustrating and demoralizing. Recognizing this reality also helps us to anticipate the ongoing challenges with conflict. It is not simply managed or resolved once, but rather, it is an ongoing process rooted in conversation, observation, and genuine commitment to improvement that can benefit from some of these strategies we have discussed so far.

12.2 The Role of Emotional Intelligence in Conflict Management

As discussed in Chapter 2, emotional intelligence is an important tool for self-understanding and self-reflection. It can be particularly important during high-stress times of conflict. Understanding how your personal psychology and individual emotional intelligence may help, or hinder, your attempts to manage, resolve, or de-escalate conflict is important. Focusing on the four emotional intelligence styles described in Chapter 2, let's examine how self-awareness of emotional intelligence can contribute positively to conflict management.

12.2.1 A Model for Understanding How Emotional Intelligence and Conflict Are Connected

Research has highlighted that conflict is a two-phase process. This model is depicted in Figure 12.1. As you see, along the X-axis is one's worldview. One's worldview can range from being very principled to very pragmatic. A principled worldview is characterized by a belief that things are either right or wrong, black or white, and that there are rarely, if ever, situations where shades of gray exist. Principled individuals have strong convictions and beliefs and stick to them, sometimes defensively. In contrast, on the other end of the X-axis, we see the pragmatic worldview.

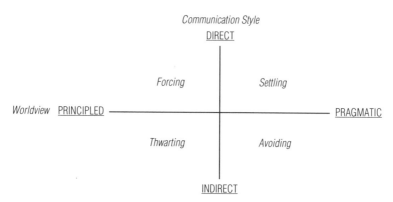

Figure 12.1. The Four Conflict Management Styles. This two-faceted model highlights that conflict is a function of two interdependent factors: your worldview and your communication style. Worldview describes the perspective you have on day-to-day life. Some of us believe things are right or wrong, black or white, whereas others believe things are generally gray. Communication style represents the way we use verbal and nonverbal messages to interact with others. Some of us are more direct, whereas others favor indirect methods. When we intersect these two processes, we have four different conflict management styles: forcers, settlers, avoiders, and thwarters.

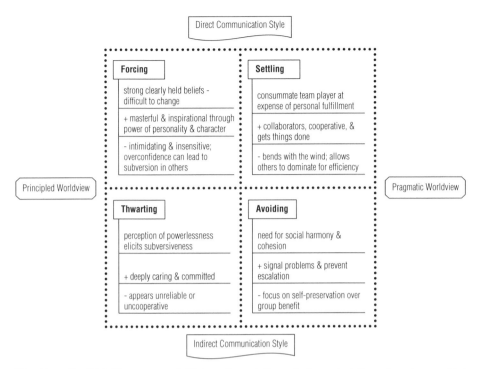

The Four Conflict Management Styles. Description of characteristics of major conflict management styles.

Those with a pragmatic worldview typically are more interested in simply getting things done, in moving forward rather than being right. They have few strongly held beliefs and tend to believe in situational ethics and problem solving; to the pragmatically inclined, most things are gray and few things are worth really fighting about. Each of us falls somewhere along the continuum of these two poles. We now intersect this dimension with the Y-axis, which depicts our interpersonal communication style. At one pole we see direct communication; direct communicators are those who speak clearly, forcefully, and typically in short, detached sentences focused on action rather than philosophy. In contrast, indirect communicators focus more on nonverbal messages and tend to use longer, more circuitous forms of communication to make their point, frequently modifying their delivery in immediate response to verbal or nonverbal cues they receive from others. This model of conflict generation maps onto the four different emotional intelligence styles, and provides us with insights into the strengths, and challenges, each style has in better managing conflict.

Convergers most frequently present in a conflict situation as forcers. Forcers exists at the intersection of direct communication and a principled worldview. This means that individuals with this dominant conflict management style tend to have strongly held, clear beliefs that are difficult to change or shape and are willing and able to use a clear and forceful style of communication to express themselves. At their best, forcers appear confident, masterful, and filled with conviction. They can be inspirational and shape a group's attitudes and beliefs through the power of their personality and character. At their worst, however, forcers can appear intimidating and insensitive to others, and are sometimes labeled as bullies because of their forceful style. The strongest forcers could benefit from simply listening more to others and giving others a chance to share their views, then authentically trying to understand these perspectives despite the forcer's preexisting beliefs. At times, the forcer may demonstrate overconfidence, which leaves them vulnerable to subversion. Subversion occurs when individuals who feel disempowered say one thing to a forcer, then behave in a different, often contradictory, way when the forcer is no longer present, and justify it by thinking, "The forcer wasn't listening to me anyway." Within a primary health care team, physicians are most frequently associated with the forcer conflict management style.

Assimilators most frequently present as settlers in conflict situations. Settlers exist at the intersection of a direct communication style and a pragmatic worldview. They share the same direct communication style as forcers, which allows them to potentially speak the same language, but with less of an interest in declaring a strong view on a subject. As a result, settlers tend to have a reputation as being pleasant, cooperative, and efficient—a consummate team player. At times, however, this reputation can come at the expense of personal fulfillment or integrity. The settler's need for efficiency and getting things done can sometimes mean they allow others to dominate over them, which can leave them feeling somewhat negative and disempowered. In some cases, this can give the impression that settlers simply bend with the wind and go along with whomever is dominant and loudest in a group. At their best, settlers are great collaborators, cooperate effectively, and get things done. At their worst, however, settlers will allow others to run rough over them and other members of a group simply in the name of efficiency. Within the primary health care team, many pharmacists—in particular many female pharmacists—tend to demonstrate this dominant conflict management style.

In conflict situations, **divergers**, with their high need for social harmony and cohesion, tend to present as avoiders. Avoiders exist at the intersection of a pragmatic worldview and an indirect communication style. In this way, they share a similar worldview to settlers but appear to speak exactly the opposite language as forcers, which may contribute to conflict escalation in some cases. Avoiders have a finely tuned radar that allows them to anticipate and predict conflict and prevent small disagreements from spiraling into open conflict. Unfortunately, at their worst, avoiders' indirect communication style and strong instinct for self-preservation means they do not communicate this clearly to others and, instead, focus on saving themselves from stress and harm rather than on a group's overall benefit. At their best, avoiders are able to signal problems early on and prevent them from escalating, but need to feel comfortable, confident, and heard in order to do this. Within a primary care health team, male nonphysician team members (e.g., pharmacists, occupational therapists, physical therapists) appear to demonstrate this conflict management style.

Finally, let's look at the thwarter style, which is most frequently associated with **accommodators,** who exist at the intersection of a principled worldview and an indirect communication style. Within the primary health care team, many nurses (male and female) demonstrate this conflict management style, as do technicians and assistants in many professions. The primary characteristic of this style is the perception of powerlessness—the belief that despite having good ideas, there is a hierarchy that frustrates them in actually getting things done. This powerlessness can lead thwarters to favor subversion as a technique: agreeing to one thing with a powerful person, then doing something different when that powerful person isn't watching. Thwarters reject the label that this is passive-aggressive behavior; instead, they may regard this as a legitimate tactic to accomplish a principled objective in an environment where they simply do not have power or control. At their best, thwarters are deeply caring and committed individuals who rarely put their own self-interest ahead of others. At their worst, thwarters can appear somewhat unreliable as team players and can be difficult to describe as cooperative.

As this review of conflict management styles illustrates, human beings have many different ways of managing and dealing with conflict. You may have noticed that each of the labels for the four conflict management styles has a somewhat negative connotation. The words *forcer, settler, avoider*, and *thwarter* are not particularly aspirational labels. This is to reinforce the notion that no one single style is better than any other, and that regardless of one's dominant style, there are opportunities to improve how we respond in difficult situations. The purpose of completing a conflict management styles inventory is to help promote self-understanding and to prompt self-reflection for personal improvement. Learning about one's own strengths and areas for improvement—and those of other conflict management styles—gives us all opportunities and options for how to manage conflict better.

12.3   Intergenerational Conflict

A common concern for many practitioners is the idea that younger colleagues and students are from a completely different generation, and consequently, the norms and rules of social engagement and interaction that used to apply may not be as relevant to them. It is important to recognize but not overemphasize the importance of intergenerational differences. Of course, today's younger generation—under the age of 30 years—has a very different life experience than those who are middle aged or older. The younger generation has grown up fully immersed within social media, technology, the Internet, and a society where public expression of private emotion is much more widely accepted than it was 30 years ago. As a result of this socialization and technology, it is natural to expect that many in this generation may respond differently to day-to-day interpersonal interactions. The younger generation, for example, has always had access to instantaneous communication through cell phones, texting, and instant messaging. They have had greater instantaneous gratification and continuous access to social networks through platforms such as Facebook, Instagram, and Snapchat. They have become accustomed to living unfiltered public lives through their social media postings. These so-called digital natives have had a significantly different life experience and socialization process than their older siblings and parents. What might be the implications of this for interpersonal communication and conflict management?

Intergenerational conflict is as inevitable as any other form of conflict. We may feel somewhat more intimidated by intergenerational conflict, of course, because we don't have the same common history or reference points when dealing with people from other generations. Several principles apply in trying to more effectively and confidently manage intergenerational conflict. First, it is important to recognize how our own life experience, socialization, and generation have shaped our personal biases and assumptions. No generation has a monopoly on the right or best way to manage a situation, and we can and should all learn from one another. Just because we did it a certain way in our generation doesn't mean another generation's approach is wrong or substandard. Second, regardless of our generation, we all have our own individual conflict management styles. Remember to apply your assessment of conflict management style to any situation, and perhaps you will find more common ground there than you may know. Third, it is important to respect and acknowledge the pressures faced by each generation. Every generation has its own unique circumstances and problems, and while this doesn't excuse bad behavior, it may help to explain it. The pressures we face as a member of our generation may unite us with our peers, but it may also make us appear whiny or self-indulgent to other generations. Understanding and respecting generational differences can be an important first step in enhancing communication and achieving the common ground we all seek—regardless of our age and stage in life.

12.4 Putting It Together

Let's revisit the case scenario at the beginning of this chapter to understand how conflict psychology and theory can help inform the kind of interpersonal communication that can manage and de-escalate conflict.

There is a lot going on in this scenario, isn't there? If we apply root cause analysis to this scenario, we can see that at the foundation, the lead doctor believes this problem started because the pharmacy didn't understand the essential need for the misoprostol to be given per vaginal insertion rather than orally, and he tried his best to communicate this. Now that it has happened a third time, he no longer believes it is a problem of information deficiency because he has provided information to address this. Therefore, he now believes it's a problem with the pharmacists and nurses themselves. They simply aren't capable or qualified to understand how important this is. As a result, it causes him to be frustrated and angry, mostly because of the suffering he knows this completely avoidable error has caused his patient. As seen in this vignette, the emotion of anger is most obviously demonstrated here, but at its core is frustration in terms of the doctor feeling helpless and wanting to figure this out.

From the pharmacist's and nurse's perspective, the root cause analysis points to role misunderstanding. This particular pharmacist wasn't there when this medication was dispensed and wasn't around when the first few errors were made, yet she is getting yelled at for something that wasn't her fault. She understands the doctor's frustration, but it isn't fair that she is bearing the brunt of it. It makes her upset, angry, and somewhat fearful because the doctor's direct communication style is so intimidating. Where do we go from here?

The doctor in this case may be demonstrating the communication style of the forcer. He is confident, clear, focused, and targeted and does not hold back criticism. He may be using the word "you" a lot in his conversation. To the pharmacist, this may sound like unfair blaming because this particular pharmacist wasn't even involved in the situation. To the doctor, "you" refers to the pharmacy and the entire profession, and he doesn't have time for niceties and nuances of politeness. His body language, posture, finger pointing, and nonverbal actions all imply self-righteousness and do not give the pharmacist many opportunities to actually engage in conversation. In contrast, the pharmacist may be a settler. She is interested and wants to solve this problem, but doesn't feel the need to apologize because she wasn't personally involved in the errors. She is trying to be a direct communicator, but in this case, her pragmatism and desire to move ahead to solutions will go nowhere until the doctor actually hears an apology as an acknowledgment of the error and its impact on his patients.

The age and gender differences of the doctor and pharmacist in this vignette may also be of relevance. The doctor—a baby boomer—may have a belief in the traditional roles of doctors and pharmacists (and even perhaps men and women). To him, it is appropriate to vent this degree of anger on someone he may view as a subordinate. To the pharmacist—a millennial—this is inappropriate. She is not a subordinate. She is a colleague and a professional on par with the physician who deserves the same respect and voice. As a millennial, she may not be accustomed to this degree of interpersonal conflict and stress because much of her experience with conflict may have been online rather than face to face. This may mean she feels both intimidated and lost in terms of how to cope with the situation. As a millennial, she likely has certain strengths and interests in terms of how to proceed in a solution—for example, by relying upon technology (such as incorporating a standardized alert flag on the misoprostol drug file to alert every pharmacist to the importance of verifying dosage formulation and route prior to dispensing the medication) rather than simply relying on memory as the doctor seems to imply.

As a settler, the pharmacist here has the potential advantage of sharing a similar direct communication style with the doctor. This might be useful to help move from impasse to common ground. For both professionals in this situation, the common ground is patient safety. They both want what is best for the patient. The pharmacist has ideas for how to prevent this from happening in the future (e.g., electronic alert to be added to misoprostol file to remind the pharmacist to double check), but it is too soon to jump to this solution. Instead, the pharmacist needs to work with the physician to find the common ground they currently lack and to find a way to break the spiral of emotion they are both currently trapped in.

The sequence in which alternatives are presented and discussed is crucial. In this situation, it will not be possible to even begin a discussion of alternatives without the pharmacist first apologizing for the error. This is challenging; it wasn't her fault, yet she is required to apologize for it. Sometimes, this is unavoidable and necessary to move forward with conflict management. As a settler, this pharmacist might not find it easy but may find it possible to apologize for something that wasn't her fault for the specific purpose of breaking the emotional spiral they find themselves in. Saying, "I'm sorry" can be incredibly powerful, and when a person hears those words, it quickly helps to de-escalate the emotional component of a conflict. It also helps to move to the next important stage, finding common ground. In this case, the common ground is clearly the patient and her needs and safety. A well-placed question by the pharmacist asking what this patient needs from the pharmacy now and what the pharmacy can do to help will be important. Allow the physician to offer his alternatives and thoughts, but be prepared for him to say insulting things like, "She needs the pharmacy to not have made this mistake again!" and to not react emotionally or defensively to such statements. Third, asking the physician what he needs from the pharmacy right now will help further establish common ground and goodwill, and will further help build the relationship with the doctor. Only then are they truly ready to engage in future preventative strategy discussions. Leaping too quickly to stage four without the first three stages consolidated may further alienate the doctor, who feels the pharmacist is not taking this seriously and does not really understand the ramifications of the error. A sequence to consider to de-escalate this conflict may be:

1. Apologize not in terms of taking personal blame but by accepting responsibility on behalf of the entire profession to ensure this does not happen again.

2. Focus on this specific patient and what this patient needs from the pharmacy right now, which will help establish common ground.

3. Focus on this colleague, this physician, and what the physician needs from the pharmacy and the pharmacist right now. This too will help establish common ground.

4. Offer alternatives and strategies for preventing this problem from occurring again.

Although this particular case happened to involve two individuals in different professions, the reality is that at some point, each practitioner is going to be blamed for another colleague's work. We may find ourselves in situations like this where suddenly we are the face of our entire profession for someone else simply because we were in the wrong place at the wrong time. We may not feel like this is our responsibility or want this kind of pressure, but this is part of what it means to be a professional. In this case, this pharmacist happened to be on duty when this situation arose; through no fault of her own, she now has a responsibility to carry forward, implement, and monitor whatever plan is decided. It is essential she does not try to pass the buck and say, "I'll check with my supervisor" or "It's not my decision to make." Such statements at such a time may inflame the physician even more and give the impression that on top of incompetence, pharmacists are all bureaucrats more interested in policies than actual patients. It is up to the pharmacist to sort out the internal procedural issues associated with what comes next. It is not the doctor's job to do this and he frankly doesn't care about this anyway. Part of apologizing also means taking responsibility for what comes next, which is now the pharmacist's job in this case. It is also her opportunity to do something positive and productive for patient care and for interprofessional relationships.

12.5 **Summary**

Managing conflict is not pleasant or easy, but it is a necessary skill for all health professionals, including pharmacists. The key to success in conflict management is self-reflection, self-assessment, and continuous self-monitoring to ensure we are being as effective as we can be in all of our interpersonal relationships. Remember that conflict begins when intellectual disagreement becomes entangled with an emotional response. The goal of conflict management is to decouple disagreement from emotion, to allow us to disagree without becoming disagreeable. Root cause analysis can help us to engage with conflicts cognitively, rather than emotionally, and can therefore help us to de-escalate an emotional spiral. Understanding your own conflict management style can help you to identify personal strengths and areas for further development with respect to interpersonal communication and conflict management. Putting it all together using a systematic process will allow you to more effectively and confidently manage conflict in day-to-day practice, which will help improve your professional satisfaction.

12.6 **Mind Map Chapter 12**

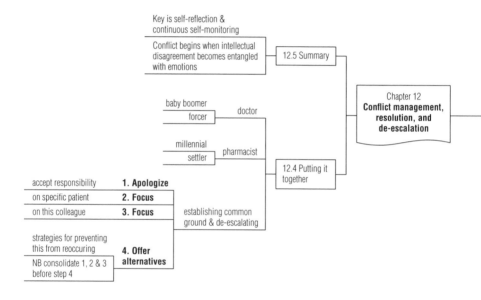

Key is self-reflection & continuous self-monitoring

Conflict begins when intellectual disagreement becomes entangled with emotions

12.5 Summary

Chapter 12
Conflict management, resolution, and de-escalation

baby boomer
forcer
doctor

millennial
settler
pharmacist

12.4 Putting it together

accept responsibility — **1. Apologize**

on specific patient — **2. Focus**

on this colleague — **3. Focus**

establishing common ground & de-escalating

strategies for preventing this from reoccuring

NB consolidate 1, 2 & 3 before step 4

4. Offer alternatives

It's happened again! Sarah, the young pharmacist working in dispensary is approached by an angry physician. The physician, an older experienced family doctor, had written a prescription for misoprostol 2 tablets per vag for a patient who had just suffered a miscarriage. The medication was dispensed by the pharmacy as "by mouth" & the patient took it as instructed on the label & by the pharmacist. As a result, the medication did not work & now the patient has to undergo a surgical procedure instead. Worse, this is the third time this exact same situation has happened in this pharmacy. After the first incident, the doctor explained the problem to the pharmacy. After the second time, he wrote it down & emailed it. Now it had happened a third time & the doctor is very, very angry. The pharmacist on duty didn't dispense the medication, wasn't around for the first two incidents, and is now caught in the wrong place at the wrong time. The first thing the doctor says in anger is, "I can't believe you pharmacists, you're more interested in making money off prescriptions than actually helping my patients. How can you keep on making this same mistake over again?"

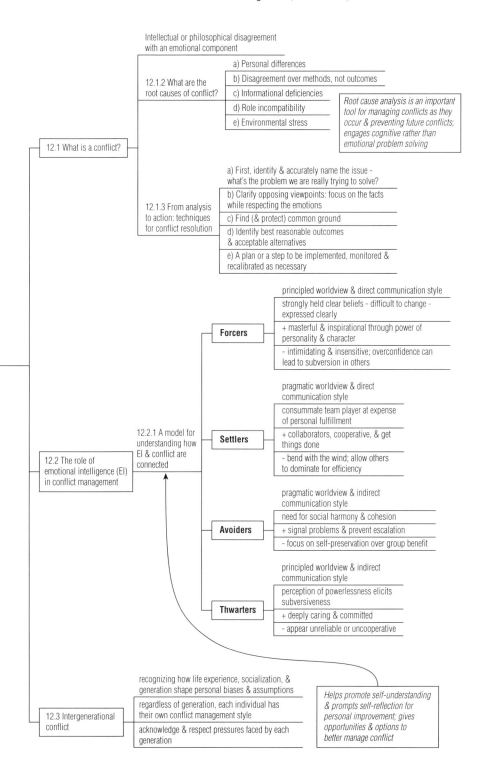

Intellectual or philosophical disagreement
with an emotional component

12.1 What is a conflict?

12.1.2 What are the root causes of conflict?
a) Personal differences
b) Disagreement over methods, not outcomes
c) Informational deficiencies
d) Role incompatibility
e) Environmental stress

Root cause analysis is an important tool for managing conflicts as they occur & preventing future conflicts; engages cognitive rather than emotional problem solving

12.1.3 From analysis to action: techniques for conflict resolution
a) First, identify & accurately name the issue - what's the problem we are really trying to solve?
b) Clarify opposing viewpoints: focus on the facts while respecting the emotions
c) Find (& protect) common ground
d) Identify best reasonable outcomes & acceptable alternatives
e) A plan or a step to be implemented, monitored & recalibrated as necessary

12.2 The role of emotional intelligence (EI) in conflict management

12.2.1 A model for understanding how EI & conflict are connected

Forcers
principled worldview & direct communication style
strongly held clear beliefs - difficult to change - expressed clearly
+ masterful & inspirational through power of personality & character
- intimidating & insensitive; overconfidence can lead to subversion in others

Settlers
pragmatic worldview & direct communication style
consummate team player at expense of personal fulfillment
+ collaborators, cooperative, & get things done
- bend with the wind; allow others to dominate for efficiency

Avoiders
pragmatic worldview & indirect communication style
need for social harmony & cohesion
+ signal problems & prevent escalation
- focus on self-preservation over group benefit

Thwarters
principled worldview & indirect communication style
perception of powerlessness elicits subversiveness
+ deeply caring & committed
- appear unreliable or uncooperative

12.3 Intergenerational conflict
recognizing how life experience, socialization, & generation shape personal biases & assumptions
regardless of generation, each individual has their own conflict management style
acknowledge & respect pressures faced by each generation

Helps promote self-understanding & prompts self-reflection for personal improvement; gives opportunities & options to better manage conflict

THE CONFLICT MANAGEMENT SCALE (CMS)

Think about a few recent situations where you have been involved in a stressful conflict with someone else. This could be a situation at work, in your personal life, or even an unexpected encounter with a stranger. Now, circle the letter in the column that best characterizes what works best for you in situations like the ones you've thought about.

When I'm involved in a conflict situation with another person...	Usually	Sometimes	Rarely	Hardly
1. I have strong beliefs about how the situation should resolve	A	D	C	B
2. It is usually because the other person has inappropriately forced their perspective	C	B	D	A
3. I am willing to compromise in order to get a resolution	B	C	A	D
4. I use many different strategies to convince them of my point of view	D	B	A	C
5. I expect that both of us will have to give and take to get to a satisfactory outcome	C	B	A	D
6. I firmly stake out and clearly explain my position	A	D	B	C
7. I am willing to "lose the battle in order to win the war"	D	A	C	B
8. It is most important to first identify all the things we both agree upon	B	D	C	A
9. I find it difficult to clearly articulate my position and reasons	C	D	B	A
10. I believe it is important to be consistent and firm with my principles	A	D	C	B
11. I avoid using the word "you" because I know it can sound inflammatory	C	B	D	A
12. I will use nonverbal communication or silence as a strategy to convey what I am thinking	D	C	B	A
13. I believe "give and take" is a cop-out	A	D	C	B
14. I feel drained and exhausted	C	B	A	D
15. I feel it is my responsibility to reach a compromise	B	C	D	A
16. I try hard not to hurt the other person's feelings	C	B	D	A
17. It is important to raise all issues immediately and get them in the open	A	B	D	C
18. I believe it is better to anticipate and prevent conflict	C	B	D	A
19. I believe "all is fair in love and war"	D	C	A	B

Now, add up the number of times you circled each letter.

A = _____   B = _____   C = _____   D = _____

Your **DOMINANT** conflict management style is the letter you circled most frequently.
Your **SECONDARY** conflict management style is the next most frequently circled letter.

A = IMPOSING

You have a direct style of communication and have strongly held beliefs and principles. You do not believe it is helpful or even necessary to avoid confrontation and instead believe that, when handled effectively and with maturity, conflict produces better results in the end. You sometimes feel frustrated that others might perceive you as a "bully" but recognize that cannot be helped; instead it is important for you to stick to your principles, articulate them clearly, and convince others of your point of view.

B = SETTLING

You have a direct communication style and are pragmatic in your beliefs and principles. While you do not like conflict, you recognize that at times it is simply unavoidable. In these circumstances, your goal is to find a way to compromise, give and take, and simply reach a solution that is palatable to everyone. As a result, you do not believe there is any benefit to sticking tenaciously to any one perspective and instead believe it is best to listen and understand what others are saying.

C = AVOIDING

You have an indirect communication style and are pragmatic in your beliefs and principles. You believe that, in most cases, conflict can and should be avoided since emotions entangled with issues frequently produces chaos. You have an ability to anticipate conflict and its emotional consequences and recognize it is best (and possible) to prevent it from erupting rather than dealing with it once it has occurred. To this end, you are particularly sensitive to nonverbal communication and are very careful in the words you choose when you speak with others.

D = THWARTING

You have an indirect communication style and have strongly held beliefs and principles. You believe that group cohesion and interpersonal connections are important and work hard to ensure that, in spite of a disagreement, people still get along with one another. You pride yourself on your ability to communicate effectively with different types of people and do not like to have emotion interfere with rational discussion of issues, even if (at times) you do become emotional during a conflict situation.

Now, as a group of individuals with the same dominant style, think about the following questions and share your opinions:

1) In your day-to-day experience, what are some of the most common reasons for conflict with other people?
2) What strategies do you find effective in identifying whether a conflict is serious or not?
3) What tactics do you use to prevent a conflict from escalating further? What tactics do you use to resolve a conflict?
4) If someone were involved in a conflict with you, what tactics would be most effective to use to "win you over"? What tactics would be less effective?

Now, share your group's discussion with members of the other groups.

For Further Reading:

Almost J, Wolff A, Stewart-Pyne A, et al. Managing and mitigating conflict in healthcare teams: an integrative review. *J Adv Nurs.* 2016;72(7):1490–1505.

Fisher R, Ury W. *Getting to Yes: Negotiating an Agreement Without Giving In.* Boston: Penguin Books; 2011.

Gregory P, Austin Z. Conflict in community pharmacy practice: the experience of pharmacists, technicians, and assistants. *Can Pharm J.* 2017;150(1):32–41.

Johansen M. Keeping the peace: conflict management strategies for nurse managers. *Nurs Manag.* 2012;43(2):50–54.

Kfouri J, Lee P. Conflict among colleagues: health care providers feel undertrained and unprepared to manage inevitable workplace conflict. *J Obstet Gynaecol Can.* 2019;41(1):15–20.

Marshall P, Robson R. Preventing and managing conflict: vital pieces in the patient safety puzzle. *Healthcare Quart.* 2005;8:39–44.

Overton A, Lowry A. Conflict management: difficult conversations with difficult people. *Clin Colon Rectal Surg.* 2013;26(4):259–264.

Saltman D, O'Dea N, Kidd M. Conflict management: a primer for doctors in training. *Postgrad Med J.* 2006;82(963):9–12.

Case Study Section

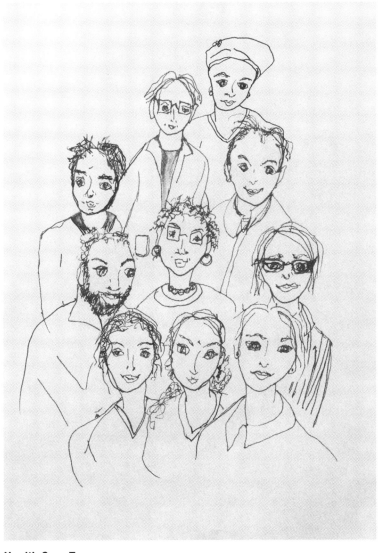

Health Care Team

1 Breaking Bad News to Patients

One of the most challenging parts of any health care professional's work involves communicating difficult, life-altering news to patients and their caregivers. Informing patients of a diagnosis, a prognosis, or the reality of their clinical situation will tax even the most experienced of health care professionals. Unfortunately, formal education rarely sufficiently prepares students for the reality of this experience. As a result, the clinician's own emotional state and response can disproportionately influence the direction of a discussion. In some cases, this might mean clinicians become unnecessarily formal or emotionally distant as a way of protecting themselves. In other cases, clinicians may become so focused on their emotional state that they do not communicate clearly and frankly, sugarcoating the truth as a way of avoiding a strong emotional response from the patient.

Breaking bad news is one of the most challenging yet important roles you will have. As with many challenging and important roles as a clinician, there is no perfect formula that applies in all situations to help guide you through this difficult situation. As has been discussed throughout this book, it is essential to understand yourself, your emotional intelligence, your strengths, your comfort areas, and your potential blind spots toward difficult conversations. Each clinician will approach a difficult conversation differently based on their own self-assessment.

For some clinicians, a structure to guide the delivery of bad news can provide both comfort and a concrete tool for both the self-reflection and self-assessment that are necessary prior to actually speaking to a patient. One of the most widely used mnemonics to support clinicians in such situations is frequently referred to as ABCDE.

A: *Advance preparation.* Ensure you have provided yourself with sufficient time to review and confirm all relevant medical, legal, and social facts and data you need, and give yourself sufficient time to emotionally prepare for this difficult conversation. Trying to break bad news to a patient within a 7-minute appointment is unfair to both the patient and to you. You will need time to gather your thoughts, decompress from other professional stresses, and allow yourself an opportunity to focus on this patient and this patient's needs. Give yourself this time and space rather than simply treat it as yet another brief interview with yet another patient.

B: *Build on your relationship.* Reflect on your previous interactions with the patient and try to identify your patient's preferences for communication and delivery of information. Find ways of connecting this conversation to other parts of the patient's life, recognizing that for many patients, the most impactful parts of receiving bad news relate to the future of their children, their families, and their social networks. Recognize the patient is embedded within a web of complex and meaningful relationships with others and try to anticipate how the bad news you are delivering may echo throughout that network.

C: *Communicate effectively.* All of the theories and skills discussed in this book will play an important role in the delivery of bad news. Determining what the patient already knows, believes, and understands of their situation is a crucial first step. Proceeding at the patient's pace—not yours—is essential. Many health professionals find themselves lapsing into formal medical jargon as a way of avoiding their own emotional response to difficult situations. This is usually not helpful for the patient and will make the conversation more difficult for you. Use clear but plain language. Avoid euphemisms (e.g., tummy problems) but also avoid overly complex language (e.g., gastrointestinal carcinoma). Building on your existing relationship with the patient, you should have a good sense of the level of language that is most appropriate for the patient. One way to achieve this is to listen and use the terms you hear the patient using. Reflecting back using the same language and terminology used by the patient can help you to ensure you are making yourself understood and that you are respecting the patient's needs.

D: *Demonstrate you care.* Of course, nonverbal communication is crucial in the delivery of bad news. Being mindful of your eye contact, body language, tone of voice, and other facets of nonverbal communication is essential. Take your cues from your patient's responses. If they appear uncomfortable with your direct eye contact, shift to indirect eye contact. If they appear to need some appropriate, gentle physical contact (e.g., a light touch on the hand or arm) be mindful of what was discussed in Chapter 7 regarding boundaries and appropriate physical contact as a form of nonverbal communication. A well-intentioned attempt to be comforting can sometimes be misinterpreted, and every individual has different needs regarding physical contact as a form of demonstrating compassion. In some cases, where the clinician feels the need to express concern through physical contact but is worried about boundaries, alternatives such as placing a comforting hand on the back or the top of the chair the patient is sitting in (rather than actually touching the back or shoulder of the patient) may be the most appropriate alternative. Sitting beside, rather than across, from a patient can also be a nonverbal way of demonstrating support and concern that does not require physical contact. Always deliver bad news in a comfortable, acoustically private, seated location.

Among the most important forms of nonverbal communication to consider will be your use of and comfort with silence. In many cases, the news you are delivering to a patient may be a shock. The patient may be in precontemplation or contemplation regarding any significant issues (see Chapters 5 and 6). As a result, patients are going to need time to process the news you are delivering. It is not the time to move quickly from delivering information to expecting the patient to start making decisions. Silence can be awkward but is an essential part of cognitive and emotional processing.

In some cases, patients may demonstrate strong, visible, emotional responses such as tears, gasps, or repeated "no, no, no" verbal patterns. In other cases, patients may cognitively and emotionally process bad news without any or with minimal outward displays of visible emotion. Be prepared for either and do not read too much into the way a patient is responding in real time. A patient who is not crying immediately may weep very soon afterward; be prepared for rapid changes during the course of a conversation. The key will be for you to respond empathetically, supportively, and authentically to whatever emotional responses your patient demonstrates. At a certain point, many patients will simply stop hearing the words you are saying, the verbal communication that tends to dominate clinicians' behaviors. Instead, your tone of voice, the expression on your face, your body language, and other nonverbal communication will be the primary way for you to communicate, share your concern, and demonstrate your support and care for your patient.

E: *Encourage, validate, and support your patient's emotional processing of the information.* As has been discussed throughout this book, human beings are hardwired to process information through emotional filters first before engaging cognitive, logical processing. This will be particularly true in the delivery of bad news. Emotional, rather than logical, processing of bad news will need to take priority, and it is essential that you support and encourage the patient in this process. Your visible or nonverbal discomfort with a patient's strong emotional response will not be helpful; for example, if a patient starts crying, standing up and saying, "Let me give you some privacy right now" and leaving the room will likely send a damaging message to the patient (i.e., that you're uncomfortable or you don't really care). You are the patient's clinician and you need to be there for the patient now, more than ever. Providing too many facts, details, or medical information too quickly, without allowing the patient sufficient time to emotionally process bad news, will be both overwhelming and, ultimately, pointless.

In a health context, bad news is usually described as information that drastically and/or negatively alters a patient's future. Patients receiving bad news often reflect back and will say, "I went to the clinic as one person and left that day as an entirely different one." The clinical activities that are part of health are important in healing, or hurting, a patient. The manner in which these clinical activities are delivered and the communication that accompanies them is just as important.

Consider the following scenario:

Stan and Gwen Johannsen arrive at the clinic. They have been asked to come in today because the team has been working with their son, Sam, who is 12 years old. For several years, Sam has been moody and difficult, losing many of his friends, aggravating his family, and performing very poorly at school. Gwen had brought Sam to the clinic thinking that perhaps attention deficit disorder or some other issue was to blame. Several of their friends and neighbors have children with this condition who responded well to medications, so the Johannsen's had prepared themselves for this. Sam had appointments with the clinic psychologist, social worker, and clinical nurse specialist as well as the physician. Gwen noticed that the simple act of having these appointments seemed to improve Sam's mood and behavior and was pleased.

At today's appointment, there is important news to convey to the family. After a thorough assessment by the team, there is a strong belief that there is no issue with attention deficit disorder. Instead, they believe that Sam is likely experiencing gender dysphoria: Sam believes that, although he is biologically male, he feels like a girl. Sam has secretly been dressing in his sister's clothes and experimenting privately with makeup. The team believes a further assessment and exploration of this is necessary and wants to involve Sam's parents and family to provide support. Through conversation with team members, Sam has indicated no one in the family yet knows; Sam wants the team's help in bringing up the subject with Stan and Gwen.

Whether this scenario warrants the heading bad news is of course debatable. For some, the existence of a possible reason for Sam's negative behavior and attitude may actually be positive insofar as it provides an opportunity to help manage the situation. Depending on the family's opinions and perspectives on the issue, the news regarding Sam's situation may not be a surprise, and it may not be an issue that triggers a strong emotional response.

Recall, however, the general definition of bad news as information that drastically and/or negatively changes a patient's future. Drastic changes are likely ahead for Sam and Sam's family; whether these are negative will depend on a wide variety of different factors influenced by the family's internal dynamics. The team has several key issues to consider, such as how best to communicate the provisional assessment to the parents (e.g., one professional, multiprofessionals, both parents together, one parent at a time, with or without the presence of Sam). First and foremost, Sam's interests, needs, and preferences must be taken into account. For example, Sam may feel that one parent is more supportive than the other and suggests that, while ultimately both parents will be informed, there should be a careful staging of who is told first.

Second, the professionals must reflect on what might work best within the family dynamic based on their previous interactions. Would multiple professionals attending a meeting with one or both parents appear intimidating? Conversely, would a single professional attempting to discuss this with the family become overwhelmed? Previous experience with this family can help identify best (or least worst) alternatives regarding delivery of the provisional assessment.

Third, the team must carefully prepare in advance where the conversation will occur. Finding an acoustically private and safe location for delivery of this news will be important to respect the family's needs. Advance preparation also should include defining what will be communicated. Understandably, the information they are communicating may be emotionally and cognitively overloading for the family or it may not be. Overloading the conversation with medical details, jargon, or asking the family to make immediate decisions will be unfair and unhelpful. What is the most important objective or outcome of this initial conversation, recognizing that there will need to be many more discussions in the future? Is the team simply interested in communicating the provisional assessment and maintaining a good relationship with both parents? Does the team need the parents to make a decision about next steps, permission for further assessment, or other medical and legal issues? Is the team concerned for Sam's safety during this time, and are they planning alternatives to protect their patient while still respecting parental rights? Each of these different issues will require a different communication approach. The team may frankly NOT know which pathway is most likely, and so might need to actually contemplate communication plans for multiple potential directions the conversation may evolve.

Issues of sexuality and gender identity can be extraordinarily sensitive and challenging, and in some cases strong emotional responses can be anticipated and must be planned for. Depending on the preexisting level of relationship between team members and the family, there may need to be high-level security and safety arrangements put in place, just in case one or both parents react very strongly and very negatively. Alternatively, ensuring availability of supports and services for the parents to support their transition from precontemplation to contemplation will also need to be considered.

As can be seen, the process for breaking bad news can be complex and requires considerable advance planning and contingency management for the many different directions that a conversation may go. In a situation such as this, the first sentence—the actual delivery of the news itself—can be the most stressful and impactful, and therefore can benefit greatly from rehearsal and planning over and beyond the setting and advance preparation issues discussed.

The first sentence will set the emotional tone for the conversation and for Sam's coming out process with his family. It is clear that transparency and honesty will be essential. Sam must be present when this conversation occurs in order to not only hear what is being said but also to observe Stan's and Gwen's reactions. What should this first sentence be?

1. "Stan, Gwen, we have some news for you regarding Sam. In our assessment as a team, Sam has told us he is feeling more like a girl than a boy and this is an issue we are going to need to explore further with him and with you both."

2. "Stan, Gwen, thanks for taking the time to meet with us. We know it's been a challenge trying to understand some of Sam's recent difficulties. In our assessment so far, we believe Sam is experiencing a condition called gender dysphoria."

3. "Stan, Gwen, let's get straight to the point. In the team's assessment of Sam over the last few weeks it's become increasingly clear that he is feeling considerable emotional distress and pain over his emotions regarding his gender. To put it plainly, Sam feels—and we agree—that he is a girl trapped in a boy's body."

4. "Stan, Gwen, the team is doing our best to help Sam understand what's happening. We have a few questions for you: Have you ever noticed or thought at all about how Sam experiences life being a boy?"

Clearly there is no single right or best way to approach this situation. Breaking news such as this to a parent requires nuance and continuous course correction during a conversation. Each of the previous alternatives have advantages and disadvantages.

1. This alternative provides the parents with a clear and unambiguous assessment of the situation without use of medical jargon. For some parents, it may be too harsh and too direct. For others, the clarity of the statement would be appreciated. It is respectful in its tone and does not try to use slang or mask the team's discomfort with inappropriate humor.

2. For some parents, the use of a medical term such as *gender dysphoria* may actually be helpful. It is not jargon, per se, but instead a diagnostic term that may reassure the parents that the team is treating this seriously and with respect. Some parents may not immediately understand what is meant by this term, so further clarification and explaining may be needed. However, by beginning with a clear diagnostic label rather than immediately talking about Sam's comfort as a boy or a girl, this may more gradually introduce the parents to the idea that this is indeed a medical issue that requires medical attention and support.

3. For some, this sentence may appear too casual or almost dismissive. The state-ment: "a girl trapped in a boy's body" almost sounds like a punch line of a joke and may be interpreted by some parents as disrespectful. For other parents, however, this crystallization of the issue may help them immediately understand what is going on and may not be interpreted by them as insulting. Importantly, in this option, "and we agree" has been used, which can be seen as a way of providing protection and medical credibility to Sam's perceptions. In some cases, this may help Sam feel better and less isolated, and may also provide the parents with reassurance that this is a medically recognized and accepted experience.

4. This approach represents an attempt to gradually elicit or draw out more in-formation from the parents. It also provides a subtle way of signaling to both parents the future direction of the conversation before specific diagnostic terms are used and labels applied. As a result, this gradualist approach may allow parents time to anticipate and emotionally prepare for the moment when the real diagnosis or assessment is stated out loud, which can provide them with a few much needed moments to gather their thoughts and better manage their emotional response.

Breaking difficult or bad news is, in essence, a series of difficult choices and decisions that must be made, and an exercise in planning multiple different pathways a conversation may evolve. Clinicians must anticipate the unanticipated, develop methods for monitoring verbal and nonverbal responses, and be ready to recalibrate the conversation accordingly. In most cases, breaking bad news is difficult because there is no clear, right way to do it. None of the four options presented really seems appropriate or correct, yet all of them have some element of value.

What then are the take-home messages for clinicians regarding breaking bad news?

- Preparation is crucial. You will face a series of conversational choices that will, in most cases, require you to rehearse, anticipate, and make a contingency plan. Allow yourself the time and space to do this preparation rather than believe you can just wing it.

- Remember the principles of the mnemonic ABCDE, which provide you with im-portant strategies and techniques to enhance your comfort in communicating bad news.

- Authenticity is essential. Being psychologically present means turning off your phone, putting away distractions, and conveying verbally and nonverbally to the patient that you are there for them and only them during this difficult time.

- The first sentence (or the sentence in which the bad news is actually conveyed) is of crucial significance and will set the template for not only the future direction of the conversation but of the relationship as a whole.

- The first sentence is not enough. Anticipating what your patient and the family might need and having ready access to suggestions, resources, and ideas (e.g., further education, mentorship, peer support groups, another appointment) are essential. Breaking bad news introduces important responsibilities for not abandoning patients and leaving them on their own.

Of all the crucial conversations health professionals have with patients, bad news is among the most important and the most difficult. Leveraging your best communication skills in this most challenging of situations is essential to providing the kind of care and support patients deserve and need.

Interested in Learning More?

Buckman R. *How to Break Bad News.* Baltimore: Johns Hopkins University Press; 1992.

Guneri P, Epstein J, Botto R. Breaking bad news in a dental care setting. *J Am Dent Assoc.* 2013;144(4):381–386.

Monden K, Gentry L, Cox T. Delivering bad news to patients. *Proc (Bayl Univ Med Cent).* 2016;29(1):101–102.

Quinn-Rosenzweig M. Breaking bad news: a guide for effective and empathetic communication. *Nurse Pract.* 2012;37(2):1–4.

CASE

2

Communicating for Patient Safety

"First, do no harm" epitomizes the ethical obligation of all health care professionals. Although health care frequently requires balancing potential risks and benefits, all health care professionals must recognize that patient safety is central and essential to practice.

The World Health Organization (WHO) defines patient safety incidents as events or circumstances that could have resulted, or did result, in unnecessary or avoidable harm to a patient. Patient safety incidents are further subdivided into two types: those that actually reached the patient and those that did not. **Harmful incidents** are patient safety incidents that result in actual harm. This term replaces previous terminology such as *adverse events* or *sentinel events*. **No-harm incidents** are patient safety incidents that reach a patient but do not result in any discernable, observable, or measureable harm. A **near miss** is a patient safety incident that does not reach the patient. This term replaces the previously used *close call*. For example, soundalike drug names may sometimes cause patient safety incidents. Consider the drug name Losec, a proprietary version of the medication omeprazole used for gastrointestinal conditions. Now consider the drug name Lasix, a proprietary version of the medication furosemide, which is used as a diuretic, most often to help control blood pressure. When spoken quickly, even by native English speakers, these two names can be confused with one another and a patient safety incident might occur. If the patient requires Losec, but due to miscommunication receives Lasix instead, several outcomes may result. If the patient receives the wrong drug from a nurse or pharmacist but recognizes that it is wrong and alerts the professional before actually taking the drug, it would be a no-harm incident. If, in contrast, the patient did not recognize the wrong drug, took it, then suffered harm because blood pressure was affected by the incorrectly administered dose of Lasix, it would be a harmful incident. Finally, if a pharmacist dispensed Lasix instead of Losec, but a nurse detected this and fixed it before it reached the patient, it would be a near miss.

There is current controversy regarding the use of *incident* versus *error* to describe patient safety events. Increasingly, the term *incident* is recommended because patient safety issues usually result from a complex interplay of factors rather than a single failure, mistake, or lapse. It is a series of small problems or failures (referred to as a cascade) that most often results in problems. For example, in the previously mentioned case, perhaps the miscommunication of Lasix and Losec occurred because workload was too high, AND there were distractions in the environment during communication, AND the drugs were stored adjacent to each other, AND one practitioner had a specific accent,

AND another practitioner had a head cold and had slightly plugged ears, etc. The accumulation of all of these seemingly unrelated issues converges in a moment to trigger the incident rather than being a simplistic single cause. Further, the word *error* sometimes can be misunderstood to mean *negligence*, *substandard*, or *inattentive*, when in fact the root cause is more complex and multifactorial. The use of a value-laden term such as *error* may also create a punitive culture or environment in which individuals fear honest disclosure and avoid discussing what happened, thereby inhibiting future learning and system quality assurance.

Patient safety relies heavily on honest, transparent, and open reporting as a vehicle for quality improvement and prevention of future incidents. As a result, it is essential that all health care providers, particularly those involved in a patient safety incident, feel supported and comfortable in honest disclosure. Health care professionals are generally well-intentioned people who want to heal, not harm. It is natural that they might feel sad, guilty, or ashamed following exposure of a patient safety incident; this can erode confidence and self-esteem and be emotionally and cognitively draining as the incident is played and replayed in their mind. Disclosure and apology can help, but so too can working diligently to understand root causes to improve quality systems to prevent similar incidents from occurring again. It is important for employers, managers, and peers to provide support, discourage idle gossip or speculation, and avoid assigning blame or isolating individuals involved in patient safety incidents. Instead, we all have a responsibility to create a culture of safety that allows individuals to feel comfortable reporting, learning from, and educating others about the causes and consequences of incidents.

Harmful patient safety incidents must always be disclosed to patients and discussed within the practice. No-harm incidents are generally disclosed and discussed. Near misses may not need to be disclosed to patients (unless there is an ongoing safety risk) but must be reported and discussed internally to ensure they do not become harmful incidents in the future.

Structured communication has been identified as an important tool to enhance quality and improve patient safety. A widely used structured communication tool is SBAR, an initialism for *situation*, *background*, *assessment*, and *recommendation*. SBAR has been demonstrated to improve patient outcomes, enhance interprofessional collaboration, and support patient safety. SBAR was first developed and used in the U.S. military, particularly on nuclear-powered submarines. Subsequently, it was used in the aviation industry, and more recently, it has been adopted across many health care organizations. The main goal of SBAR is to reduce communication problems affecting patient safety that are attributable to seemingly simple differences in communication styles between health care professionals.

From a patient safety perspective, SBAR reduces variability, enhances efficiency, and encourages consistency and promptness in communication because of its standardized, structured format. It also helps ensure that key pieces of information are not overlooked or forgotten, or that some information is disproportionately emphasized or overdiscussed at the expense of other pieces of important information.

Situation: When communicating in complex, interruption-driven, and high-stress environments (such as health care), there is a strong need for clarity and concision. The situation part of SBAR is important because it provides a focused and concise description of what is going on and why health care professionals are actually needed. Learning to clearly state a problem—rather than simply reporting emotions, feelings, or experiences—is essential. Insofar as these emotions, feelings, or experiences are in fact a part of the problem, they should of course be reported; however, in practice, the emphasis in situation is on medical, objectively verifiable details relevant to immediate needs. If you are not familiar to or known to the person you are communicating with, it is equally essential to introduce yourself and to provide your title and your role. This should be done whether you are meeting face to face, on the telephone, virtually, or in writing (i.e., documenting in a chart or sending a note or email to another clinician). It wastes time and causes confusion if partners in a conversation do not know who the other is. Key pieces of patient-specific information to communicate in the situation include the patient's name, age, sex, and current chief complaint. Finally, it is important to provide a succinct status update about the patient's current condition (e.g., "experiencing difficulty breathing right now"). Concision is important in presenting the situation; experienced practitioners can deliver a situation report in less than 20 seconds, which significantly enhances efficiency and clarity of communication.

Background: The next step in the SBAR process focuses on background. The objective here is to identify and provide relevant medical details associated with the current chief complaint. Details here may include past medical history, medications, relevant social history, allergies and intolerances, most recent laboratory test results, most recent vital signs, and/or vital signs outside of normal or expected parameters, etc. It is essential to prepare to deliver this background section of the conversation; do not waste precious time actively flipping through a patient's chart or toggling through computer screens while in the middle of the conversation. This wastes everyone's time and gives the impression of lack of preparedness. Instead, collect and organize relevant background information before engaging in a conversation to enhance quality, concision, and efficiency of communication.

Assessment: This third stage of the SBAR process allows the health care professional to exercise professional judgment in interpreting the situation and background. An assessment need not be definitive and certain; in many cases, assessments are nothing more than initial suspicions or hunches. If this is the case, however, it is essential to communicate this so the receiver of communication does not misinterpret or assume you are more confident of your assessment than you actually are. Initial assessments provide a useful starting point for further investigations and discussion, but must be appropriately contextualized so as not to potentially lead to patient safety incidents. Finding the right balance between educated hunches and outright guesswork or speculation can be challenging; your intuition and experience can be valuable in deciding what to say during the assessment, but it must be grounded in both your clinical self-confidence and best evidence-informed judgment.

Recommendation: The recommendation stage of SBAR is in many ways the most important and difficult because it requires the rapid integration of a large amount of patient-specific clinical data, professional experience and judgment, and evidence regarding treatment options. Recommendations should be clear and prioritized so the listener understands what you believe are priorities. Some novice practitioners try to avoid making decisions or taking responsibility by simply providing a series of options with no indication of which is most important or impactful. This style of communication is profoundly unhelpful and should be avoided. Instead, a systematic list in order of priority of what should be done in what sequence (and a brief explanation of why) should be used. Other clinicians may or may not agree with this list or make other decisions, but at least they will know and respect your thinking and clinical problem-solving process. Explicit statements about what is required, how urgent, and what next steps or actions should be taken should be the structure of the recommendation section.

As can be seen, the SBAR approach favors a certain kind of clinician, the problem-oriented rather than story-oriented individual. Although SBAR may or may not be appropriate in all health care contexts, it is still an essential communication skill to acquire and be able to use, whether or not you are problem or story oriented in your clinical reasoning.

Consider the following case:

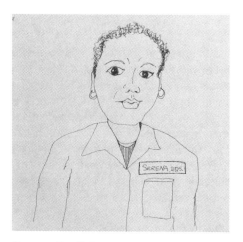

Serena, Dentist

Serena is a community dentist. Today, her patient Chantal Cummins has come into the practice complaining of an extremely sore tooth and sharp, shooting pain. Upon investigation, Serena determines there is damage to the tooth itself and a full extraction and root canal procedure will be required. Serena consults the treatment guidelines and notes that antibiotic prophylaxis prior to the procedure does not appear necessary because Chantal has no risk factors. She has no listed allergies and is currently being treated for asthma that is not very well controlled. To help manage the pain prior to the surgery, Serena recommends Chantal use an over-the-counter analgesic such as acetaminophen as needed. Chantal goes home; her daughter has some ibuprofen that she uses for menstrual cramps and offers them to Chantal to control the dental pain. Chantal takes several doses within 8 hours to deal with the pain but notices increased shortness of breath and wheezing that alarms her. She goes to the pharmacy to ask what to do and the pharmacist (Binoo) contacts Serena.

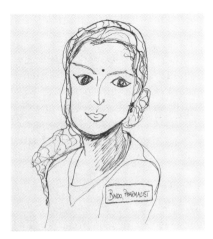

Binoo, Pharmacist

Binoo:	Hello, Dr. McGundy? This is Binoo the pharmacist at Community Drug Store down the street from you. *[Note: Introduce name, role, and location.]*
Serena:	Yes, hello, Binoo—please, call me Serena. What can I do for you?
Binoo:	Your patent Ms. Cummins is here with me right now.
Serena:	Oh, is she asking you about painkillers? I'd suggested she get some acetaminophen to help with her tooth pain.
Binoo:	She's here because she went home and took some of her ibuprofen and now she's having difficulty breathing without her salbutamol inhaler and of course is very concerned and upset. *[Situation]*
Serena:	Oh no.
Binoo:	When she went home, her daughter gave her some ibuprofen tablets to take for the pain. As best as I can tell, she took 600 mg every 3 hours for three doses, a total of 1800 mg. She's had recent trouble with her asthma, with two flare-ups and visits to the emergency department in the last month alone. They've told her to up the dose of salbutamol and that worked. This time before she went back to the emergency department, she came to see me to see if that would work. *[Background]*
Serena:	What happened?
Binoo:	Best as I can tell, that large dose of ibuprofen may have triggered bronchospasm since she is quite vulnerable right now. Before calling you, I suggested she take the extra doses of salbutamol. That's worked already and she is breathing easier and is calming down. She will likely need to take a few more additional doses of the salbutamol to keep ahead of things and to keep her breathing stable. However, her tooth pain is quite severe. Those high doses of ibuprofen didn't do the job. *[Assessment]*

Serena: That's good to know. I'm glad her breathing is stabilizing.

Binoo: She should be okay. You may want to make a note that she should not take ibuprofen or any NSAID medication because of her asthma. I think she just assumed that ibuprofen and acetaminophen were the same thing. I've let her know they're not and to avoid all NSAIDs in the future. For now, however, she'll need something stronger for her tooth pain. I noticed she's taken acetaminophen with codeine in the past and that's helped, but you'll need to give me a prescription of course. *[Recommendation]*

Serena: Yes, you're right. That's okay with her asthma?

Binoo: She's taken it before for a short period of time with no difficulties.

Serena: Okay, I'm just on my way home anyway, so I will drop it off for you now and see Ms. Cummins while I'm there. I'll be over in less than 5 minutes. Thanks for calling!

When spoken, this entire conversation would take less than 90 seconds, and yet an enormous amount of critical patient safety information was discussed in a concise and focused manner. The advantage of SBAR is in providing a structure to guide conversation efficiently while ensuring critical pieces of information are not overlooked.

SBAR can also be used in situations where patient safety incidents have not yet occurred, but where a practitioner has concerns and wants to communicate them to other team members.

Consider the following case:

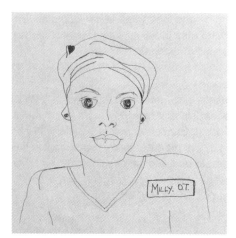
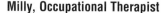

Milly, Occupational Therapist

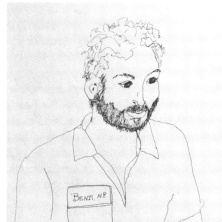

Benji, Nurse Practitioner

Milly, the occupational therapist, is working with Mr. Bains, a recently widowed 65-year-old man with a variety of health-related issues. He has arthritis, a recent ostomy, early symptoms of Parkinson disease, and he is also losing his vision due to macular degeneration. He lives alone in a suburban house, with no family members or friends close by. Given his social isolation,

Milly has been asked to meet with him to discuss activities of daily living associated with navigating a large suburban house with stairs. In conversation, Milly notes that he appears very down: He does not maintain eye contact, mumbles frequently, does not express any interest, sighs frequently, and occasionally interjects hopeless thoughts such as "What's the point?" and "No one cares." Milly suspects that Mr. Bains may be suffering from depression and is concerned for his safety, but she recognizes this diagnosis is beyond her scope of practice. She needs to connect with Mr. Bains' primary care provider Benji, the nurse practitioner, to discuss this further.

Both Milly and Benji are busy professionals juggling multiple responsibilities. Milly has identified a potential issue that, in her professional judgment, warrants further exploration and investigation. The SBAR technique can be a useful way of structuring the conversation to enhance clarity and focus. Prior to the conversation with Benji, Milly reviews Mr. Bains's chart to gather relevant information for efficient presentation. Milly sees Benji in a corridor in the practice and recognizes this is an important opportunity to alert him to her concerns regarding Mr. Bains through a face-to-face hallway conversation.

Milly:	Benji, do you have a few moments? I wanted to speak with you about your patient Mr. Bains.
Benji:	Yeah, sure. I'm just on my way to a family meeting but I have a minute or two. What's up?
Milly:	I just met with Mr Bains. I'm concerned about his emotional and psychological status. I see in the chart that he has not seen a counselor or psychologist since his wife died, and I think this might be an issue we need to deal with sooner rather than later. *[Situation]*
Benji:	Hmm. I haven't seen him in a few weeks but don't recall that issue the last time he came in.
Milly:	He's juggling a lot. His arthritis seems to be flaring and he is having difficulty doing simple things like opening jars right now. Worse, he is struggling to manage his ostomy, and this is making him even more socially isolated than usual. It's also dawning on him that his Parkinson disease is getting worse and he told me he doesn't know how he is going to cope on his own with all of this. *[Background—only relevant information for current discussion, not a full or comprehensive presentation of patient's history.]*
Benji:	Poor guy. That's awful.
Milly:	I think he's just coming to terms now with his wife's death and how he has no one else close by to help him anymore. He is sounding hopeless and resigned to his future, and I wonder if he might be depressed or anxious. *[Assessment]*
Benji:	That would make sense.

Milly: I think you should meet with him as soon as possible. He's here now, so if you can find some time to check in that would be great. He might need a referral to a counselor or social worker. Here's the referral form and list of consultants we've used before that are close to where he lives. I think even if you just drop by now to say hello, that would perk him up a lot. He really connects to you. *[Recommendation]*

Benji: Okay, let's go say hello now. Thanks for the form and the list of consultants. That'll save me a few minutes, and maybe I can get this paperwork done now so he doesn't need to wait too long. Really appreciate this. Thanks, Milly!

In summary, patient safety is the first and most important job of every health professional. Effective communication is crucial for patient safety. Structured communication such as SBAR can provide a common foundation across teams and diverse health professionals to ensure critical information is communicated clearly, effectively, and efficiently and that patients are safeguarded.

Interested in Learning More?

Beckett C, Kipnis G. Collaborative communication: integrating SBAR to improve quality/patient safety outcomes. *J Healthc Qual.* 2009;31(5):19–28.

Dunsford J. Structured communication: improving patient safety with SBAR. *Nurs Womens Health.* 2009;13(5):384–390.

Shahid S, Thomas S. Situation, background, assessment, recommendation (SBAR) communication tool for handoff in health care—a narrative review. *Saf Health.* 2018;4(7).

Tews M, Liu J, Treat R. Situation-background-assessment-recommendation (SBAR) and emergency medicine residents' learning of case presentation skills. *J Grad Med Educ.* 2012;4(3):370–373.

Woodhall L, Vertacnik L, McLaughlin M. Implementation of the SBAR communication technique in a tertiary centre. *J Emerg Nurs.* 2008;34(4):314–317.

3 | Communicating When Language May Be a Barrier

In our increasingly multicultural and multilingual communities, there may be many circumstances where verbal communication may be challenging due to barriers experienced by both English and non-English speakers alike. Importantly, many people who speak English as a second, third, or fourth language have no difficulty at all communicating in English. Conversely, those who speak only English may sometimes have difficulty communicating with other English speakers due to accents, word choice, or pattern of speech. A language barrier is, by definition, a two-way street. Both people in the conversation may struggle and find it difficult trying to communicate with each other, and consequently, both need to adjust and adapt their delivery and receipt of communication in order to move forward.

Each interaction between people is unique, but certain principles regarding verbal communication across language barriers can be useful to consider.

Pronounce your words correctly, but do not exaggerate or overemphasize them. Depending on the region in which you learned to speak English, certain words may commonly be pronounced differently. For example, those who grew up in the Canadian city of Toronto sometimes pronounce their hometown as "Trawno". In some places, the word *nuclear* is pronounced "nucular," and in other places the term *y'all* connotes a collection of individuals. In all three cases, those from that geographical area will likely understand what was meant, but the mispronunciation can cause confusion and irritation for others (native and non-native English speakers alike). Pronouncing words carefully, as they were intended, rather than lapsing into verbal shortcuts can enhance understanding and reduce the effects of a language barrier. Importantly, overexaggerated pronunciation can be equally unhelpful. Saying, "To-RON-to" in an overly enunciated tone begins to sound insulting or dismissive, and can introduce another kind of barrier into interpersonal communication.

Do not simply speak louder to compensate. A language barrier is not a physical ability limitation. Simply saying the same thing louder will not help another person understand your intention more clearly, and in some cases will actually appear as an insult. Equally important, of course, is that you do not speak too quietly. A moderate volume and a clear tone are important, but by themselves may not be sufficient to address all language-related communication barriers.

Allow your face to be fully visible. Experienced non-native English speakers acquire an impressive ability to derive vocabulary and context by integrating watching and listening. Even if they do not understand every word that is spoken, by observing lips and faces, they may be able to piece together more of the conversation. In a complex and nuanced way, observing lips can help one to decipher words, and observing faces can help fill in the blanks with respect to tone, intensity, and meaning of conversations. Looking downward, talking into a clipboard or table computer, or holding your hands over your face can deprive the other person of these important visual cues that can help address a language-related barrier.

Minimize use of slang contractions. The enormous flexibility of the English language can sometimes be a handicap, even for native English speakers. For example, the ability to run together words into a single sound bite can cause confusion. Think of the New Yorker who might say "fuggedaboutit" almost as one word rather than "forget about it." Similarly, many native English speakers casually say "djwanna?" instead of "do you want to?" These elided verbal contractions can be very confusing and worsen language barriers.

Use the simplest and clearest words possible. Complex terminology can be a barrier for both native and non-native English speakers. Medical terminology such as *gastrointestinal* or *psychomotor* will be a barrier for many. Using the simplest but most important term to convey your meaning will help minimize verbal language barriers in many case.

Be conscious of the frequency with which you use fillers such as "uh" or "hmm." Unconscious use of filler words is common in English, but many of these filler words can sound similar to real words (e.g., "hmm" can be mistaken for "him"). Some fillers are also confusingly similar: Think of how acoustically or aurally similar "uh-huh" and "uh-uh" are—fillers that are completely opposite to one another. If you mean "uh-huh," simply say "yes" to avoid a language barrier or misunderstanding.

Be conscious that there are many different types of English spoken around the world. Considering the reach of the English language, it is not a surprise that there are many variations of it, so that even native English speakers may not understand one another all the time. For example, in Caribbean English, it is not uncommon to pronounce the word *ask* as "aks," or use regional colloquialisms such as "botheration" when describing someone who bothers you. Often, context can help us to decipher meaning correctly, but equally important, respecting the full range of English that exist is important.

Be polite and listen before you speak. Many people who are comfortable speaking with one another fall into the habit of finishing each other's sentences. Whether this is charming and comforting, or irritating and annoying, will be up to you. Where language barriers exist, this speech pattern can be profoundly unhelpful. Indeed, some non-native English speakers will be simultaneously listening and translating what you are saying, and will therefore need time to do so. An interruption-driven speaking pattern is not only rude, but it can also be overwhelming.

Be patient and try. Sincere efforts to understand one another are most frequently rewarded by not only a better level of communication but also by a mutual sense of respect and warmth between people. Remember, a communication barrier works both ways, and both individuals must compromise and find ways of navigating it together.

Techniques such as these may be helpful in supporting better communication in challenging situations where individuals do not speak the same language. Of course, it is essential to also be attentive to nonverbal cues to gauge how effectively your messages are being received and how they are being interpreted, and to recalibrate your delivery as required.

Consider the following situation:

A new patient to your clinic is being seen by a team member. This individual speaks limited English. As best as the triage nurse can tell, the patient is suffering from intense, cyclical abdominal pain but no clear cause has yet been identified. Think about the following conversation and how effective it might be in terms of helping this patient who is in pain (and therefore experiencing both physical and psychological distress) and who cannot communicate fully in the language used by the health care professional.

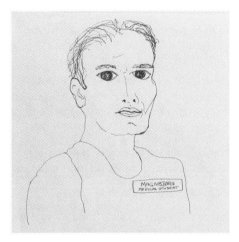

Magnbjorg, Third-Year Student

Magnbjorg (a student in 3rd year): Hello, Mr. Cuellar? (Note: He pronounces it "queller.")

Patient: Yes. Cuellar. (Note: He pronounces it "quay-ar.")

Magnbjorg: Okay. My name is Magnbjorg, I'm going to be looking after you today. I just need to ask you a few questions. Would that be okay?

Mr. Cuellar: Ma . . . Manye?

Magnbjorg: Yes, I'm Magnbjorg. So, I can ask you some questions?

Mr. Cuellar: (no verbal response, but patient further furrows brow, squints eyes, and tilts head slightly to the side)

Magnbjorg: Okay, let's go ahead. (pause, then slightly louder) I said, let's go ahead, okay?

Mr. Cuellar: Okay? (grimacing and shaking head slightly)

Magnbjorg: (getting frustrated, sighing audibly and drooping shoulders) Okay. So I see here you are having some abdominal pain? Can you tell me more about it?

Mr. Cuellar:	(no verbal response, but shifts back in seat slightly, looking quizzical, sighing heavily, slight frown on mouth)
Magnbjorg:	(with a forced smile) Pain? You're having abdominal pain? How severe is it? (starts pointing vigorously at patient's abdomen)
Mr. Cuellar:	Oh. (starts removing shirt)
Magnbjorg:	(a bit panicked now) No, no, you don't need to take your shirt off yet. I just need to ask . . . your abdominal pain? How severe is it? When did it start?
Mr. Cuellar:	(still removing shirt)
Magnbjorg:	(moves in to stop patient from unbuttoning shirt)
Mr. Cuellar:	(puzzled and surprised facial expression) No?
Magnbjorg:	(firmly with a stern, paternalistic face) No, not yet, I need to ask you some questions first. (then louder) I need to ask you some questions first. Sir, what language do you speak? (pause, then louder, and overly enunciated) What language do you speak? Spanish? Italian?
Mr. Cuellar:	(some relief despite the pain he is currently experiencing, happy to finally be able understand something) No, no. Portugal.
Magnbjorg:	Ah, Portuguese! Hola! Como esta usted?
Mr. Cuellar:	(smiling slightly, finding this ham-fisted attempt at communication vaguely humorous) Muy bien. But no, not Española. Portuguese.
Magnbjorg:	(somewhat self-satisfied at belief that communication has finally occurred) Oh, okay. We don't have one of those interpreters here. Let's just skip the questions, go ahead and take your shirt off now and let me see if I can figure out what's going on here.
Mr. Cuellar:	(not verbally responding, now just getting tired of Magnbjorg)
Magnbjorg:	Shirt? (motions to unbutton and remove) Take off.
Mr. Cuellar:	(resigned and still in pain) Oh, okay.

Clearly, this is not the most effective interaction between patient and health care professional. Magnbjorg (whose family of origin is Norwegian) has tried to follow a systematic approach to patient care but was frustrated by a lack of responsiveness from the patient, and as a result, has concluded the only way forward is to move directly to physical assessment. Unfortunately, this means enormous amounts of vital information (e.g., onset and duration of pain symptoms, severity of pain, what has been tried to relieve the pain) will go unasked and unanswered, which may fundamentally and negatively influence the assessment, diagnosis, and treatment. The patient is also feeling overwhelmed. He already is in pain and in distress, but now the fear associated with not being able to understand and communicate during this difficult time will amplify his physical symptoms considerably.

What are some things that Magnbjorg should have done to enhance the conversation and improve the flow of communication? If the student had followed some of the ideas presented at the beginning of this chapter, a very different interaction may have evolved. First and prior to even meeting the patient, it would have been helpful if the triage nurse had specifically communicated to Magnbjorg (in person or by documenting in the chart) the language issues faced by Mr. Cuellar. Anticipating and planning for a conversation in such a situation can be very helpful, rather than being caught off guard and having to respond rapidly in real time.

Had Magnbjorg been aware of the language issue, and perhaps specifically been made aware that Mr. Cuellar is a Portuguese speaker, he might have been able to identify an interpreter to support the interview or (if no one was available) downloaded a series of Portuguese phrases from the Internet or use Google Translate to enhance the conversation. In such a case, Magnbjorg could ask his questions in Portuguese, and Mr. Cuellar could respond in English or nonverbally. Importantly, this shifts the center of the conversation to Mr. Cuellar and gives him options for communicating, rather than resting all conversational control in Magnbjorg's hands. Although this model of communication is undoubtedly slow, time consuming, and not perfect, it is clearly more effective than the conversational pattern we saw.

Being able to read a few phrases in the patient's own language can be incredibly comforting for a patient in distress, and signifies both respect and a sincere attempt to help the patient. In such situations, it will likely not be possible to undertake the same level of comprehensive assessment as might be possible with a fluent English speaker. Magnbjorg will need to exercise his clinical judgment to determine what are the most essential questions he needs to ask and to find ways of communicating. Increasingly, many practitioners will rely on freely available Web-based software (e.g., Google Translate) and, rather than ask questions, bring the patient to the computer and type in questions, allowing the patient to type out responses in his or her own language. Simply because a person does not speak fluent English does not mean he or she is unfamiliar with the Internet or how to use a computer. Using technology to intermediate a conversation when a live translator is not available is also an option to consider.

Let's rewind this conversation and try to incorporate some of the ideas in this chapter.

Magnbjorg: Hello, Mr. Cuellar?

Mr. Cuellar: Yes. Cuellar.

Magnbjorg: (translated from Portuguese, reading from tablet) Thank you, Mr. Cuellar. (Note: He pronounces it "quay-ar") How are you?

Mr. Cuellar: (surprised and relieved) Portuguese!

Magnbjorg: (translated from Portuguese, reading from tablet) I'm sorry I cannot speak Portuguese, but we can use this computer and together try to speak. Is that okay?

Mr. Cullar: (in English) Yes, yes, okay. Thank you.

Magnbjorg: (translated from Portuguese, reading from tablet) I'm sorry I will need to speak slowly. Show me where you are in pain.

Mr. Cuellar: (points to the right of navel, but then using palm does circular sweeping gestures all around the abdomen)

Magnbjorg: (taking a moment to type into tablet to translate) Does it hurt here (pointing to right of navel) or does it hurt everywhere in this area (making circular motion around abdomen)?

Mr. Cuellar: (holds up two digits to signify both)

Magnbjorg: (taking a moment to type into tablet to translate) When did the pain start today? (points to wrist watch)

Mr. Cuellar: (points to 6 on the watch face)

Magnbjorg: 6 AM this morning? (taking a moment to type into tablet to translate then repeats in Portuguese)

Mr. Cuellar: Yes, morning.

Magnbjorg: (in English) Were you sleeping? (makes a sleeping gesture with hands and head)

Mr. Cuellar: Yes, sleeping. *Depois senti dor.* (Portuguese for "then I felt pain" and simulates sharp pain grimace with face)

Magnbjorg: (muttering to self, while documenting in patient chart) Sudden onset of pain first thing this morning. (takes a moment to type into tablet to translate) How much pain are you feeling right now?

Mr. Cuellar: (does not speak, but grimaces and winces to indicate he is experiencing a great deal of pain right now)

As can be seen, this format of conversation, although not optimal, is certainly preferred to the previous format. It is taking a long time to gather information from the patient, and requires the health care professional to be constantly vigilant and interpret the patient's nonverbal cues. The entire conversation will be longer and more exhausting for both the patient and the practitioner, but in the end, they will exchange much more information because both parties have made a concerted effort to try to communicate as best as possible under the circumstances.

In some cases, it may be possible to involve a professional interpreter or a family member who can act as an intermediary between the patient and the health care professional. One of the major reasons for substandard health care for recent immigrants or those who do not speak English is the failure of health care professionals to take the time to learn how to work with interpreters to make sure best possible communication is occurring. When working with an interpreter, it is useful to consider the following points:

Ascertain the interpreter's qualifications. If a trained professional interpreter is available, they will likely need no instructions or reminders about confidentiality or the process of triadic (i.e., three-way) patient interviewing. They will also be capable of culturally interpreting the patient's meaning and intentions, not simply their words, and this can save time and prevent misunderstanding. If a nonprofessional, such as a hospital employee or volunteer in the department, is acting as an interpreter, it will be necessary to explain this process more thoroughly and, in particular, issues related to confidentiality and respect.

Prior to meeting with the patient, it may be useful to brief the interpreter with the information you already have, and how you wish to proceed during the interaction. Remember that many non–health care professionals may not be familiar or comfortable with the patient–practitioner interview process, particularly in acute situations. In addition, family members working as interpreters may also have their own emotions or concerns they are grappling with, and consequently, this may have an impact on the nature and quality of the interaction. Again, a professional interpreter will have greater skills to manage these issues and should be relied on if available.

During the actual interview and interactions with the patient, face and speak directly to the patient so you can observe nonverbal responses yourself. The interpreter should translate exactly what is said by both parties rather than assuming the patient (or the professional) might not understand what is being communicated. Again, when family members are relied on to provide translation they may, in a well-intentioned way, edit what is being said. Reminding family members of the importance of a full and accurate translation of everything being said will be important.

Use brief sentences wherever possible to allow the interview to proceed more quickly. Complex sentences or compound phrases involving multiple clauses connected by "and" or "or" are simply more difficult to translate and will take more time.

Be alert to signs that information is not being translated accurately. For example, if the patient provides a long response to a question and there is verbal interaction between interpreter and patient, and the only thing you hear from the interpreter is "fine," this suggests something may have been edited. It is appropriate and necessary to ask the interpreter for further clarification and specific details of what transpired before "fine" was given as the answer.

Simply because an interpreter is present, do not overlook nonverbal communication projected by the patient. This will continue to be an important source of information that you can translate and interpret for yourself with no intermediary required. It can also provide an important second check on the translation. If the interpreter's translation does not align with your observations and assessment of nonverbal messages and cues, ask further questions.

Every conversation is as unique as the two people involved. The techniques Magnbjorg used in this scenario may or may not work with other patients. The key is to simply try as many different ways as possible to facilitate understanding and communication by leveraging technology, use of nonverbal cues, hand gestures, pantomime, drawings, or whatever tools you have available. In the first scenario, Magnbjorg concluded that he could not communicate with the patient and was willing to simply proceed to the physical examination without conversation. In the process, he missed out on vital information that could have enhanced the quality of the assessment and the treatment outcomes for the patient. Avoiding the tendency to quickly assume a conversation is not possible and being willing to invest the time and energy required to be creative in finding alternative ways of communicating is essential. Not only will it assist you in your work as a practitioner, but also it will help build your relationship with the patient.

Interested in Learning More?

Alborn J, McKinney K. Use of and interaction with medical interpreters. *Am J Health Syst Pharm.* 2014;71(12):1044–1048.

Greyu B, Donaldson H. Why do we not use trained interpreters for all patients with limited English proficiency? Is there a place for using family members? *Aust J Prim Health.* 2011;17: 240–249.

Hadziabdic E, Hjelm K. Working with interpreters: practical advice for use of an interpreter in healthcare. *Int J Evid Based Healthc.* 2013;11(1):69–76.

Juckett G, Unger K. Appropriate use of medical interpreters. *Am Fam Physician* 2014;90(7): 476–480.

Karliner L, Jacobs E, Chen A, Mutha S. Do professional interpreters improve clinical care for patients with limited English proficiency? A systematic review of the literature. *Health Serv Res.* 2007;42(2):727–254.

Ku L, Flores G. Pay now or pay later: providing interpreter services in health care. *Health Aff (Millwood).* 2005;24(2):435–444.

4

Communication and Cognitive Bias

Cognitive bias is one of the most important and underrecognized factors influencing interprofessional, person-centered care. Cognitive bias influences and affects the way all people—patients, their caregivers, families, health care professionals, managers, and policy makers—process information from the external environment and how they subsequently make decisions.

These biases—sometimes referred to as *heuristics* or *cognitive shortcuts*—are a core feature of human thinking and perception and help us to manage the important problems associated with information overload in our environment. Consider all the different sources and pieces of information that surround you from moment to moment. Next, consider how during a single interpersonal interaction you are simultaneously receiving and processing a diverse array of emotional, cognitive, verbal, and nonverbal cues and signals, some of which, frankly, will be contradictory and many of which may be unclear or ambiguous. Human beings have evolved the capacity to cope with this informational environment by relying heavily on these cognitive shortcuts to help us better manage four core problems associated with complexity and ambiguity in our environment. They include (1) too much information of all different sorts, which prevents us from truly paying attention and focusing; (2) insufficient meaning associated with all this information, making it difficult for us to accurately and effectively prioritize all this information; (3) the situational need and desire to act and respond quickly to information in our environment, which forces us to truncate any sort of deliberative thinking process; and (4) the need to determine what is worthy of being learned (i.e., what pieces of information in the external world can we safely ignore or disregard and what is actually important and worth remembering).

Cognitive bias governs almost all of our day-to-day interactions with others, yet for most of us, these biases are hidden from consciousness. Most of us are simply unaware of these biases and how they influence our thinking, behavior, and actions. Even highly educated and well-intentioned health care professionals are susceptible to having their behavior skewed or altered because of unconscious responses directed by cognitive bias. Psychologists suggest that the single most important first step in gaining greater control over these biases and their influence on our behavior is to understand them and be able to name them accurately as they influence our thinking and perception. For health professionals, it is essential to understand that cognitive biases—our own, our colleagues', and our patients'—all will have a direct influence on communication, and as a result, we need to develop work-around strategies in order to more effectively communicate, negotiate, and interact with others.

Some cognitive biases will have a greater influence on your communications plans than others. The following are a list of some of the most important and impactful cognitive biases of which you should be aware and recognize.

Anchoring: When we anchor, we disproportionately and inappropriately rely too heavily on one piece of information amid many other pieces of information. We anchor our subsequent decisions based on that first piece and give it far more influence than makes sense in the context. This is sometimes referred to as the first impression problem. When we have a negative first impression of someone, anchoring may result and that person will have a difficult time recovering. Logically, we should know that a poor first impression could easily be followed by a positive second, third, or fourth impression, yet many of us will assume the first piece of information we have about someone else is the entire story and cognitively will no longer be open to changing our opinion.

Availability: The availability cascade describes the tendency to believe information that is repeated over and over again, regardless of whether it is true or not. Increasingly, with the rise of social media, people can easily and repeatedly be exposed to so-called *alternative facts*, and the simple repeating of these statements begins to create the perception that they are true even if they are not. Commonly held truisms (e.g., drink eight cups of water a day, you'll catch a cold if you go outside with wet hair in the winter) are examples of the availability cascade. There's no real evidence to back up these statements, yet people have heard them over and over again and, consequently, assume they are true and in turn continue to perpetuate these statements themselves.

The bandwagon effect: This describes the tendency to act and think just like other members of your tribe. Social desirability describes the psychological need to want to fit in and connect with those we define as peers. A cognitive shortcut to doing this is to actually start to think like them and absorb group norms and expectations. This cognitive bias has been used to explain, in part, the rise of hyperpartisanship in politics right now.

Base rate fallacy: This cognitive bias describes our tendency to deliberately overlook or ignore any statistical evidence that conflicts with a preexisting belief. For example, when confronted with statistics related to climate change, some people may say, "But it was so cold last winter here, so therefore, climate change isn't real." Ignoring statistical evidence and basing belief only on personal experience is an important cognitive bias, particularly in a health care context, where people may consistently underestimate their risk for disease or illness.

Confirmation bias: Human beings have the less-than-charming tendency to want to prove themselves right and will actively seek to do this through fixating on information and focusing on people who reinforce, rather than challenge, their beliefs. Again, social media makes it extremely easy to only connect with like-minded people and to surround oneself with confirmatory data only, further reinforcing incorrect thinking. For example, a person who doesn't want to quit smoking might find other people who keep smoking and say, "Well, none of them is in the hospital, so how bad can smoking be?"

Illusory truth effects: This cognitive bias is the tendency to believe that truth should always be simple, uncomplicated, and require little intellectual energy to decipher.

Simple, sweeping statements have the veneer of truth because they are easily digested. Complexity and ambiguity are therefore seen as ways of hoodwinking or fooling people and can consequently be disregarded as false. Of course, in reality, many things in life are messy, complex, and ambiguous and take intellectual effort to understand, and these things are in fact truthful and accurate.

Representativeness: This is the tendency to judge something (or someone) as belonging to a group, class, or category based on a limited number of characteristics that are not actually truly or fully representative. For example, in many health care professional education programs, the only time gay or lesbian people are discussed and so identified is in the context of management or treatment of sexually transmitted diseases, as though they never get colds, athlete's foot, or other conditions all human beings experience. This may result in some health professionals developing the erroneous association that the only thing they need to be concerned about with LGBTQ+ individuals is related to sexual health, which, of course, is false.

There are many other cognitive biases that have been named and identified. For health care professionals, it is less important to memorize a list and definitions than it is to understand how such biases influence thinking and behavior, and to develop communication strategies that will allow you to manage and overcome such biases in communication with others.

Consider the following scenario:

> *A well-dressed, articulate middle-aged businessman, Ed, comes to the clinic for assessment of a nonspecific set of symptoms including fever, sore throat, a rash, swollen lymph nodes, fatigue, and some unusual ulcers in his mouth. Ed is married with three children and has a successful career in business. None of his other family members are demonstrating any similar symptoms. In conversation, Ed is pleasant, humorous, highly engaged, and interested in how he is being examined and assessed.*

Many health professionals examining a patient such as Ed might never stop to think that these symptoms he is demonstrating might be consistent with early symptoms of HIV, and as a result, there may be a delay in getting blood work and tests done. Why? The representativeness and base rate fallacy biases, coupled with anchoring, will make many professionals assume that anyone who is a well-dressed, articulate, middle-aged businessman named Ed surely would not or could not be involved with anything that could expose him to HIV infection.

Consider an alternative scenario:

> *Dreselda is an energetic and flamboyant young African American who is a successful drag performance artist who prefers to be addressed as* zhe *rather than* she *or* he. *Dreselda tours nationally, has been on TV, and is well known for being "out there" in terms of style. Zhe is often in gossip papers doing notorious things. Today, zhe has come to the clinic complaining of a fever, sore throat, a rash, swollen lymph nodes, fatigue, and some unusual ulcers in the mouth.*

A health professional examining Dreselda may more readily leap to an assumption that these symptoms are related to a sexually transmitted condition or substance abuse issues, even if in reality, Dreselda is too exhausted from having a successful media career to do anything other than fall asleep at 9:30 PM every night. Again, cognitive bias may influence thinking and behavior and may adversely influence the care both Dreselda and Ed receive.

What communication techniques should health professionals use to minimize the influence of cognitive bias in their own practice?

Be conscious of and avoid use of stereotypes in day-to-day language. As the case of Ed and Dreselda suggest, it is important to not assume all members of a group are interchangeable. Simply because Dreselda prefers to be addressed as "zhe" doesn't mean that zhe is at a higher risk for sexually transmitted disease than Ed.

Use person-first language. A small but important change in word choice can help remind everyone of the influence of cognitive bias in thinking and decision making. For example, saying "autistic children" places the emphasis on the condition, rather than saying "children who have autism." When we use person-first language, it sends an important signal that we think of individuals as people, rather than a list of medical conditions.

Be conscious of how individuals' identities (e.g., race, gender) are communicated. Why, in the description of Dreselda, was it necessary to include the term *African American* in the description? How did that influence, alter, or affect perception, assessment, diagnosis, and treatment? Why was race not mentioned in the description of Ed? Use of identity as a tool for categorization in verbal communication will adversely influence and amplify expression of cognitive bias, particularly through representativeness and anchoring. Unless it is actually medically relevant, necessary, and important, verbal categorization based on identities should be minimized.

Use inclusive language. Inclusive language involves careful attention to avoid the use of stereotypical gendered terms such as *manpower*, *guys*, or *fireman* and instead using gender neutral alternatives, such as *workforce*, *people*, or *firefighter*. Although some may decry the so-called political correctness associated with this kind of inclusive language, its purpose is to demonstrate civility and to reduce the risk of cognitive bias being reinforced through language use and word choice.

Cognitive bias is an important issue in many practitioner–patient conversations. Consider the following scenario:

Meredith has been recently diagnosed with irregular heartbeats and heart rhythm, resulting in occasional episodes of fainting, weakness, and confusion. Her health care team believes this is a serious condition, but one that can be managed through use of prescription medications focused on regularizing her heartbeat and rhythm. Eventually, a pacemaker or other surgery may be required. Meredith is extremely resistant to Western medicine, and in fact only visited the clinic at the insistence of her daughter. In receiving the prescriptions for medicines, Meredith has indicated she will not take these and instead has discovered through her online social media communities that a combination of vitamin C and magnesium along with a diet rich in fish will work wonders.

It may be easy and convenient to simply dismiss Meredith as flaky. Health care professionals know that arrhythmias are serious and potentially life-threatening conditions that should not be managed with vitamins, minerals, and diet alone. How might Meredith have arrived at her beliefs? Clearly, a series of cognitive biases are adversely influencing her decisions, including anchoring, confirmation, and availability. What should her health care team do to reorient her thinking in this case while still being respectful and maintaining a positive relationship?

In addressing cognitive bias, it is important to recognize that communication that is dismissive, insulting, or threatening will only serve to reinforce, rather than reduce, the bias. Saying, "Who are these people online who are telling you this, and what do they know? They're not experts like us," will have the inadvertent effect of activating the bandwagon effect. Attempting to use medical evidence and statistics regarding mortality and morbidity associated with untreated arrhythmias will not address the base rate fallacy or the confirmation bias. Attempting to refute cognitive bias with facts and information alone will rarely be successful.

Instead, consider the following approach.

Health care professional:	So, Meredith, I understand you are thinking about not using the medications prescribed, and instead there's another regimen you'd like to try?
Meredith:	Yes, that's right. I've been doing a lot of reading and talking to experts.
Health care professional:	That's interesting, tell me more. Who are these experts?
Meredith:	Well, I belong to a group online that is working to expose the pharmaceutical industry for all the scams they perpetrate. They have publications about how you can use all natural products to manage almost every medical condition, including mine.
Health care professional:	I'm not familiar with these publications. Can you point me to them?
Meredith:	I have some printed copies here you can look at. See?
Health care professional:	Are these publications from people you know? Friends or family?
Meredith:	Oh no, I've never met any of these people personally, just on the Internet. But I'm sure they're very reliable, top-drawer people if they can produce documents like this.
Health care professional:	Hmm. So when you read these, what conclusions do you draw for yourself?
Meredith:	Well, of course that medications cause more harm than good! And I shouldn't—no one should be taking them.
Health care professional:	What does your daughter say about this?

Meredith:	She probably thinks I'm nuts, but what can you do?
Health care professional:	Well, we've all met your daughter a few times now. She seems very concerned about your health.
Meredith:	Well, sure, but she doesn't know what's best for me.
Health care professional:	She may not KNOW what's best for you, but she really WANTS what's best for you.
Meredith:	I guess so. I never thought about it that way.
Health care professional:	All of us here want what's best for you.
Meredith:	I know. You're all just lovely people.
Health care professional:	Thank you! That means so much to hear that from you. Sometimes we just never know if we are making a difference.
Meredith:	Well, you've been so kind and so wonderful with me.
Health care professional:	I'm glad you think so. We really want you to be as healthy as possible and we really do our best.
Meredith:	I know.
Health care professional:	So, let's talk a bit more then about these medications and what you might think about finding a way to include them with the other options you are reading about.

It's not clear how Meredith might respond to this invitation from the health care professional, but there are some important advances that this conversation has triggered. One important communication technique that can be successful in challenging cognitive biases is to find ways of triggering mild cognitive dissonance. In reminding Meredith that her daughter cares about her and the health care team wants what's best for her, it reinforces the point that people who actually know her (versus the people on social media who don't know her) have a different opinion of the medications. Leveraging strong personal relationships as a way of triggering cognitive dissonance may provide a jolt to Meredith sufficient to have her start to question her assumptions and biases. Further, by suggesting Meredith might be able to find a way of keeping her social media friends happy by taking relatively innocuous substances like vitamin C and magnesium and eating fish, in addition to taking the prescribed medications, provides Meredith with a face-saving way of keeping all the important people in her life happy with her decision. Cognitive dissonance can be a powerful tool for indirectly challenging cognitive biases, and will generally be more effective than direct confrontation, debate, or argument. It may require both parties to find common ground and compromise. Presumably, both Meredith's daughter and the health care professional would prefer it if Meredith didn't involve herself at all with the social media group, but that may not be a realistic objective right now. Instead, it is important to pick your battles carefully and focus on the core objective of finding ways to convince Meredith to take the medication that was initially prescribed.

Recently, social psychologists have identified an important emerging communication technique that is being amplified through use of social media. *Firehosing* is the term used to describe communication that is presented repeatedly and with significant force. Whether the communication is true or false seems not to matter to many people: Information that is provided frequently, with great confidence, and at great volume and intensity starts to take on the character of truth for many people. Firehosing is particularly prevalent online. Individuals may be firehosed into being convinced that scientifically valid and medically necessary interventions (such as vaccinations) are false due to the cognitive bias evoked through intensity and repetition of messaging. In part, firehosing works because it appeals to a specific need or concern of the individual (e.g., "I need to keep my child safe"), and it may contain a kernel of truth or correspond to a random observation made by a patient (e.g., "My neighbor's kid got a vaccine and got really sick afterward"). Of course, random observations and kernels of truth are not the same as medical or scientific evidence. This may make some individuals particularly susceptible to firehosing and can make challenging the cognitive bias particularly difficult.

Cognitive bias is an important consideration, and developing a communication plan to effectively manage one's own biases and those that may influence others' decision making is important. General principles of effective communication, including empathizing, active listening, use of reflective questions, and assuming a listening rather than telling orientation, will all be helpful. Gentle ways of triggering mild cognitive dissonance may be an effective way to address cognitive bias indirectly, where open disagreement, argument, or debate may actually shut down communication and negatively impact relationships.

Interested in Learning More?

Bhatti A. Cognitive bias in clinical practice—nurturing healthy skepticism among medical students. *Adv Med Educ Pract*. 2018;9:235–237.

Burgess D, van Ryn M, Dovidio J, Saha S. Reducing racial bias among health care providers: lessons from social-cognitive psychology. *J Gen Intern Med*. 2007;22(6):883–887.

Gladwell M. *Blink: The Power of Thinking Without Thinking*. Boston: Back Bay Books; 2007.

Royce C, Hayes M, Schwartzstein R. Teaching critical thinking: a case for instruction in cognitive biases to reduce diagnostic errors and improve patient safety. *Acad Med*. 2019;94(2): 187–194.

Saposnik G, Redelmeier D, Ruff C, Tobler P. Cognitive biases associated with medical decisions: a systematic review. *BMC Med Inform Decis Mak*. 2016;16:138.

Stone J, Moskowitz G. Non-conscious bias in medical decision making; what can be done to reduce it? *Med Educ*. 2011;45(8):768–776.

Sullivan E, Schofield S. Cognitive bias in clinical medicine. *J R Coll Physicians Edinb*. 2018;48:225–232.

White-Means S, Zhiyong D, Hufstader M, Brown L. Cultural competency, race, and skin tone bias among pharmacy, nursing, and medical students: implications for addressing health disparities. *Med Care Res Rev*. 2009;66(4):436–455.

5

Communication in Virtual Team Settings

Interprofessional person-centered care can occur in a variety of different ways. Most traditionally, it has occurred within a geographically contained space, such as a clinic or hospital. In this setting, different professionals interact with one another in the same unit, floor, or building and physically see (i.e., meet and assess) patients in a face-to-face manner. Increasingly, however, nontraditional team structures are emerging in which health professionals may not be physically or geographically colocated, and in which patients connect virtually or electronically to different health care providers using tele-medicine, Web-based, or mobile applications and technologies. For example, a family physician may never "see" or directly interact face to face with a pharmacist, yet may develop a strong professional relationship related to pharmacotherapy questions over the phone, by email, or fax. When people never see each other physically and never have an opportunity to bump into one another in a common hallway, how do trust, collegiality, and entitativity (the sense of psychologically belonging to the same team) evolve?

Much of the research and experience related to communication and psychology in health care has been undertaken in traditional face-to-face environments, yet today and in the years ahead, the increasing prevalence of virtual health care delivery will introduce new challenges and opportunities for health care professionals, patients, and their families and caregivers. Learning to communicate effectively and efficiently within a virtual, technologically mediated environment introduces many variations on the themes discussed in this book, and ensuring best possible quality health care when face-to-face interactions are rare or nonexistent requires a new series of skills and competencies.

Virtual teams are groups of geographically or time-dispersed (asynchronous) in-dividuals who connect through information and telecommunication technologies to ac-complish specific goals and complete specific tasks. The fundamentals of success for virtual teams are not that different from that of traditional teams, but there are many more variables that must be considered and accounted for. Beyond simple logistics associated with asynchronous communication, unreliable technologies, or unsteady Web-based connections, as well as potentially different time zones, lots of travel, among others, there are substantial issues of human psychology that have to be managed related to how we learn to trust, rely, and grow connected to one another.

Communication Challenges in Virtual Teams

For all teams, good and effective communication is one of the most important essential components of success. Within teams, individuals and their leaders must manage and nurture communication patterns that foster cohesion and enhance a sense of belonging and importance that will allow for full interdependency and interaction. Poor and ineffective communication will make individual team members more likely to have weak or absent commitment to one another, feel overwhelmed and overloaded with responsibilities, have a lack of professional and social purpose in their work, and ultimately increases risks of absenteeism, errors, and misinformation being disseminated. Where professionals need to communicate virtually with patients, without benefit of physically seeing them, interpersonal connections can easily be lost and the patient or client can easily transform into the customer or consumer.

The single biggest issue facing virtual teams and virtual patient–practitioner interactions is the absence of or significant change in the quality of nonverbal communication. As noted previously, verbal communication conveys just a small part of the overall and complete meaning of what we intend to communicate. Nonverbal cues such as tone of voice, vocal emphasis, hand gestures, pauses, facial expressions, etc., are what make interpersonal communications rich, nuanced, and meaningful. With the proliferation of emoticons in electronic messages and extra care and attention paid to specific words used in correspondence such as email or text messages, it is becoming increasingly possible to mitigate some of the risks associated with virtual teamwork and communication. Everyone has stories (some of them humorous, some of them terrifying) of how a poorly worded or erroneously autofilled email or text triggered inadvertent blowback from the recipient. Within the context of virtual teams, such situations may pose interpersonal problems but may also have the real risk of causing serious errors.

Another important risk associated with virtual teams is the tendency for all team members to fall back on stereotyped images of other team members. When members of a group do not have the time or opportunity to get to know one another as individuals, they will naturally use cognitive shortcuts (heuristics) to better understand one another and predict each other's expected behaviors. As a result, each team member may be seen as an arch-stereotype of his or her profession, rather than as a fully rounded human being who happens to have a specific professional designation and set of professional experiences, knowledge, and skills. Stereotyping most frequently relies on inaccurate and inappropriate preconceptions of other people based on superficial characteristics such as age, gender, place of geographical origin, professional designation, etc. When this happens, and we are forced to rely on stereotypes as a way of knowing each other, we cannot help but filter information through these biases, which in turn will result in the potential of a broad range of misinterpretations and miscommunication.

A third risk associated with virtual teams is the potential for a high level of anonymity and diffusion of responsibility. When we are neither seen nor known by other people, this can trigger the belief that we are somehow insulated from sharing responsibility for the group's outcomes, and that someone else is in charge. Virtual teams can produce conditions where each professional stereotypes themselves and their own role, and rather than thinking creatively and collaboratively, each professional reverts to the most narrow and basic of scope of practice expectation. In such settings, there may be less of a tendency to want to find common ground, achieve consensus, and authentically engage in discussion to find agreement; in the most difficult of cases, virtual teams can actually become more polarized, more angry with one another, and more dysfunctional than face-to-face teams, who may have a greater incentive to cooperate simply because they are all in the same room. The same principle applies with practitioner–patient interactions. Across Skype, email, or texts, there may be a tendency for both patients and their professionals to become less personable, more argumentative, and ultimately, less caring about what each other is saying.

Given the increasing prevalence of virtual teams in health care and technologically mediated interactions with patients and caregivers, how can we all be better and more effective communicators? Some key strategies include the following.

1. **Be clear in terms of structures.**
   The root cause of most problems in virtual, interprofessional, person-centered care relates to uncertainty or ambiguity: Team members are uncertain as to what they are supposed to do, what tasks they are sharing, and what responsibilities they each and collectively have, and patients are uncertain as to who is doing what. A first important way of dealing with these problems of ambiguity is to ensure there are clear structures in place—for example, job descriptions for team members, policies and procedures around what to do if technology isn't working properly, how telephone-based conversations will operate, who will be host, team leader, or traffic cop to ensure orderly conversation, etc. Many of these issues are spontaneously resolved in face-to-face communications through nonverbal cues and messaging, but it can be more complicated in virtual team settings and should be explicitly addressed as soon as possible.

2. **Be explicit about expectations and norms.**
   Virtual teams may appear to be more efficient and convenient for everyone, but this may not immediately translate into saving time. It is essential that there is leadership and clarity around expectations for appropriate behavior; for example, many virtual teams suffer from the reality that, protected from view from others, some team members may wile away time on a conference call with each other by surfing the Internet and not actually paying attention to the conversation. In other cases, virtual team members may simply assume they are required to report what they have done, rather than truly interact and engage in productive discussion and creative and collaborative problem solving. A simple verbal statement such as "Let's all turn away from our computers right now and focus on this telephone call so we can be productive" or "We need everyone to be firing on all pistons right now because this is a complex situation we have so we all have something to contribute" may be needed. Importantly, unless the virtual team has a preestablished structure that empowers and enables someone (i.e., the team leader) to say such things, it may be left unsaid, and consequently, team functioning may be compromised.

3. **Recognize trust is central to teamwork and interpersonal relationships.**
   One of the greatest challenges in virtual teamwork and health care is that individuals who do not know one another personally may have difficulty trusting

one another. Trust is essential in human relationships to help manage risks of uncertainty: Trust reduces our inherent risk aversion related to things over which we have little or no control, in particular the risk that other people on the team are not pulling their weight. Where people have no preexisting—or have no opportunity to develop—personal relationships alongside their professional relationships, it is frankly difficult to build trust, and this can compromise both teamwork and practitioner–patient interactions. One way to manage this is to be pragmatic about expectations: Early in the life of a virtual team, or a virtual practitioner–patient interaction, expectations may be unrealistically high. It is essential to manage these expectations appropriately and gently guide them down to something more realistic. It is also helpful to ensure the first few tasks or jobs of a virtual team or virtual interaction are relatively safe and achievable to help foster a sense of mutual trust. Having succeeded early in a virtual team can establish a foundation for future success.

4. **There is really no substitute for face-to-face interactions.**
   Despite the advances in information technologies, human psychology has not evolved as quickly. Where virtual teams and virtual care have been most successful and effective, there is usually a strong, preexisting interpersonal relationship and communication pattern that has been fostered from face-to-face interactions. Once face-to-face interactions have established a foundation of mutual trust and respect, virtual teams and virtual care and be introduced to enhance efficiency of communication provided there continues to be periodic opportunities to reconnect face to face to continue to nurture the interpersonal relationship. The most challenging situations occur when virtual teams or virtual practitioner–patient interactions must be used without any prior face-to-face interactions or any possibility that in the near future the individuals will actually meet one another. In the absence of previous in-person experience with one another, there are simply too many gaps in mutual awareness and understanding, which of necessity, will be filled through stereotypes and cognitive biases.

   Ideally, then, virtual teams and virtual care do not replace in-person meetings and health care delivery, but are simply an additional alternative mode for communicating. Where there is no possibility of face-to-face interactions before virtual meetings, it is important to be realistic and modest in terms of what success is possible given the psychological barriers to trust formation discussed previously.

5. **Facilitate social connection and communication.**
   Technology eliminates, filters, or distorts nonverbal communication and thereby introduces limitations on the process of getting to know one another, which in turn can affect the quality of relationships, trust, and human connection. It may be possible to partially compensate for this reality by ensuring opportunities for virtual team members and virtual patient–practitioner dyads to have at least some informal, unstructured opportunities to get to know each other as people by sharing feelings, opinions, personal news, or things that are not necessarily related to specific jobs or professional tasks. Social communication of this sort, although it will still be bereft of nonverbal cues, can at least partially start to

replace nonverbal communication that exists in face-to-face interactions. For example, some virtual teams begin meetings by having a contest in which each team member tells the best joke they've heard this week, or have team members who are geographically separated describe the weather. Small attempts to ensure personal connection can provide important positive dividends in team functioning and communication.

6. **Use words to clarify.**
Most virtual communication will rely heavily on words, whether typed (in email or text) or spoken (in videoconferencing). Learning to use words to clarify meaning, rather than relying on nonverbal cues, can be difficult and awkward, but it is important to help minimize misunderstanding. In telephone- or Skype-based conversations, one of the most challenging issues to deal with is silence or non-responsiveness. In face-to-face conversations, silence is paired with a nonverbal cue that helps us to recognize whether the other person is angry, shocked, surprised, or simply thinking about what's been said. In virtual settings, it may be necessary to explicitly ask, "You haven't responded yet; how are you feeling about what I just said?" Similarly, if you were expecting a longer or more detailed response in an email, and all you received was "Fine," it may be important to use words to clarify what this means by responding, "Thanks. Could I ask you to expand a bit on 'fine' so I have a better sense of what you are thinking?" Again, in face-to-face conversations, we can use nonverbal cues to gauge what "fine" really means. In virtual settings, we may need to ask explicit questions to arrive at this same conclusion.

Visual-based technologies such as Skype may give the appearance of mitigating the loss of nonverbal cues more than text-based technologies such as email; however, it is important to be aware of how videoconferencing and teleconferencing can distort or amplify nonverbals. With time and experience, you will learn how this distortion and amplification works on an individual basis with colleagues on the other side of the phone or computer monitor, but in the interim, using carefully crafted words to clarify unexpected responses or silences can be very helpful.

Word-based technologies such as email and texting introduce unique challenges for communication among team members and with patients. Although the productivity and efficiency gains associated with these technologies have been significant, there may also be inadvertent consequences that have arisen that diminish the quality of interpersonal communication. When using email and texting, consider the following principles to enhance communication.

1. **Be clear and concise.**
Not only will you save time in composing messages, but also your audience will appreciate it. Rather than use sentences, consider using bullet points to convey dense facts and information. There is an inverse relationships between the length of an email or the volume of text included and the way it is received by the other person. Overly long and wordy emails are frequently ignored or referred for later reading. It is sometimes said that "if someone is asking you the time,

don't explain to them how to build a clock." Email and text work best when you get to the point and answer directly.

2. **Always double-check a message before hitting send.**
   While spellcheck and other online services exist, they are not perfect. Written messages with spelling or grammatical errors can cause misinterpretation, lead to error, or perhaps result in the recipient being underwhelmed by your skills and losing confidence in your abilities. Simply rereading your messages before hitting send will catch the vast majority of errors and prevent errors.

3. **Do not just reply; include information about what you're replying to.**
   Most people receive hundreds of emails a day or week. As a result, it is quite likely they may not remember the exact question they asked you when you respond. It is good practice to copy the portion of the email you received with a specific request, paste it into your response, then give your answer. For example, if a nurse emailed a physician with the question, "Should we be sending a sample to the lab for testing, or just go ahead and give antibiotics to treat empirically?" an email response such as "Treat" is unclear. Instead, copying and pasting "give antibiotics to treat empirically" as the response provides the most direct and unambiguous response to the question possible.

4. **Subject lines matter.**
   We are all overwhelmed with email and texts, and sometimes messages ricochet between individuals and within groups for several weeks, so subject lines provide an important tool for categorizing messages and keeping things organized. They also facilitate searching for a message after the fact if necessary. A subject line also indicates to your message recipient that your message is important, legitimate, and may increase the likelihood they open it immediately, rather than leave it unread until a more convenient time exists. Vague subject lines such as "hey!" or " 'sup?" should not be used.

5. **Set a delay on sending emails.**
   The anonymity of text-based virtual communication can sometimes lull us into believing our emotional responses do not matter. Many people have fired off immediate, angry emails to others in the heat of the moment, only to regret it the second they hit the send button. If you are upset by the content of a message, try to delay responding for 24 hours to allow an opportunity for you to regain your composure. Many email programs allow users to set a 5- or 10-minute delay time. Once you hit send, your message actually stays in your inbox for 5 to 10 minutes before being sent, allowing you an all-important opportunity to recall it before it has even been sent. This can be particularly important if there is a risk of "reply all" in an email being triggered, a message intended for an individual inadvertently sent to a larger group.

6. **Don't assume everyone understands your shortcuts and abbreviations.**
   Similar to chart-based documentation in health care, shortcuts and abbreviations can lead to misunderstandings in text or email communication. If you are not an efficient typist or do not have skills using a phone-based keyboard, consider using the now commonly available dictation function that converts words

to text to avoid having to use shortcuts and abbreviations. For example, sending a text to a patient that says "take it prn" will cause confusion. Explaining what "prn" means and how "as necessary" actually applies in the patient's specific case is essential and will prevent misunderstanding and errors.

7. **Use humor carefully.**

   Although humor is an important way of building relationships and establishing interpersonal chemistry, it may be interpreted differently than intended in texts and emails, particularly if you do not already have a strong preexisting relationship with the other person. Common acronyms used among friends, such as LMAO, may be inappropriate or offensive. Cutesy shortcuts and deliberate misspellings, such as LOL or OMG, can be off-putting in professional and health care contexts. The key is to know your audience and to not assume they will be charmed by your wit. If in doubt, leave it out, and save your humor for another time or context where it may be easier to rely on nonverbal communication to support your delivery.

In reading this chapter, it may be tempting to assume virtual teams and health care delivery are too problematic and therefore best avoided. In today's and tomorrow's world, this is increasingly unlikely. Rather than avoid technologically mediated interactions with others, learning to prevent problems, or manage them should they arise, is more valuable.

Consider the following scenario:

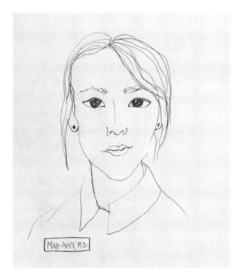 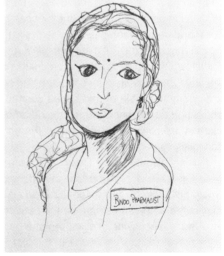

Mah-Ahn, Family Physician   **Binoo, Pharmacist**

Mah-Ahn is a family physician who routinely texts with her patients to provide them with information and updates, and to answer questions. One of her patients, Chadrigah, has just texted her saying his pharmacist sent an email saying he should stop taking the drug he normally uses for high blood pressure and use another one instead. Mah-Ahn does not know the pharmacist but asks Chadrigah to keep taking the medication that was initially pre-scribed. A few moments later, Chadrigah texts back to say the pharmacist won't give him the prescribed medication. Mah-Ahn is very annoyed by the presumption of the pharmacist, but is busy and can't call. Instead, she sends a text back to Chadrigah asking him to tell the pharmacist to follow the initial order. Chadrigah shows the text to Binoo, the pharmacist at the drug store, who in turn is irritated by Mah-Ahn's tone in the message and responds in a fax to the doctor's office, "Hey, I'm just doing my job," implying Mah-Ahn is not doing her job.

This scenario highlights the limitations of virtual communication, particularly when individuals do not know each other well. In this situation, the patient has been put in the middle in what appears to be an interprofessional disagreement and potential conflict. What is not obvious in this case, because there are no nonverbal cues and no three-way communication between Mah-Ahn, Binoo, and Chadrigah, is that the real problem here is that the original prescription medication is not available due to a backorder situation. Recently, there have been many cases of medications that are simply not available be-cause of supply chain issues; pharmacies may not be able to secure certain medications due to production problems, delivery issues, or other difficulties and, as a result, patients might not be able to get the medications they are used to taking. In such situations, the pharmacist will usually work with the prescriber to identify a short-term alternative to ensure therapeutic goals are met even if this might mean temporarily (or permanently) changing the initially prescribed medication. Regrettably, this is an increasingly common situation in primary care, but one that can be managed with effective communication and collaboration between patient, pharmacist, and prescriber.

In this scenario, all three people were busy speaking to only one other person, and not all together to each other. As a result, miscommunication proliferated, ultimately lead-ing to vaguely insulting messages being sent, which risks escalating into a conflict. The anonymity of email- or text-based communication, coupled with the fact that Mah-Ahn and Binoo do not know each other, is amplified by the role of the patient as the interme-diary in the communication, rather than having the professionals speaking directly and collegially to one another.

It is obvious that if Binoo and Mah-Ahn had simply communicated directly—by phone, fax, email, or in person—about the drug shortage problem, this misunderstanding would not have occurred. Ideally, Binoo, Mah-Ahn, and Chadrigah would have all com-municated at the same time so the patient was also aware of the problem and could be involved in discussing alternatives and options for changing the medication. What might have prevented this situation? In the first instance, Binoo could have communicated di-rectly with Mah-Ahn rather than having Chadrigah act as the intermediary. In the second instance, upon receipt of Chadrigah's text, Mah-Ahn should have communicated directly with Binoo rather than having the patient relay her response. Perhaps most importantly, because drug shortages are not a new or surprising problem, it would be useful for Binoo's pharmacy and Mah-Ahn's practice to have a structure in place to ensure that when drug shortages do occur there is a process that can be followed to prevent miscom-munication and to expedite a solution. For example, the pharmacy sends an email or a preprinted form to the physician's office outlining the problem and proposing alternatives based on what medications are available in stock, with a recommendation based on the patient's unique circumstances. In this way, technological communication and virtual teamwork could facilitate better patient care rather than triggering conflict.

In this scenario, miscommunication resulted in stereotyping (i.e., the pharmacist should follow the doctor's order or the doctor is a know-it-all who should focus on doing her job better) that unnecessarily and emotionally escalated tension between the professionals and with the patient. Rapid escalation and amplification of emotional responses are a risk in virtual communication because nonverbal cues that can help buffer such escalation are not present. This miscommunication highlights challenges associated with virtual teams and health care, but also signposts potential opportunities to better use technologies to enhance communication and provide better care to patients.

Interested in Learning More?

Dixon R. Enhancing primary care through online communication. *Health Aff (Millwood).* 2010;29(7):1364–1369.

Katz S, Moyer C. The emerging role of online communication between patients and their providers. *J Gen Intern Med.* 2004;19(9):978–983.

Neville C. Telehealth: a balanced look at incorporating this technology into practice. *Sage Open.* 2018;4:1–5.

Shaffer K, Speakman E. Using technology to enhance interprofessional collaborative practice: creating virtual clinical opportunities by implementing Google Docs and Google Hangouts in clinical rounding. *Collab Healthc.* 2014;5(1): Article 2.

Terrasse M, Gorin M, Sisti D. Social media, e-health and medical ethics. *Hastings Cent Rep.* 2019;49(1):24–33.

Torous J, Hsin H. Empowering the digital therapeutic relationship: virtual clinics for digital health interventions. *NPJ Digit Med.* 2018;1:16.

Tuckson R, Edmunds M, Hodgkins M. Telehealth: special report. *N Engl J Med.* 2017;377: 1585–1592.

Dealing with Grief:
What to Say When You
Don't Know What to Say

Among the most difficult conversations health care professionals will have will be those involving death and dying. Few topics trigger as much personal emotion for health care professionals as witnessing the grief of another person. Many practitioners feel they have a duty to remain stoic, objective, and detached despite the personal emotional responses they may be experiencing. Some practitioners feel able to share grief with their patients or clients. It is essential to recognize there is no right, perfect, or one-size-fits-all answer to the question of how you as a practitioner can or should help someone manage grief. Each person and family is different, and sometimes grief cannot be managed. It must be honored, experienced, and simply respected.

In times of grief and loss, it is tempting to believe there is a script or formula that can be used to relieve the practitioner of the strain of having to determine how best to deal with a strongly emotional and difficult situation. There is no formula, and the attempt to rely on a formula will backfire, giving the appearance of lack of interest or worse. Instead, learning to discern and respond to your own personal emotional responses, acquiring a comfort in witnessing strong emotion, and not feeling this is a problem you can or should solve is essential.

Elisabeth Kübler-Ross highlighted a model for understanding the emotional progression that many individuals navigate as they grieve, although this model has been criticized for not being sufficiently culturally sensitive, and presenting an overly linear explanation for the complex psychological and adaptive processes associated with grieving, death, or dying. Her model suggests there are five distinct and interconnected stages through which individuals progress: denial, anger, bargaining, depression, and eventually, acceptance. Each person's trajectory will differ and the way each of these stages will display themselves will also be different. The notion that acceptance is both an objective and a possibility associated with grief has become engrained in our society, despite evidence that it may or may not be true. Although this model may be overly simplistic and nonrepresentative, it does provide a useful tool for understanding there are many stages and phases to grieving, that grieving will involve strong emotions that are uncomfortable to witness, and that it is a process requiring time and understanding from those who support the grieving individual. Attempts to create prefabricated statements in response to each phase of the process are both disrespectful and unhelpful, despite the appeal this may have for the health care professional who is struggling with his or her own discomfort in providing support.

Authenticity, empathy, and perhaps most importantly, presence, are required. Even when you do not have the words or do not know what to say, paying attention and being fully present—not distracted or not consumed by your own discomfort—are among the most helpful things for those who are grieving. In some cases, some practitioners may simply not have the emotional capacity to manage this. The cognitive and emotional load associated with another's grief is intense, and if this is something that exceeds your capacity, it is essential that you understand this about yourself and determine different ways to provide support to the best of your ability. In many cases, an understanding of your own emotional intelligence will be an important guide to help you. For example, strong assimilators, with their preference for structure and planning, may find they are best suited to help grieving people and family members manage complex legal processes, which can be extremely stressful to sort out. An assimilator with the capacity to focus on details and get things done can be a comfort. In contrast, strong divergers may have a more natural inclination toward being able to witness others' grief and be present during difficult emotional times. Their capacity for understanding and quiet support can be hugely important. Strong convergers, with their bias toward action, may find they are best able to support grief through providing a strong and steady presence and being a pillar of strength during difficult times. Accommodators may find themselves wanting to do things and keep busy in a meaningful way by, for example, cooking meals, mowing lawns, and helping take care of activities of daily living as a way of relieving the burden on grieving individuals and family members. There is no single right or best way for any of us to support people through grief. Your emotional intelligence can be a useful guide in helping you be as authentic and present as you can be, and as you are capable of being.

We often struggle to say the right thing, but in many cases, there may not be any right words to express. Instead, nonverbal support, including eye contact, appropriate and gentle physical contact (an arm around the shoulder, holding a hand), and a gentle tone of voice, can provide both reassurance and support regardless of words that may or may not be said.

Sadly, in your personal and professional life, you will become all too familiar with grief. It is an unavoidable part of being both a practitioner and a human being. Being patient with yourself and your responses and focusing on your own, authentic, and genuine methods for providing support as best as you can will be most important and helpful.

Consider the following scenario:

The Cavanaughs have been patients at your clinic for several years. Mrs. Cavanaugh, after a valiant struggle with cancer, recently died. It was a difficult and painful passing, despite everyone's best attempts to provide palliative care and support. Mr. Cavanaugh is now alone; the couple had no children and their family lives out of town. You were close to the family after having spent so many years as part of their care team. You attended the funeral and were personally quite moved by it. Today, Mr. Cavanaugh has come to the clinic. He is generally healthy but now appears lost. He is tidy and well dressed, and appears holding a large brown paper bag. He sees you, smiles, and thanks you for coming to his wife's funeral. He then says, "I know these medications are so expensive and, well, I want to make sure someone else who really needs them can benefit from them now that we don't need them anymore. You will make sure someone who is in need, who really, really can benefit, will get these, right?"

Of course, from a legal perspective, a clinic cannot accept and repurpose medications that have already been dispensed for another patient. There is no way to ensure the safety and quality of medicines that have been stored in a person's house for a period of time. Mr. Cavanaugh's generous and thoughtful gesture, thinking of others even now, during his time of grief, commands both respect and may even trigger strong emotional responses in you. What can you say? What should you do?

1. Do you simply say "thank you" and accept the medications graciously, knowing full well you will dispose of them and not abide by Mr. Cavanaugh's request? Do you tell a well-intentioned white lie?

2. Do you gently let him know that you can take the medications so they are out of the house, but regulations prohibit repurposing drugs and avoid the guilt of telling a lie by crushing Mr. Cavanaugh's generous gesture?

3. Do you offer to sit with him, share reflections with him about this wife, then gently redirect him so he actually does not make this request any more, a subtle and understandable form of manipulation to avoid telling a lie or crushing his generous gesture?

Clearly, in a situation like this, there is no right or good answer. In large part, your response is going to need to be a function of who you are as a person—your emotional intelligence, your level of connection to the Cavanaugh family, your present emotional and cognitive state of mind, and the load you are experiencing.

Is it acceptable to lie to the patient and say thank you and pretend you are going to repurpose the medications, even if you know you cannot? This is a difficult question to answer, because truth telling is integral to the work of health professionals. Although it may be perfectly understandable in this circumstance, and although it is perhaps the path of least resistance and the option that has the least level of immediate emotional complexity and intensity, some people may be concerned about the slippery slope it enables in terms of trusting relationships between practitioners and patients. What if Mr. Cavanaugh returns in a few weeks and asks to speak to the family that received the medications? Do you tell another lie and say you're not allowed to disclose that? What if he later finds out that this was not legal in the first place. Perhaps he will understand you were just being kind, but if it establishes that you (for the best of reasons and intentions) lied to him, how will it affect your relationship in the future?

Similarly, if you select option 2 and tell the truth, what kind of an immediate emotional impact might that have on Mr. Cavanaugh? Many people might believe that telling the truth, no matter how gently right now, is actually cruel and unnecessary. Although truth telling is of course important and an expectation for health care professionals, should there not be some flexibility in difficult times such as this?

Although objectively and rationally, option 3 may be the most appropriate, or the least worst, alternative, how realistic is it that you or most health care professionals have both the communication skills, time, and cognitive and emotional capacity available to engage in this kind of important conversation? And what might this kind of conversation look like?

In most cases, this kind of conversation may begin as an invitation for Mr. Cavanaugh to talk or not, depending on how he feels. Learning to observe and interpret his nonverbal cues (e.g., eye contact, teary eyes, body language, sighs) as well as his verbal signals, and applying all your effective listening and empathy skills as best and authentically as you can to allow him to direct the flow of the interaction, is important. You may or may not ever get to the point where you discuss the bag of medications, but in the interim, if you are able to engage and connect with him during this difficult time, you may be providing the most important care a practitioner can ever provide.

Mr. Cavanaugh:	"I know these medications are so expensive and, well, I want to make sure someone else who really needs them can benefit from them now that we don't need them anymore. You will make sure someone who is in need, who really, really can benefit, will get these, right?"
Health care professional (HCP):	Mr. Cavanaugh. I'm so pleased to see you. Do you have a few minutes? Let's go into the office to sit down.
Mr. Cavanaugh:	Okay. I have nothing but time on my hands these days.
HCP:	Come in . . . sit down. Can I get you anything? A glass of water? A cup of tea?
Mr. Cavanaugh:	No, no, I don't want to be a bother. I know how busy you all are. You do such important work here.
HCP:	You are not bothering at all! I'm really happy to see you today. I have been thinking a lot about you, about your wife.
Mr. Cavanaugh:	That's so sweet of you, thank you, thank you.
HCP:	She was a really amazing person.
Mr. Cavanaugh:	Yes, yes. I . . . I miss her so much.
HCP:	How are you holding up?
Mr. Cavanaugh:	It's, well, I don't know. I can't sleep at night.
HCP:	Take your time. I really want to know.
Mr. Cavanaugh:	I . . . I just don't know what to do anymore. She, my wife . . . she was everything to me.
HCP:	(Says nothing, simply waits)
Mr. Cavanaugh:	I'm . . . I will be okay. But for now, I just really want to know that someone else can benefit from these expensive medications. You'll take them and give them to someone who really needs them right?
HCP:	(gently, maintaining sympathetic eye contact throughout) Thank you so much for your generous offer and thinking of other people right now. That is so kind of you. This may be difficult to hear, but we actually aren't allowed to pass medications on from one patient to another patient. There are . . .

Mr. Cavanaugh:	Why not? I mean, they're perfectly good still.
HCP:	Of course they are. But many patients will feel uncomfortable knowing the medications they are taking have not been stored or controlled by a health care professional before they take them. We have safeguards in place to make sure medications are stored at the right temperature, in safe conditions, in sealed containers, and for so many patients that is important as it lets them sleep easy at night knowing what they are taking is safe.
Mr. Cavanaugh:	But I haven't done anything bad to the medications!
HCP:	Of course, I know that. But not everyone is as thoughtful and kind and careful as you, Mr. Cavanaugh, so the rule is in place to protect everyone. Does that make sense?
Mr. Cavanaugh:	I guess so, but it just seems so wasteful, and I really want to help someone else.
HCP:	Maybe we can talk about other ways you might want to help?

The conversation may carry forward from here. Importantly, in this scenario, the health care professional did several things.

1. Grief is not a problem to be solved, certainly not a problem to be solved by this health care professional. There were times where a health care professional, feeling emotionally overwhelmed, may try to step in and suggest, "Would you like a sleeping pill?" This is premature at this stage in the conversation; of course he will be having difficulty sleeping given his recent loss, but the question of whether medicating it is appropriate will require a different sort of medical assessment, not simply an empathetic conversation.

2. The professional was present and engaged, inviting Mr. Cavanaugh to speak, and indicating interest by saying, "I really want to know" and asking open-ended questions like "How are you holding up?"

3. At a very emotional point in the conversation when the professional didn't know what to say, nothing was said. Silence and presence, rather than idle chatter or a nervous attempt to fill in conversation were avoided, and this too is a concrete demonstration of empathy and presence.

Should a situation such as this arise in your professional practice, please do not simply pick up this book and attempt to replicate this conversation. What makes this conversation unique is the specific chemistry, history, and connection between Mr. Cavanaugh and the fictitious health care professional depicted here. Authenticity, engagement, and presence cannot be lifted from a textbook; however, principles related to the examples listed previously can be useful to help guide you in applying your emotional intelligence, your personhood, and your compassion to help support someone to the best of your ability.

Mind Map Case 6

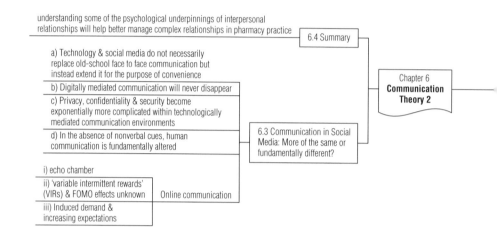

understanding some of the psychological underpinnings of interpersonal
relationships will help better manage complex relationships in pharmacy practice

6.4 Summary

a) Technology & social media do not necessarily
replace old-school face to face communication but
instead extend it for the purpose of convenience

b) Digitally mediated communication will never disappear

c) Privacy, confidentiality & security become
exponentially more complicated within technologically
mediated communication environments

d) In the absence of nonverbal cues, human
communication is fundamentally altered

i) echo chamber

ii) 'variable intermittent rewards'
(VIRs) & FOMO effects unknown   Online communication

iii) Induced demand &
increasing expectations

6.3 Communication in Social
Media: More of the same or
fundamentally different?

Chapter 6
**Communication
Theory 2**

Mind Map for Emotional Intelligence

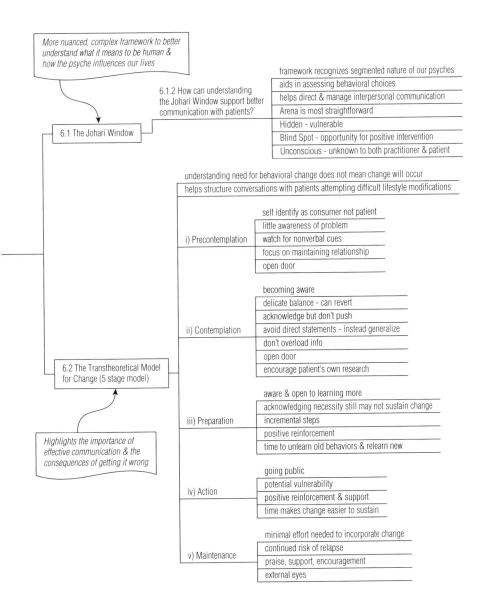

More nuanced, complex framework to better understand what it means to be human & how the psyche influences our lives

6.1 The Johari Window

6.1.2 How can understanding the Johari Window support better communication with patients?

framework recognizes segmented nature of our psyches

aids in assessing behavioral choices

helps direct & manage interpersonal communication

Arena is most straightforward

Hidden - vulnerable

Blind Spot - opportunity for positive intervention

Unconscious - unknown to both practitioner & patient

6.2 The Transtheoretical Model for Change (5 stage model)

Highlights the importance of effective communication & the consequences of getting it wrong

understanding need for behavioral change does not mean change will occur

helps structure conversations with patients attempting difficult lifestyle modifications

i) Precontemplation
- self identify as consumer not patient
- little awareness of problem
- watch for nonverbal cues
- focus on maintaining relationship
- open door

ii) Contemplation
- becoming aware
- delicate balance - can revert
- acknowledge but don't push
- avoid direct statements - instead generalize
- don't overload info
- open door
- encourage patient's own research

iii) Preparation
- aware & open to learning more
- acknowledging necessity still may not sustain change
- incremental steps
- positive reinforcement
- time to unlearn old behaviors & relearn new

iv) Action
- going public
- potential vulnerability
- positive reinforcement & support
- time makes change easier to sustain

v) Maintenance
- minimal effort needed to incorporate change
- continued risk of relapse
- praise, support, encouragement
- external eyes

Interested in Learning More?

Bruce C. Helping patients, families, caregivers, and physicians in the grieving process. *J Am Ostopath Assoc*. 2007;107(12 Suppl 7):ES33–40.

Corless I, Limbo R, Bousso R, et al. Language of grief: a model for understanding the expressions of the bereaved. *Health Psychol Behav Med*. 2014;2(1):132–143.

Devine M. *It's OK That You're Not OK: Meeting Grief and Loss in a Culture That Doesn't Understand*. Boulder, CO: Sounds True; 2017.

Kutner J, Kilbourn K. Bereavement: addressing challenges faced by advanced cancer patients, their caregivers, and their physicians. *Prim Care*. 2009;36(4):825–844.

Love A. Progress in understanding grief, complicated grief and caring for the bereaved. *Contemp Nurse*. 2007;27(1):73–83.

Ray E, ed. *Health Communication in Practice: A Case Study Approach*. Mahwah, NJ: Lawrence Erlbaum Associates Publisher; 2005.

Stajduhar K, Martin W, Cairns M. What makes grief difficult? Perspectives from bereaved family caregivers and healthcare providers of advanced cancer patients. *Palliat Support Care*. 2010;8(3):277–289.

CASE

7

Dementia: Communication with Patients and Their Caregivers

Dementia is a general term used to describe a broad array of symptoms associated with disorders affecting the brain. Symptoms may include memory loss, problems with everyday problem solving, difficulty in speaking and retrieving words (including the names of loved ones), and challenges in decoding verbal and nonverbal messages sent by others. Dementia is a progressive condition in which gradual deterioration of functioning occurs over a period of time. Those closest to an individual with dementia may not even recognize this decline because it can occur so gradually. Instead, individuals who only periodically interact with the individual may be the first to actually notice and become concerned about the symptoms of cognitive decline that are the hallmark of dementia.

The cognitive decline associated with dementia may express itself in different ways. Most frequently, memory loss is accompanied by difficulty in finding or communicating words, and difficulty with activities involving visual or spatial skills (e.g., driving or parking a car). Further symptoms may include challenges with coordination and motor function, confusion and disorientation, and difficulty with planning or organizing activities of any sort. Complexity and ambiguity within a situation may further worsen the experience and can trigger strong, sometimes frightening psychological responses and changes, including depression, anxiety, agitation, hallucinations, or paranoia.

Exact causes of dementia remain unclear, but in general, dementia appears to be the result of damage to or loss of nerve cells and their connections within the brain. Specific symptoms and the expression of dementia will vary from person to person, based on the specific area of the brain that is damaged. In many cases, dementia is referred to as a progressive, irreversible condition. Alzheimer disease is the most common type of dementia and is related to an accumulation of plaques that damage healthy neurons and the fibers connecting them. Vascular dementia is another common type; this is usually the result of damage to the vessels that supply blood to the brain. The most common symptoms of vascular dementia will include difficulties with everyday problem solving, slowed thinking, inability to focus, and difficulty in organizing oneself. Other forms or causes of dementia include Lewy body dementia and frontotemporal dementia.

Age is described as a risk factor for dementia; one's risk of developing dementia increases with age, especially after 65 years old. Importantly, dementia is NOT simply a normal and expected part of aging. It is a condition that requires medical management and support even though no cure currently exists. Family history is also a risk factor for developing the condition; however, many people with a family history of dementia will never develop symptoms, and many people without a family history do, making it difficult to define the familial and genetic issues involved. Modifiable risk factors for dementia include poor diet, lack of exercise, smoking, and heavy use of alcohol, all of which increase risk of developing dementia. Certain cardiovascular health conditions, including high blood pressure, elevated cholesterol and build up of fat on arterial walls, and a personal history of diabetes also may be risk factors.

With an aging population and increasing prevalence of dementia, many techniques to help prevent dementia or slow its progress have been proposed. The success of these interventions may be limited and vary considerably from person to person, and include mental stimulation (such as reading, solving puzzles, and playing word games); regular physical activity of 150 minutes per week or more; regular social activity and interaction; addressing lifestyle risk factors such as smoking and drinking; maintaining a healthy diet; and sufficient, consistent, and good quality sleep.

For many families, dementia is a particularly painful and difficult condition to manage. In almost all aspects of human life, communication is the primary way in which relationships are formed, maintained, and nurtured. Dementia robs individuals of their ability to remember, speak, and understand, and it can therefore rob them of the relationships they need to sustain them.

How Does Dementia Affect the Ability to Communicate?

As dementia progresses and harms or destroys brain cells, a significant cardinal symptom may emerge: aphasia. Aphasia describes the loss of ability to find words, to speak, and to understand speech of others. Aphasia typically worsens as the disease evolves, but this process can take years to manifest. In early stages of dementia, individuals appear capable of carrying on normal conversations, but will sometimes simply struggle to find words, or forget a word, or use the wrong word. Occasionally, the word that is forgotten will be the name of a loved one. Such communication hiccups are frequently dismissed as a normal sign of aging, although it is not necessarily so. As the condition evolves, individuals may start to confuse the meaning of words and confidently use inappropriate or inaccurate nouns or verbs. An important stage in the evolution of the condition occurs when individuals have a difficult time holding multiple ideas in their heads at once, and as a result, they may start to jump incoherently from topic to topic without completing a sentence. At this stage, there is frequently an accompanying decrease in the ability to understand the conversation of others, particularly if the other person speaks quickly, in a high-pitched voice, has an accent, or uses complex words and speech patterns.

Communication is central to human life and relationships, and the loss of ability to speak and understand is devastating for patients, their families, and caregivers. Moreover, as communication recedes, relationships become difficult to sustain or maintain and confusion, misunderstanding, resentment, and anger can build, especially if dementia is also accompanied by other health- or mobility-related issues that are time consuming and challenging to manage.

How Can Health Care Professionals Communicate More Effectively with Patients with Dementia?

Understanding the causes, symptoms, and trajectory of dementia can be helpful in guiding discussions and interactions with patients, their families, and caregivers. An overarching principle in communication with patients with dementia is to remember to demonstrate authentic kindness and patience. As the ability to decipher verbal communication recedes, there may be increased reliance on the most basic of nonverbal cues such as tone of voice and a smile. These will become essential tools for communication, especially in later stages of the condition. No comprehensive road map for communicating with patients with dementia exists; instead, a series of potential techniques have been proposed, some of which may work to a greater or lesser degree for a specific patient. As a result, it is important for the health care professional to remember to be patient and kind, to be willing to invest the time and energy in experimenting with different techniques to find what works best, and to be aware that simply because a technique works today, there is no guarantee it will work tomorrow. Examples of techniques that can be used include the following:

1. Use music and, in particular, songs as a way of communicating. Music and melodies are often coded and stored in a part of the brain that may be unaffected by dementia. People with dementia often remember, recognize, and respond to songs even in advanced stages, and this can be used to provide comfort, trigger positive memories, and provide support during times of stress.

2. Learn some phrases in the patient's primary language. As dementia progresses and language production is compromised, some individuals find that they gradually lose the ability to speak their second or third language, and instead will revert to the first language they learned to speak. In some cases, this can be particularly painful and tragic because adult children or grandchildren may not speak the same first language and may therefore have difficulties communicating. If it is possible, encourage adult children and grandchildren to prepare to speak as much of the patient's first language as possible, and try to learn a few words and phrases yourself.

3. Avoid external or environmental distractions. People with dementia are particularly susceptible to being overwhelmed by environmental and background noise. Seemingly simple things like background music, a radio playing in the background, or a television in the basement can cause distress and compromise the patient's ability to think, speak, and understand. When interacting with patients with dementia, avoid time-pressured, interruption-driven environments and instead find a quiet, acoustically private space where both you and your patient can focus on one another.

4. Be sensitive to the way you first approach and are seen by the patient. Approaching a patient from the side or the rear can trigger anxiety or aggression because it is an unexpected surprise. Wherever possible, plan on meeting and greeting the patient face-on, and allow sufficient time for your presence to be

noticed and processed before engaging in actual conversation. Never assume the patient remembers your name or your role. Introducing yourself and your job title, and referring to the patient by his or her name routinely is important, even if it may feel awkward to you.

5. Anticipate verbal mix-ups and avoid overcorrecting. Listening carefully to what the patient is saying and allowing sufficient time for the patient to search, find, and form words are essential. Avoid the temptation to finish sentences and to constantly correct when the wrong word is used; this is a game that you can never win.

6. Enunciate clearly; speak slowly; avoid jargon, slang, and short forms; and use formal pronunciation and grammar. Although this may appear stilted and unnatural to you and those observing you, this may facilitate greater understanding. Avoid the temptation to simply speak louder, unless of course the patient with dementia is also suffering from hearing loss.

7. Consider the essential and most important things to communicate to the patient. The ability to process multiple ideas and complex concepts is severely compromised with dementia, particularly in later stages. As a result, health care professionals need to consider carefully what are the essential things to communicate, rather than trying to say everything all at once. Focus on one idea, problem, or issue at a time and allow the individual to digest this thoroughly before moving on to something else. Avoid presenting multiple ideas at the same appointment or meeting; instead, schedule frequent follow-up visits to discuss multiple issues rather than trying to include everything all at once.

8. Be conscious of the tendency to want to test the individual. Seemingly simple questions such as "Do you remember when you were a little girl?" may seem like a gentle invitation to reminisce, but to a patient with dementia, it may feel like a test that they are failing. Try to emphasize successes and positive accomplishments; for example, if someone is attempting to tie their shoelace and is not succeeding, avoid saying, "No, that's not the way you do it" and instead say, "Let's try it this way." Words such as *no* and *not* convey strong nonverbal cues associated with negativity and failure, and this will likely create a negative emotional response that can be difficult to manage. Being careful to phrase things in a positive way is more helpful for self-esteem and empowerment.

9. Avoid infantilizing those with dementia and treating them like they are children. It may be expected that the challenges associated with communicating with a patient with dementia may cause exasperation, irritation, and leave you feeling like you are the parent or caregiver of a child; however, acting on this impulse and actually treating a patient with dementia like a child is both profoundly unhelpful and highly insulting. Avoid using baby-talk speech or tone of voice or using patronizing sentences that are diminishing or dismissive.

Communication with nonverbal cues—including hand gestures, facial expressions, eye contact, body language, and touch will become increasingly more important over time as the symptoms of dementia advance and the condition progresses. Learning to be comfortable expressing yourself nonverbally and relying on nonverbal cues can be challenging for both the patient and the health care professional. Depending on your comfort level and the specifics of the situation, nonverbal demonstrations of empathy, care, and concern may include a warm smile, holding a patient's hand, putting an arm around a shoulder, or even giving a hug. It is essential to be mindful of the patient's comfort levels and boundaries associated with physical contact, but in many cases, when words are failing, there can be incredible value to nonverbal communication in keeping people connected with one another.

Learning to Listen to a Patient with Dementia

Effective listening is a cornerstone of person-centered care. For patients with dementia, listening may require a variety of additional techniques and approaches to accommodate for the natural progression of the condition. A key variable to consider is time. Most health professionals work in busy, time-pressured practices and are accustomed to a 5- to 7-minute appointment time slot. This may simply not work or be practical with a patient with dementia. These patients will require your focused and uninterrupted time and attention. Be prepared, in the course of listening, to repeat what you have just heard, ask questions, wait a moment, then ask the same question again. Assuming that a patient with dementia can be simply slotted into a typical appointment schedule will likely result in frustration for both you and the patient. Give these people the time, patience, and kindness they need and deserve.

Effective listening in this context also means empowering patients and helping to boost their self-confidence. During the decline phase of dementia, many patients are consciously or subconsciously aware of how they are being seen by others, and as a result, may experience great embarrassment at how they are perceived by others. This will adversely impact their self-confidence and can easily lead to a downward spiral, psychologically and emotionally. Encouraging the patient to speak, letting them know they should take their time, and highlighting to them that you are actually interested in what they have to say can have a hugely important role in enhancing self-confidence and allowing people to feel better about themselves.

It will become readily apparent that arguing with someone who has dementia is not only pointless, but also counterproductive. In some cases, dementia may produce a form of disinhibition in which patients will say things that range from slightly racy to downright offensive. There is no point in trying to fix or debate them; even if you disagree or are offended, try as best as possible to simply redirect the conversation, change the subject, and move forward. It will be important to prioritize which battles you can actually engage in with a likelihood of a successful outcome.

As our society ages and individuals live longer, cognitive decline and dementia will become more common. As health care professionals, and human beings ourselves, it is essential that we learn the skills necessary to communicate effectively despite the limitations and barriers dementia introduces in both interpersonal communication and in building relationships. Key considerations include kindness and patience, and the recognition that additional time and undivided attention will be required to fully support and help your patients with dementia be as comfortable as possible.

Interested in Learning More?

Bayles K, Kaszniak A, Tomoeda C. *Communication and Cognition in Normal Aging and Dementia.* Boston: Little, Brown and Company; 1987.

Egan M, Berube D, Racine G, Leonard C, Rochon E. Methods to enhance verbal communication between individuals with Alzheimer's disease and their formal and informal caregivers: a systematic review. *Int J Alzheimers Dis.* 2010;2010.

Ellis M, Astell A. Communicating with people living with dementia who are nonverbal. *PLoS One.* 2018;13(4):e0196489.

Kindell J, Keady J, Sage K, Wilkinson R. Everyday conversation in dementia: a review of the literature to inform research and practice. *Int J Lang Commun Disord.* 2017;52(4):392–406.

Stanyon M, Griffiths A, Thomas S, Gordon A. The facilitators of communication with people with dementia in a care setting: an interview study with healthcare workers. *Age Ageing.* 2016;45(1):164–170.

Weirather R. Communication strategies to assist comprehension in dementia. *Hawaii Med J.* 2010;69(3):72–74.

CASE

8

Disagreement Without Being Disagreeable: When Team Members Differ

Interprofessional, person-centered care is premised on the notion that different professionals, with different knowledge and skills, can bring multiple perspectives on complex issues and collectively will provide better and more effective health care than any single individual practitioner. The value of collaboration, respectful listening, and balancing multiple perspectives is greater than the operational or logistics issues associated with corralling busy and strong-minded professionals together.

In some circumstances, multiple perspectives and strong-minded opinions can lead to substantial disagreement. Learning to manage professional differences of opinion without becoming disagreeable or triggering conflict is an important skill to develop in team-based settings.

Consider the following scenario:

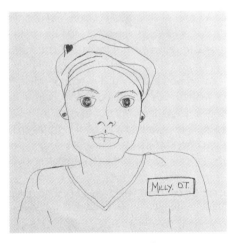

Milly, Occupational Therapist

Mrs. Mary Seto is a 79-year-old patient with complex care needs. She suffers from a variety of medical issues, including an irreversible, progressive, and debilitating neuromuscular condition that is both incredibly painful and makes it impossible for Mary to have any control over her motor functions.

Her pain is reasonably well managed with high doses of opioid analgesics, but this results in haziness and altered cognition that further impairs her ability to have any sort of satisfactory interaction with her family members. She is clearly suffering, physically, emotionally, psychologically, and existentially. Milly is her occupational therapist and has worked closely with her to try to help her be as comfortable as possible at home; she has refused to be placed in an extended health care institution. Over multiple conversations over many months, Milly has come to learn that Mary is calmly and clearly asking for her, and the health care team's, help to die. Although Milly is not qualified to assess this, she believes Mary is lucid enough to clearly understand the dimensions of her current situation. Mary is suffering and has concluded that she has no quality of life and no reasonable prospect for improvement or recovery. Medical aid in dying (MAID) is legal in this jurisdiction, and Mary has clearly asked Milly for her help to start this process. With a heavy heart, but great sympathy and understanding for her situation, Milly brings this forward at a team meeting to discuss further. She has worked with this team for many years and considers her colleagues to be friends. She is surprised by the reactions; half of her colleagues are adamantly opposed to MAID, believing it signifies failure of health care delivery and indicating that for personal moral reasons, they cannot be part of this process. The other half are not only entirely supportive of MAID, but immediately recognize that Mary is in need of their care and services to end her life painlessly, with dignity, and on her own terms. Although Milly expected some disagreement, she never anticipated the strength of opinions on both sides. Worse, each side cannot believe the other side could call themselves health care professionals and believe what they do about medical aid in dying.

In many jurisdictions around the world, it is now possible for health care professionals to support patients' wishes with respect to medical aid in dying. The list of countries, states, and provinces that allow for MAID continues to grow, as does general public acceptance of this process. Importantly, this growing public and legislative acceptance is relatively new. Until recently, MAID was thought by many to be equivalent to suicide, something that has historically been viewed negatively by lawmakers and religious leaders alike.

Growing public acceptance, however, does not mean universal approval. Among the general public, politicians, lawmakers, and health care professionals, vigorous debate surrounding MAID continues. Those in favor of MAID highlight the intensely personal decision-making process patients undertake when requesting help in dying with dignity. They note that there are operational safeguards in place and in legislation to ensure no individual is forced or coerced to ask for MAID by uncaring and unscrupulous family members, and that a thorough assessment of psychological competency to make such a decision occurs to ensure mental illness (such as depression) or other deficits are not interfering with clear and cogent reasoning. Health professionals, in particular, argue they have a duty to prevent suffering and support autonomous decision making by patients. As a result, it should be both the duty and responsibility of caring health professionals to provide dignified and medically appropriate end-of-life interventions. Conversely, other health professionals, although they may or may not agree in principle on the idea of MAID, have strong personal moral objections in being the instrument of accelerated un-natural death for any patient. This perspective may or may not be informed by religious conviction, but it is almost always based on a belief that health care professionals strive to heal and that MAID represents a failure of health care delivery. Rather than succumb to the path of least resistance, we must all work harder to alleviate suffering, restore func-tioning, and help patients live, rather than die, with dignity.

There are, of course, other controversial issues health care teams have faced in the past that can sometimes threaten their ability to function. Issues related to reproductive health, including women's choices around abortion, can rip apart the closest of friends, families, and health care teams. As MAID becomes legally available in more jurisdic-tions around the world, these tensions continue to grow. Arguably, MAID is different than many other issues because death is the one common denominator for every human being. As individual people, all health care professionals will need to deal with issues related to MAID in their personal lives. Unlike, for example, reproductive health issues or gender identity issues, every health professional will have a personal and emotional response to and stake in the evolution of MAID-related practices. Such personal in-vestment heightens the emotional nature of the discussion itself and can more easily lead to disagreement and conflict escalation. In jurisdictions that adopted MAID, an interesting trend has been observed on occasion. Although in some cases, practitioners can simply agree to disagree, allowing those who are willing to provide MAID services to do so while simultaneously ensuring no one who is opposed to MAID on personal or moral grounds is forced to participate (or quit their job), the irreversible nature of MAID appears to provoke striking polarization among team members. As Milly's case illustrates, strong opinions can sometimes lead colleagues to say regrettable things to one another such as, "You call yourself a health care professional and THAT'S what you think about MAID???"

It is clear from the case description that Milly, both personally and professionally, is supportive of MAID in medically appropriate circumstances. It appears that Mary rep-resents such a medically appropriate circumstance from both a legislative and clinical perspective. Milly also recognizes that this issue risks fracturing her successful and well-functioning interprofessional practice. There is little space for neutrality with respect to MAID, nor are their easy opportunities to accept and affirm both sides of this debate. Milly feels a sense of responsibility to Mary to continue to advocate on her behalf with the team and to begin the process of psychological and clinical assessment to determine whether Mary meets legislative requirements for MAID. She also feels a sense of respon-sibility as the person who brought this forward to the team to find common ground across all the professionals and to respect disagreement without being disagreeable. How can she best proceed in this situation?

First, it is essential to turn down the emotional heat (e.g., resentment, name-calling, disrespect) this issue has generated. When colleagues start saying, "I can't believe you think this, what's wrong with you?" this is a major sign of organizational dysfunction. Further, when one group, no matter how well intentioned, attempts to impose its moral beliefs on the entire group, this can lead to significant tension. Perhaps understandably, those who oppose MAID do not want to be seen to be part of a practice that provides this service and equally understandably, those who support MAID do not want to be seen to be part of a practice that withholds this legally available service to patients who need it. In the middle of course is Mary, who must trust that her health care professionals will do what is in her best interest and will respect her desires and wishes.

At this particularly divisive team meeting, where no middle ground seems possible and where everyone seems to have strong opinions on the issue, what should Milly do to balance all these contradictory and competing concerns? Mediation is a technique used in diverse settings that allows individuals and groups to try to work through difficult, seemingly impossible differences of beliefs, opinions, or morals. There is no formula or road map for effective mediation. Instead, it is an art that requires empathy, effective listening, and the careful application of a variety of techniques or tactics in a nuanced way to help each side see the other side's perspective in the hopes of ultimately finding an acceptable middle ground. For Milly, thinking about and applying some of these tactics may be one way of moving the discussion forward for the team, while honoring her professional and personal commitments to Mary.

Common techniques used by mediators include the following.

Naming the elephant in the room and speaking openly about it. Difficult situations often arise because individuals have an initially strong emotional response to something, thereby blocking any opportunity to engage cognitively or logically with an issue. In the context of MAID, making a strong principled statement about the rightness or wrongness of it in a public meeting with team members present can make it difficult to later climb down from such a pronouncement and find compromise. Instead, there may be a psychological need to further double down on the initially strong opinion, further escalating disagreement and conflict. Expert mediators help opposing sides clearly articulate—in logical, cognitive terms, not emotional ones—where the sources of disagreement occur. Learning to speak openly and logically about why there is disagreement, rather than reverting to name calling, insults, or other emotional response, is absolutely essential to move the process forward.

Caucusing is a technique that can potentially be risky, but when applied by a skilled mediator, has great potential in helping move beyond an impasse. Caucusing is a process where those who have substantially similar views on a disagreement are free to meet together privately to discuss the situation without fear that what they say may be held against them in the future. The risk of caucusing is that it can potentially create group think; those who may have only been mildly opposed to MAID may become even more strident in their beliefs if they spend considerable time with other colleagues who already have strong opinions, and in the process, important, swayable, and moderate opinion makers may be lost. At its best, however, caucusing allows a group to talk itself through their opinions and actually start to engage in some reality checking with like-minded individuals. The power of like-minded peers to help change opinions and beliefs is significant, and with a skilled mediator present who can gently nudge or redirect caucus conversation in a more productive manner, it may be possible to start to establish the building blocks of a consensus. Importantly, in this case, Milly may NOT be the best mediator, because she appears to already have declared which side she is on. If no one else is available to be a mediator, it may be possible for Milly to serve this role, but she will have to be very careful to fully disclose her preexisting views and beliefs, work strenuously to avoid the judgment of others, and minimize her use of what-about hypothetical questioning, which can give the appearance of bias.

Shuttle diplomacy can be an effective tool for mediation when entrenched factions have caucused and are no closer to conflict de-escalation or consensus building. In shuttle diplomacy, a trusted, neutral mediator physically moves between the groups, presenting each group with the other's ideas, messages, thoughts, and trial balloons for moving forward through the disagreement. In shuttle diplomacy, it is essential that those within each caucus remain separated from each other and that only a trusted, neutral mediator shuttles between the groups. This is an important technique to prevent escalation and reintroduce emotional tension into the discussion with the mere presence of someone from the other side. In this situation, Milly may or may not be able to act in this role. If she has previously made strong statements that are supportive of MAID or has advocated vigorously for Mary, it is unlikely she will be trusted or believed by those opposed. In contrast, if instead she has focused on more neutral, generally acceptable elements of this case (e.g., managing Mary's pain, providing psychosocial and spiritual care and support), it may be possible for her to serve as trusted mediator for both sides. In many cases such as this, however, the team or organization may realize they have little choice but to bring in an external, respected third-party mediator for shuttle diplomacy, a person who is respected by both sides but whose personal views on the issue are either unknown or are truly neutral.

Generating alternative points of view. When those in disagreement with one another become entrenched in their views, they are at high risk of confirmation bias. Confirmation bias is the human tendency to actively seek out opinions and perspectives that align with one's own, while equally and actively ignoring, diminishing, or insulting those who have opposite opinions. A skilled mediator can help caucus groups to see the other side's perspective once the group itself has clearly established its own positions and perspectives. The simple question, "What do you think the other group is saying right now?" can help open a discussion about alternative ways of viewing a situation. Once again, a skilled mediator should be present to help keep this discussion respectful, focused, and on track. In generating alternative points of view, the caucus group can reality test their initial positions and ideas, some of which will fail, which ultimately may make it easier to reach a consensus.

Some highly skilled mediators have claimed success using the risky technique of *exaggeration*. This is not a technique to be used lightly or in an amateurish way, because there is a real possibility it could backfire spectacularly and further escalate disagreements and conflicts. Exaggeration is a technique in which the mediator encourages caucus groups or individuals to upwardly amplify and distort their beliefs as much as possible. For example, a group opposed to MAID may be encouraged to build on the slippery slope argument that once you start helping needful patients like Mary, how can we possibly say no to a patient whose dog just died and they are very upset? This is patently ridiculous and, frankly, insulting to compare Mary's situation to this what-about hypothetical. It is the act of hearing oneself make such ridiculous extensions during exaggeration that can, sometimes, with the help of a skilled mediator, lead individuals in a caucus to start to recognize the extremity of their views and lay the foundation for a compromise or consensus.

Finding common ground is by far the most important and impactful technique used by mediators and nonmediators alike. Common ground represents those things we can all agree on. Hearing oneself agree with the other side provides a window into what compromise can look like and helps us to better understand the value of trying to find such compromise. Unlike many of the other techniques noted previously, finding common ground can be undertaken without a neutral third-party mediator. Some argue that it is more authentic and, therefore, more effective when it is spontaneously generated by those on opposite sides of an issue. In this case, what is the common ground both sides can agree to focus on? Mary, her needs, her health, her wishes, and what the team is and is not doing to support her in this time. Rather than debating an abstract philosophical issue such as "MAID: Are you for or against?" focusing on a real, pragmatic, and important case (Mary and what we must do to help her now) can help to reduce the emotional intensity of the discussion and help both sides to see a path forward together. What might Milly suggest in terms of common ground? Perhaps a psychological assessment to better understand Mary's current state of mind. This can be invaluable information to support clinical decision making regardless of one's perspective on MAID. It may end up being supportive of those who want to provide MAID in this case, or it may not be if it is determined that Mary has diminished cognitive capacity. In either case, the common ground associated with undertaking this psychological assessment represents the team working collectively together and focused on a patient's immediate needs in a pragmatic way. Another example may be to focus on comfort measures to provide Mary with greater physical, emotional, or psychosocial support. Regardless of one's philosophical views on MAID, such supportive measures will be impactful for Mary and will be well received by the entire team. Common ground does not solve all problems or overcome all disagreements. It does, however, provide a small window of opportunity for a team in sharp disagreement to actually hear themselves agreeing, see themselves collaborating, and start to imagine how such seemingly small steps—all focused on a real patient's immediate needs rather than a philosophical disagreement—can be so much more meaningful.

Clearly, there is no simple answer or straightforward road map to solve problems that arise from moral objections or disagreements associated with a difficult issue such as MAID. Importantly, the objective may not be to have everyone agree or to prevent disagreement in the first place. Instead, the use of foundational communication skills related to empathy, active listening, reflective questioning, and simple respect for differences in opinion are the best that can be achieved. In a situation such as this, if the team disagreement continues to escalate, there may be no viable alternative other than bringing in a skilled, third-party, neutral mediator to apply some of these techniques to bring about greater cohesion. As a first crucial step, with or without an external mediator, the entire group needs to start to work toward finding common ground. Focusing on the immediate needs of Mary and finding sources of agreement, rather than disagreement, will not solve all this team's issues but may help them to establish a foundation for further respectful dialogue and discussion in the future.

Interested in Learning More?

Apker J, Propp K, Zabava Ford W, Hofmeister N. Collaboration, credibility, compassion and coordination: professional nurse communication skill sets in health care team interactions. *J Prof Nurs.* 2006;22(3):180–189.

Bowman K. Communication, negotiation, and mediation: dealing with conflict in end of life decisions. *J Palliat Care.* 2000;16 Suppl:S17–23.

Brown J, Lewis L, Ellis K, Stewart M, Freeman T, Kasperski M. Conflict on interprofessional primary health care teams—can it be resolved? *J Interprof Care.* 2011;25(1):4–10.

Cullati S, Bochatay N, Maitre F, et al. When team conflicts threaten quality of care: a student of health care professionals' experiences and perceptions. *Mayo Clin Proc Innov Qual Outcomes.* 2019;3(1):43–51.

Kim S, Bochatay N, Relyea-Chew A, et al. Individual, interpersonal, and organizational factors of healthcare conflict: a scoping review. *J Interprof Care.* 2017;31(3):282–290.

Liberman A, Rotarius T, Kendall L. Alternative dispute resolution: a conflict management tool in health care. *Health Care Superv.* 1997;16(2):9–20.

Matheson C, Robertson H, Elliott A, Iversen L, Murchie P. Resilience of primary healthcare professionals working in challenging environments: a focus group study. *Br J Gen Pract.* 2016;66(648):e507–515.

McKenzie D. The role of mediation in resolving workplace relationship conflict. *Int J Law Psychiatry.* 2015;39:52–59.

Ramsay M. Conflict in the health care workplace. *Proc (Bayl Univ Med Cent).* 2001;14(2): 138–139.

Disclosing Errors: Communicating and Being Open with Patients and Families

Medical incidents are an unfortunate and, at times, catastrophic reality. Although health professionals and teams work diligently to provide safe and effective care, errors or omissions resulting in harm to patients may still occur. Many people are affected by medical incidents, including patients, their families, other health care professionals, other patients, and the broader community who may begin to lose trust. It is sometimes said that patients do not necessarily expect perfection, but they do deserve honesty, justice, transparency, accountability, and compassion. When things go wrong, it is essential that those who are affected know what happened, know what changes will be made to prevent it from happening in the future, and hear two important words compassionately and sincerely delivered: "I'm sorry."

All health care teams and professionals should accept nothing less than the safest possible care. This means fully implementing and utilizing best possible evidence-based prevention strategies for avoidable harm and fostering a culture of open communication at all levels. The Canadian Patient Safety Institute has noted that: "Good healthcare starts with good communication" (Hannawa 2014).

Consider the following scenario:

Tricia Halliday is a vibrant, active, and educated person and an opera singer with a burgeoning career. For the past 10 years, she has been receiving treatment for hypothyroidism. Her condition has been well managed using medications. At a routine recent visit to the clinic, her laboratory tests indicated there was a need to increase her current dose of levothyroxine from 0.025 mg daily to 0.0375 mg daily to help manage some emerging hypothyroid symptoms. A medical intern, Garth, being supervised by a team physician, Mah-Ahn, discussed the case with the Tricia's primary care provider, Benji, a nurse practitioner. Garth reviewed the patient's chart and recent laboratory work, then wrote a new prescription, in error, for levothyroxine 0.125 mg instead of levothyroxine 0.0125 mg. During the conversation with the nurse practitioner, the intern had said "0.0125 mg," and had documented this in the chart that was reviewed by the physician, but neither the nurse practitioner nor the physician actually checked the computer-generated prescription provided by the intern to Tricia. As a result, she went to her usual pharmacy with a new prescription for levothyroxine 0.125 mg, with instructions to add this new tablet to the existing levothyroxine 0.025 mg dose she had been taking for many months. The pharmacy dispensed a 3-month supply. It was only at the time of refill, 3 months later, that the error was uncovered. As a result, for 3 months, Tricia had been receiving levothyroxine 0.125 mg daily, rather than the intended dose of levothyroxine 0.0375 mg, 4 times the dose she was supposed to get.

From a clinical and therapeutic perspective, this medical incident-related overdose is of course potentially problematic. Levothyroxine overdose can produce symptoms of overactive thyroid including fatigue, sensitivity to heat, increased appetite and sweating, along with confusion and disorientation. From a practical perspective, this medical error will require Tricia to undertake a series of unnecessary additional medical tests and attend additional appointments to ensure she is safe. From a personal perspective, being exposed to this overdose of levothyroxine for 3 months may have caused Tricia to experience unnecessary and unusual new symptoms that perhaps she misinterpreted as premenopause, the flu, depression, or something else. From a trust perspective, the fact that so many different professionals missed this seemingly simple decimal place error might make Tricia much less likely to believe in medical expertise in the future. Compared to other medical errors, this particular situation, fortunately, may not result in a catastrophic outcome, but it is still serious, still an error, and still an important communication challenge and opportunity for the team involved.

As the team meets to discuss how to proceed in this case, there are important principles that should underpin their next steps:

1. Person-centered care means that there is no such thing as a small error. For the person who is the innocent victim of medical error, there will always be concern, worry, symptoms, and other issues that are serious. Dismissing a decimal place error as insignificant, or suggesting that it was *only* four times the appropriate dose is both disrespectful and profoundly off-putting for the person who is on the receiving end of the error.

2. Patients have the right to know what has happened to them and to be as actively involved in the planning and decision making surrounding their ongoing care as they choose to be.

3. Disclosure of all incidents is essential, even in the event that there are few immediate symptoms or problems, or no long-term consequences, disclosure is essential at fostering trust that is integral to the patient–practitioner relationship. Disclosure itself must be respectful, honest, transparent, and open.

4. Patients need to know that individual practitioners, the health care team, and the entire system has learned from this mistake and will enact systems to prevent a future error of this sort from happening again. The consolation in knowing other patients will be protected in the near future can be of considerable solace to those who are innocent victims of medical error.

Disclosure is central to the process of managing incidents in health care. At minimum, disclosure must include:

*   The facts about what happened, presented clearly and in plain language, in an organized, systematic, chronological manner with a minimum of medical jargon

- The specific steps that were taken once the incident was discovered and what will be done in the short, medium, and long term to minimize specific harm for the patient

- A clear statement from the individual health care provider(s) involved and the health care team or organization that they are sincerely sorry for what has happened

- A clear indication of what changes will be implemented to prevent this kind of situation happening again in the future to another innocent patient

Disclosure is the best way of preventing patients, their families, and the broader community from becoming anxious, fearful, or losing trust in the health care system and in medical professionals. Some practitioners may be fearful of disclosure, believing—wrongly—that disclosure may actually increase the chances of litigation, complaints, or a lawsuit of some sort. In the vast majority of cases, disclosure actually decreases these risks because patients feel more respected and do not feel necessary facts are withheld or being hidden. In the event that litigation does occur, effective communication and disclosure may help protect the health care professional or team from the highest available sanctions by demonstrating accountability and responsibility.

Disclosure conversations can be extremely stressful for all involved, but can be facilitated through application of most of the principles discussed in this book. Empathy and person-centeredness will be essential for a successful conversation. In addition, careful planning of a conversation will be essential and should include the following.

- Clinical supports to manage short, medium, and long-term actual or potential risks associated with the incident. This will include, for example, ensuring appropriate clinical investigations and tests, timely reporting of results, ongoing monitoring and follow-up, and clear instructions to minimize chances for confusion.

- Creating a respectful environment for the initial conversation. This will include ensuring acoustic privacy, allowing sufficient time for the patient to internalize and digest the news and to ask questions, respect for the emotional response the patient may demonstrate, and application of effective listening skills. Professionals involved in the conversation must be prepared and rehearse what will be said and how it will be said. This is not the time to improvise or wing it. In many cases, it can be extremely helpful to have another, knowledgeable, and trusted team member who was NOT involved in the incident in any way to be present to provide both practical and emotional support to both the patient and the team members involved.

- Initiate emotional and psychological supports. Patients and their families should play the key role in identifying what supports (e.g., family, friends, spiritual or religious leaders) are most valuable in the specific situation, and the professional and/or team should work to help access these supports. Other nonteam professionals, including social workers, counselors, psychologists, or occupational therapists, may also be mobilized to provide such support based on the patient's preferences and needs.

- Identify practical supports that are of value to the patient. For example, facilitate access to the patient's chart so the patient and family members and others so authorized can review the care provided, offer to provide reimbursement for reasonable expenses associated with the error and its disclosure (e.g., offer to pay for parking, lab test costs), provide access to space within the clinic or health care facility for the family to meet to discuss and come to terms with the disclosure, provide medical and drug information resources to help educate patients and family members about the situation, etc.

Expense reimbursement is often controversial and misunderstood. The intent of reimbursing reasonable expenses is NOT to compensate the patient directly for any harm resulting, but instead relates to the organization and/or professional taking responsibility for its actions. Although every incident is different, examples of reasonable expenses that may warrant reimbursement include travel expenses, parking, meals, child care, photocopying of medical records, accommodations, laboratory tests for follow-up purposes, etc. Offering reimbursement for these types of expenses demonstrates both care and concern. Equally, however, it is important to understand and define in advance nonreimbursable expenses (such as continuing care costs, long-term care requirements, or funeral costs). Each situation is different, and each health care team has different resources available; defining limits of reasonable reimbursement up-front is difficult but essential.

Any disclosure conversation should begin with a clear and authentic apology—a genuine expression of being sorry for what has happened. The actual words "I'm sorry" need to be used because they are important. Using "we" (as opposed to "I") may appear to deflect responsibility, and words such as "regret" do not have the same emotional connotation as "I'm sorry." An early and clear apology is often the only pathway by which a damaged patient–practitioner relationship can be restored.

In summary, preparation is essential prior to any disclosure conversation and must, at minimum, cover the following points:

- Who will attend the initial conversation? Who will lead it? Who will be the designated contact person for the monitoring and follow-up process? Who will provide support to both the patient and to the practitioners involved?

- What are the facts that are known and will be discussed?

- Where will the conversation take place?

- When will the meeting occur (as soon in time after discovery and investigation as feasible)?

- Why are we having this disclosure conversation?

- How will the disclosure be discussed?

To answer the last question (How will the disclosure be discussed?), several key steps are required and include:

- Clearly provide facts, using straightforward words and phrases.

- Explain the proposed care plan and what steps come next in the monitoring and follow-up process.

- Avoid speculation, second-guessing, or innuendo. Stick with the known facts only.

- Authentically and honestly express regret.

- As best as possible, describe what the patient can reasonably expect to happen next.

- Make arrangements to ensure follow-ups (e.g., lab tests, referrals to specialists) are as simple as possible for the patient.

- Clearly indicate who the main point of contact will be for management and follow-up.

- Document what was discussed and decided to avoid future uncertainty or ambiguity.

Let's return to the initial case and consider how a disclosure conversation might occur.

To begin, the primary care clinic has asked Zander, the team pharmacist, to attend the meeting with Tricia. Zander was not involved in dispensing the medication and was not involved in the error in any way; however, as a pharmacist, he is knowledgeable about medications and side effects, and as a team member, he has a preexisting positive relationship with Tricia. Zander, Mah-Ahn (the physician), Benji (the nurse practitioner), and Garth (the intern) are all prepared to attend this meeting. Initially, so as to not overwhelm or intimidate Tricia, Mah-Ahn is meeting with her alone.

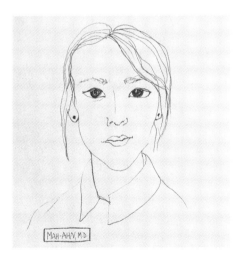

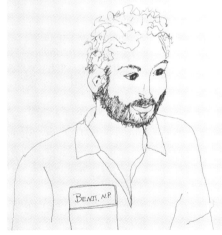

Mah-Ahn, Physician   **Benji, Nurse Practitioner**

Mah-Ahn: Hi, Tricia. Thanks for coming in to see me today. *(Note: It is important for the disclosure conversation to ensure a senior, most responsible health care professional leads the initial discussion, to provide reassurance to patient.)*

Tricia: No problem, but I must say, I'm a bit worried. You haven't called me in like this ever before and I usually just see your student. What's wrong?

Mah-Ahn: I know it must have been stressful for you. I was able to change a few appointments to see you as quickly as possible. *(Note: Acknowledging the patient's stress and highlighting efforts to minimize time delay in meeting helps establish care and concern.)* I've asked you in today to let you know about an incident we just learned about. I'm very sorry about this, but we made a mistake with your last prescription for thyroid medication. *(Note: Rather than prolonging the conversation, it is sometimes helpful to get straight to the point, directly and clearly. Importantly, beginning the conversation with an apology can also help set the best possible tone to convey this difficult news.)*

Tricia: Oh no. What . . . what happened?

Mah-Ahn: Garth, our intern who met with you, made a mistake writing your prescription for the levothyroxine. Neither Benji, your nurse practitioner, nor I reviewed the prescription before it was given to you. *(Note: This is a clear and succinct description of error without immediately burdening patient with specific details and complexities regarding decimal points and mathematical errors.)*

Tricia: (a bit stunned) Oh.

Mah-Ahn: The pharmacist at the drug store you normally go to discovered this error *[Note: Some sources suggest NOT using the word "error" in a context such as this as it may be misunderstood as suggesting negligence or lack of attention; others, however, endorse using this word because it is clear and immediately understood by most patients]* when you went to get a refill yesterday, and called us about it. *(Note: Here is an additional factual clarification to help Tricia understand HOW the incident was discovered.)*

Tricia: Okay. What does this all mean?

Mah-Ahn: It means you've been getting too much of the thyroid medication for the last 3 months. *(Note: Here is a brief but clear summary of the problem, without trying to dilute or hide the issue behind unnecessary details at this point.)*

Tricia: How much more? *(Note: In asking this question, Tricia has signaled she requires more factual information to assist with processing this news. She is engaging her cognitive, rather than emotional, self at this point, opening an invitation for Mah-Ahn to respond accordingly. Had Tricia signaled a more emotional response, such as "I can't believe you let this happen! I trusted you with my health!" the conversation would of course go in a different direction.)*

Mah-Ahn: We think you received four times as much thyroxine as we'd intended. *(Note: This clear, focused summary is more helpful than the details of how the error occurred and what mathematical combination of doses lead to the situation. These details can be discussed later as needed.)* I have some information here you can read later. I want to reassure you that while this error is serious, I don't think you are at risk of any kind of long-term problem or complication because of this. *(Note: Use of "I" as opposed to "we" in this sentence provides assurance of personal responsibility and accountability and may be more comforting to patient at this time.)*

Tricia: Four times too much! That sounds like a lot. How do you know for sure I'm going to be okay?

Mah-Ahn: I want to send you for some blood tests to confirm. I've got the forms here, and results will be expedited. I've also spoken with the lab and they can see you immediately. *(Note: She provided a practical strategy and helpful support for the important and immediate next step.)* That will help us to determine what has happened and what might be likely to happen next. I know how inconvenient and difficult some of these tests can be. I'm sorry about this. But I do think this is the most important thing we can do now to determine the impact of this mistake.

Tricia: Of course, fine, I'll do this, I want to know too. (Now getting angry) I just don't understand why this happened to me.

Mah-Ahn: It was a mistake. I've asked Garth, the intern, along with Benji, your nurse practitioner, if they could join us, so all three of us can apologize for what happened, and explain it to you. If you're okay with that, I can ask them to come in.

Tricia: Yes, I'd like to talk to them, especially Garth! I can't believe he did this. You know, I worried about his competence the first time I met him.

Mah-Ahn: This is difficult, and believe me, they are both very upset and very sorry about this too, and really want to have a chance to meet with you to apologize in person. I've also asked our team pharmacist, Zander, if he could sit in on this conversation.

Tricia: Zander! I used to like him so much. Was he involved in this too?

Mah-Ahn: No, not at all actually. He was on vacation when this happened. However, he is our medication expert and he can help explain what's happened and answer your questions.

Tricia: That would be good. I . . . I don't even know where to start.

Mah-Ahn: Would you like a few minutes to yourself before I ask the others to join us? *(Note: Mah-Ahn is reflecting Tricia's comment and emotional state, and providing an option.)* Take whatever time you need.

Tricia: I'm just so . . . I just can't believe this happened. I used to trust you so much!

Mah-Ahn: I am so sorry about this mistake. And I want you to know that my colleagues and I will do everything we can to try to earn your trust again. I will be with you throughout this process to make sure you get the best care possible. *(Note: Avoid responding defensively to emotionally charged statement and assume a forward-looking focus in the conversation. Commit to personally being primary contact during this monitoring and follow-up process.)* For now, what would be best for you? Would you like me to stay or give you some time to process this on your own? Or would you like to meet with the others now? *(Note: Provide options and allow patient to determine next stage in disclosure process.)*

This is clearly a difficult conversation, and equally a difficult conversation to fully depict within a written sample in a textbook. The emotion and nonverbal cues being sent and received by the patient and practitioner are in many ways more important than the words spoken. Nonetheless, the words do matter. Mah-Ahn has started the process of conversation with Tricia by highlighting several key points:

- Apologizing and taking personal responsibility for the situation

- Describing immediate next steps (e.g., laboratory tests)

- Providing options to the patient for further disclosure conversation

- Allowing the patient opportunities to express both emotional concern and distress

- Focusing on the future and her desire to re-earn the patient's trust

All health professionals will at some point be involved in and lead a disclosure conversation such as this. Each conversation will be different and will take its own course. Recognizing that effective disclosure must be built on principles such as trust, honesty, and transparency and utilize foundational communication skills such as empathy and effective listening will help such conversations be as effective as possible given the difficulties inherent in such situations.

Interested in Learning More?

Chamberlain C, Koniaris L, Wu, A, Pawlik T. Disclosure of nonharmful medical errors and other events. *Arch Surg.* 2012;147(3):282–286.

Hannawa A. Disclosing medical errors to patients: effects of nonverbal involvement. *Patient Educ Couns.* 2014;94(3):310–313.

Hannawa A, Shigemoto Y, Little T. Medical errors: disclosure styles, interpersonal forgiveness and outcomes. *Soc Sci Med.* 2016;156:29–38.

Mazor K, Reed G, Yood R, Fischer M, Baril J, Gurwitz J. Disclosure of medical errors: what factors influence how patients respond? *J Gen Intern Med.* 2006;21(7):704–710.

Mazor K, Simon S, Yood R, et al. Health plan members' views about disclosure of medical errors. *Ann Intern Med.* 2004;140(6):409–418.

Petronio S. Disclosing medical mistakes: a communication management plan for physicians. *Perm J*. 2013;17(2):73–79.

Rosner F, Berger J, Kark P, Potash J, Bennett A. Disclosure and prevention of medical errors. *Arch Intern Med*. 200;160(14):2089–2092.

Wu A, Huang I, Stokes S, Pronovost P. Disclosing medical errors to patients—it's not what you way, it's what they hear. *J Gen Intern Med*. 2009;24(9):1012–1017.

CASE

10

"But He Doesn't Want to Share His Marbles!": Challenges When Professionals Simply Don't Want to Collaborate

Interprofessional, person-focused care works best when all practitioners are ready and willing to learn with, from, and about one another. Although this model is now commonly taught in schools and clinical training programs, there are many practitioners who were educated and who have practiced for many years in an older model of hierarchical care using a differentiation of labor structure (see Chapter 3).

Consider the following scenario:

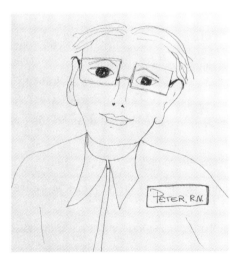

Peter, nurse practitioner

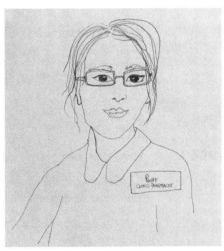

Ruby, pharmacist

> *Peter is an experienced nurse who has worked in primary care for almost 35 years. Peter believes nursing is a noble profession, and that nurses work best when they follow directions from physicians and other more senior professionals. Ruby just qualified as a pharmacist and is now part of the primary care team, and is accustomed to a more collaborative model of practice in which all practitioners share information and work to their maximum scope of practice. For Ruby, this means she will monitor patients' responses to*

drug therapy and independently modify doses based on laboratory values, informing the initial prescriber and the rest of the team of what has occurred through her documentation. Today, she is looking for some recent laboratory data about a patient named Mrs. Corrascenti.

Ruby:	Hey Peter, how are you doing?
Peter:	Great, thanks.
Ruby:	Where's Mrs. Corrascenti's most recent test results?
Peter:	I just got through with her. I haven't had time to put it in the chart yet. Crazy day!
Ruby:	She's still here and I need to get her most recent blood pressure, vitals, all that.
Peter:	Why?
Ruby:	I need to adjust her medication doses before she leaves today.
Peter:	You're doing that now? Not Dr. Singh?
Ruby:	Yeah, it's just faster and easier, and well, that's my training, right? Do you have the BP?
Peter:	Um . . . yeah. I gotta get this form done for Dr. Anderton first, then I'll be right on it.
Ruby:	But Mrs. Corrascenti is just waiting for me to adjust the dose so she can get her ride home.
Peter:	Yeah, but I gotta get this insurance stuff done first.
Ruby:	Can't that wait? Okay, just tell me the BP and vitals and I'll go on that before you document in the chart.
Peter:	Listen, I don't . . . I have to get that from my log book but it's not here, it's in the office.
Ruby:	Seriously?
Peter:	Yes. Seriously.
Ruby:	Okay, then I guess Mrs. Corrascenti will just need to wait. I hope she doesn't miss her ride home or anything. That would be bad, don't you think?

What went wrong in this conversation? Although it did not spill over into frank conflict or confrontation, it is clear, even when only reading the words and not observing non-verbal messaging, that this is not a positive, collaborative conversation. What might have been done differently?

Ruby: Hey Peter, how are you doing?	*Positive opening, use of open-ended question, and addressing colleague by name to establish collegial relationship.*
Peter: Great, thanks.	*Truncated response: Is he busy, irritated, or distracted? No invitation from Peter to follow-up with Ruby to ask about her day.*
Ruby: Where's Mrs. Corrascenti's most recent test results?	*Direct question with no acknowledgment of her interrupting Peter by, for example, saying, "Sorry to bother you" or "I see you're busy." No attempt at summarizing, paraphrasing, or empathizing and therefore no indication of attempt to build rapport, relationship, or trust.*
Peter: I just got through with her. I haven't had time to put it in the chart yet. Crazy day!	*Did not respond verbally to the question. Could that be hinting at or a nonverbal suggestion of a problem? He does provide an opening to follow-up on what a busy day it has been for him, but gives no indication (other than workload) as to why he is unwilling to share results.*
Ruby: She's still here and I need to get her most recent blood pressure, vitals, all that.	*Does not respond to Peter's emotional statement regarding his "crazy day." Did she not hear what he was saying or is she simply overlooking it to focus on her own immediate concerns? In either case, it suggests lack of engagement and responsiveness, which interferes with communication and their relationship.*
Peter: Why?	*Very direct statement. Asking why can be interpreted as aggressive. Is he threatening or questioning Ruby's professional competency and skill? His nonverbal tone will be crucial to differentiating what was meant.*
Ruby: I need to adjust her medication doses before she leaves today.	*Responds directly to question; if delivered in a defensive tone, is she escalating tension? If delivered in an exasperated tone, does this indicate lack of respect for Peter (i.e., HE can't do this important job, only SHE can)?*
Peter: You're doing that now? Not Dr. Singh?	*Nonverbals will be crucial here: Is this simply an information gap, or does Peter not trust this new, young pharmacist to do this important job? Either way, tone will likely be negative and escalation is likely.*

Ruby: Yeah, it's just faster and easier, and well, that's my training, right? Do you have the BP?	*Becoming defensive in responding. If tone is sharp and nonverbal posture (e.g., gestures, facial expression, position of arms) is pinched or closed, is Ruby irritated or angry? Closes with direct request using "you." Could this be threatening? Would "Could I get the BP please?" be better?*
Peter: Um . . . yeah. I gotta get this form done for Dr. Anderton first, then I'll be right on it.	*Seems dismissive and reinforcing physician-centered hierarchy, favoring the doctor's needs over Ruby's. If tone is at all dismissive, it will be interpreted very negatively. Choice of words ("I'll be right on it") could be interpreted as sarcasm.*
Ruby: But Mrs. Corrascenti is just waiting for me to adjust the dose so she can get her ride home.	*No empathy demonstrated for Peter's workload or his concerns. Immediately focused on her own needs, although using the patient's concern as a form of common ground.*
Peter: Yeah, but I gotta get this insurance stuff done first.	*Reaching an impasse: For the last two rounds of conversation, neither party has said anything new, which suggests each person is getting further entrenched in their position and a positive resolution may be difficult to achieve unless something is done quickly to break the downward negative spiral.*
Ruby: Can't that wait? Okay . . . just tell me the BP and vitals and I'll go on that before you document in the chart.	*Exasperation has escalated to irritation. Asking, "Can't that wait?" signals she thinks Peter doesn't know how to do his job properly. At this point, tone and nonverbals will be all-important, and both parties are interpreting each other emotionally rather than cognitively. Use of directives such as "just tell me" reinforces Peter's negative emotional opinion of her.*
Peter: Listen, I don't . . . I have to get that from my log book but it's not here, it's in the office.	*Important verbal insertion ("Listen") provides clue that Peter believes Ruby is not listening to him and this is upsetting, resulting in his intransigence. Is comment regarding log book subconsciously designed to further inflame and provoke rather than productively solve the problem and address the impasse?*
Ruby: Seriously?	*Frank sarcasm. No nonverbals or tone can compensate for use of this word at this point in the context. The conversation is now over and each side is entrenched, hostile, and not open to resolution.*

Peter: Yes. Seriously.	*Marked escalation, with frank verbal hostility and aggression from both parties now. Depending on nonverbals and tone, this could become outright conflict very quickly.*
Ruby: Okay, then I guess Mrs. Corrascenti will just need to wait. I hope she doesn't miss her ride home or anything. That would be bad, don't you think?	*Ruby moves to de-escalate but does so using sarcasm, and co-opting the patient's best interest as her own responsibility, not Peter's. No attempt to bring Peter into a more collaborative stance and no recognition of how the situation has escalated so quickly and so badly.*

As can be seen, a real-time conversation such as this would only take 1 to 2 minutes to complete, but in that time, a significant and negative emotional tone has grown between these two colleagues that will make future collaborations and relationship difficult to achieve. Long after this particular incident is passed, the emotional memory of this interaction will taint each other's views of one another.

How could this have been managed more effectively?

Sentence 3: Although direct communication and getting to the point may work for some people, clearly this does not suit Peter. Ruby's direct statement could have been framed as a polite question instead. For example, "Sorry to bother you. I can see you're really busy, but I was wondering if I could get the patient's latest lab data?" If delivered with sincerity, a positive tone, and appropriate nonverbals, this may have established a more collegial and civil dialogue to follow.

Sentence 6: Peter's direct, somewhat challenging question of "Why?" is easily open to misinterpretation. A single word response to sentence 5 sounds either deliberately provocative and confrontational or simply petulant. In either case, it comes across to Ruby as being dismissive, as though he believes she doesn't DESERVE to have this information because she is not qualified to do anything with it. Although this may not be his intention at all, it is most likely the way she heard it and her emotional response to this will be swift and negative. Instead of a single word response, he could have said, "Okay. I really need to get this insurance form done right now, could I get this for you in 5 minutes?" Assessing Ruby's immediate need for the information and demonstrating openness to her request and respect for her role, while also indicating his competing workload demands may have been less confrontational.

Sentence 8: "You're doing that now?" could have different meanings depending on the emphasis and tone. If the emphasis was on "you're," it would suggest Peter is surprised that a pharmacist is doing this job and doesn't think that's appropriate. If the emphasis was on "now," it would suggest the focus is on the specific timing of the job, not Ruby's competency to do the job itself. The addition of "not Dr. Singh" could similarly be misinterpreted. Is this diminishing Ruby and her profession, and reinforcing a physician's power in the hierarchy? Perhaps it was simply an information gap, because Peter was lead to believe Dr. Singh would make the dose adjustments. Alternatively, depending on tone and body language, it could come across that Peter believes that only physicians are qualified to do this task, which would be a broad insult to Ruby and her professional education and status. Regardless, the ambiguity in word choice used by Peter leaves it open to Ruby's emotional interpretation as to what he intends and truly means. Far better for Peter to clearly state, "I thought Dr. Singh wanted to adjust the doses himself. I wasn't aware that you were going to be doing that," or "Did you want to wait until we get all the laboratory data back from the lab before adjusting the doses? All I have are the blood pressure readings I just took. Will that be enough for you to do your work?"

Sentences 15 and 16: By this point in the conversation, conflict escalation has occurred in earnest. A simple question like "Seriously?" can be delivered in a way that is dripping with sarcasm and contempt, and the emotional tone will be what the receiver responds to and escalates. Although the conversation does not appear to be heading toward outright hostility, there is clearly tension and high emotions on both sides, and this does not bode well for collaboration now or in the near future. Rather than try to be funny or sarcastic by saying, "Seriously?" Ruby could have simply said, "All right, I will let the patient know we will be a few more minutes," and walk away to allow emotions to settle down. Rather than say, "Yes. Seriously" in response, Peter could have highlighted the urgency of the task he was faced with and apologized that he couldn't do everything at once.

Importantly, team-based miscommunication and interprofessional tension can sometimes be addressed through team-building activities focused on better understanding of one another's emotional intelligence and/or conflict management styles. In this example of conflict, it appears as though Ruby is behaving as a settler, favoring direct communication and a pragmatic worldview, whereas Peter is likely a thwarter, favoring indirect communication and a principled worldview. Ruby appears to be more of a converger and Peter is likely more of an assimilator. This may further complicate interactions given foundational differences between these individuals. Recognizing one another's conflict management and emotional intelligence styles can help colleagues better anticipate how best to communicate and interact with one another in challenging situations such as this.

A short conversation such as this illustrates how a reasonable request can quickly lead to misunderstanding, resentment, and an interprofessional problem. Had both Peter and Ruby used empathy, truly listened, been clearer in what they were saying, and applied their understanding of communication theory and applied psychology to this conversation, it would not have escalated in this unfortunate manner. And Mrs. Corrascenti may have been able to get her ride home after all!

Interesting in Learning More?

Bosch B, Mansell H. Interprofessional collaboration in health care: lessons to be learned from competitive sports. *Can Pharm J.* 2015;148(4):176–179.

Clements D, Dault M, Priest A. Effective teamwork in healthcare: research and reality. *Healthc Pap.* 2007;7:26–34.

Gougeon L, Johnson J, Morse H. Interprofessional collaboration in health care teams for the maintenance of community dwelling seniors health and well being in Canada: a systematic review of trials. *J Interprof Educ Pract.* 2017;7:29–37.

Mayo A, Williams-Woolley A. Teamwork in health care: maximizing collective intelligence via inclusive collaboration and open communication. *AMA J Ethics*. 2016;18(9):933–940.

O'Daniel M, Rosenstein A. Professional communication and team collaboration. In: Hughes R, ed. *Patient Safety and Quality: An Evidence Based Handbook for Nurses*. Rockville, MD: Agency for Healthcare Research and Quality; 2008.

Saint-Pierre C, Herskovic V, Sepulveda M. Multidisciplinary collaboration in primary care: a systematic review. *Fam Prac*. 2018;35(2):132–141.

Whitehead CM, Whitehead C, McLaughlin G, Austin Z. Harmonious healthcare teams: what healthcare professionals can and cannot learn from chamber musicians. *J Res Interprof Pract Educ*. 2014;4(1). doi.org/10/22230/jripe/2014v4n1a169.

11

Providing Person-Centered Care When You Don't Agree with a Person's Choices

Person-centered care is a philosophy of health care practice that recognizes the centrality of autonomy and self-determination at the heart of the clinician–client (or practitioner–patient) relationship. Sadly, the history of health care practice provides many regrettable examples of health care practitioners who have used their education, their status, and their power to dominate patients and to have them undergo tests or procedures they had reservations about. Today, we recognize the importance of all recipients of health care being as informed as possible regarding benefits, risks, costs, and consequences of their decisions, and for health care professionals to respect and support informed, autonomous decision making.

At times, however, this can produce conflict or cognitive dissonance when practitioners disagree (sometimes strongly) with decisions made by their patients and clients.

Consider the following scenario:

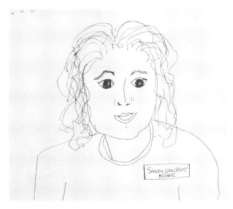

Sandy, Midwife

Mathilda Colangelo is a new mother visiting the Health Baby Clinic for an educational session and for a first check-up following her delivery. Mathilda is married, well-educated, and was thrilled about the birth of her first child, Milo. The pregnancy and delivery were uneventful; Mathilda was extremely careful in what she ate and the physical activities she pursued, and completely abstained from alcohol, coffee, and all other drugs to ensure the healthiest possible pregnancy. Milo was born with no complications and is thriving with his family. Today, during an education session with Sandy, the clinic midwife, the topic of routine infant vaccination arose. Mathilda chose her words carefully, but clearly indicated she and her husband had done much reading and discussion and ultimately decided that the risks of vaccination outweighed the benefits for their son, and as a result, they would not be having him vaccinated ever. In conversation, the midwife learns that the reading and discussion the Colangelo's have undertaken are with dubious, non–evidence-based sources, and when she tries to point this out, Mathilda dismisses Sandy by saying,"Well, of course I know you HAVE to say that and try to convince me to get Milo vaccinated, but you seem pretty intelligent so I'm sure you don't really believe it either, do you?"

One of the most vexing problems for any clinician is managing situations where patients' behaviors run contrary to best medical evidence and may actually be harmful in the short or long term. In some cases, there may be some explanation for this behavior. For example, it actually IS very difficult to quit smoking or lose weight, so it may be somewhat understandable if patients resist these suggestions to modify their behavior or if they are unsuccessful in their attempts. In other cases, however, health care professionals may have a difficult time understanding why patients do what they do, and this difficulty will often spill over into poor communication and negative conversations. For example, patients who repeatedly take very unsafe risks with sex or those who repeatedly engage in high-risk sports activities can be difficult to work with because the common sense or logic of their behavior is lost on the professional. As a result, it becomes difficult to find common ground with which to have a discussion.

Recently, there has been a significant and disturbing increase in the number of parents (like the Colangelo's) who consciously and deliberately refuse to have their infants and children vaccinated against formerly common childhood infectious diseases such as measles, mumps, or rubella. Contrary (perhaps) to expectations, studies suggest these parents are most typically upper middle class, generally well educated, and most often employed and integrated into their communities. At first glance, most evidence-informed practitioners will simply not be able to understand or accept this. How could such people deprive their children of the single most important and effective public health intervention of the 20th and 21st centuries? The evidence is clear, strong, and irrefutable: Vaccinations have had a tremendous and significant positive benefit on health, wellness, and society as a whole. The parents refusing vaccinations SHOULD be the kind that understand and respond positively to evidence such as this, yet sometimes they do not. In some cases, there may be a misguided religious objection to vaccinations despite the fact that virtually every single major recognized religious group and leader supports compulsory universal vaccination. How can health professionals, like Sandy the midwife, understand Mathilda's thinking and behavior, and try to customize communication and conversation to help convince her to do what is best for Milo?

An influential theory, sometimes called public understanding of science or public awareness of science, and more recently referred to as public engagement with science and technology can provide helpful insights into such behaviors to help Sandy work with Mathilda. First, it is important to recognize and acknowledge that people like Mathilda who are skeptical of medical evidence are not deficient, stupid, or evil. It is sobering for health professionals to note the large number of times in the recent past where the best possible medical evidence turned out to be actually wrong; for example, in the 1990s, it was considered best practice for all menopausal women to receive hormone replacement therapy to manage symptoms based on the evidence available at the time. During this period, many women were skeptical. How could a naturally occurring event (menopause), which EVERY women of a certain age would experience, be considered a disease or a situation that warranted use of high potency medications? Although the majority of middle-aged women remained silently skeptical, but did as they were told and took the medications, a few were vocal and challenged the received wisdom and orthodoxy of the day, refusing to take the medications and pushing researchers to examine this issue further. A decade later, they were vindicated; hormone replacement therapy was shown to NOT be necessary, helpful, or indicated for all women, and in fact, in some studies, it was shown to have actually contributed to harm. Other high-profile examples, for example, the use of thalidomide in the 1960s to treat pregnancy-induced morning sickness, leading to many cases of birth defects, should cause all health care professionals to remain humble in the face of any skepticism shown by patients.

The public's understanding of science is influenced by many sources. Health professionals, who are generally strangers, somewhat aloof and remote, and who may not have strong relationships with patients, are only one sometimes less significant source of facts and information. Today, when "truth" is found on the Internet, through social media, and in complex networks of friends and acquaintances, it is challenging to know how to address a situation such as Mathilda's. Unfortunately, in most cases, health care professionals become angry or insulted when their recommendations for care are challenged or ignored, and this emotional response can lead them to become dismissive to the patient and write them off as uneducated or dim-witted. Worse, health professionals may project this so-called deficit model on to the patients themselves, through less than professional communication and interaction. Some practitioners respond that they have neither the time nor patience to manage deliberately self-inflicted harmful behaviors, that adults need to be more responsible for themselves (and their children) and not believe every crackpot theory they read online. In return, a skeptical patient may see this kind of imperious behavior as further evidence that health care professionals are know-it-alls who don't deserve to be listened to because they were wrong about thalidomide and they were wrong about hormone replacement therapy, so why can't they admit they might also be wrong about vaccinations? This tit-for-tat escalation of defensiveness and hurt feelings ultimately leads to an impasse and fractured professional relationships, which of course is bad for everyone.

In the situation involving Milo, Sandy is well advised to manage her initial negative emotional response to Mathilda's beliefs and her provocative statements, and to avoid immediately launching into a telling mode.

Mathilda: Well, of course I know you HAVE to say that and try to convince me to get Milo vaccinated, but you seem pretty intelligent so I'm sure you don't really believe it either, do you?

Sandy: Of course I believe in vaccines. I have had all three of my kids vaccinated and keep them up to date. It's the safest and best way to prevent these preventable illnesses.

Mathilda: No, it isn't. I've been reading this book by a Professor Wakefield and he says. . .

Sandy: Wakefield? Don't you know he has been completely discredited as a researcher? His work is completely bogus.

Mathilda: What? No, I don't think so, besides, you know there's hardly ever any cases of these measles or mumps, and who even knows what rubella is, so what's the need anyway?

Sandy: The only reason we don't see these preventable illnesses is because they've been prevented by the vaccines, and the vaccines only work if everybody—including you, me, my kids, and Milo—get vaccinated.

Mathilda: So you'd want me to expose my baby to the pain of an injection, just so somebody else's kid won't get sick? We will always protect Milo, he is not going to get sick. We keep the house spotless, don't have pets, eat organic food, and wear hypoallergenic clothes.

Sandy: That's not how these diseases spread. You can't keep Milo bubble wrapped forever and if you don't vaccinate him now, not only is he at risk, he is putting other kids and the whole community at risk. And believe me, vaccinations don't hurt that much. You can give him some sugar water to drink or. . .

Mathilda: Sugar?? Are you crazy? My child is not getting processed sugar just to withstand a vaccine he doesn't even need in the first place!

As we can see, this conversation is not going well, and is perilously close to an impasse. There is a real risk that Sandy, who has been factually accurate in conveying information regarding vaccinations, will lose Mathilda, and in fact, Mathilda may never return to this clinic again, thereby depriving Milo of both his vaccination and important postnatal care. What should Sandy have done differently?

First, Sandy assumed Mathilda's beliefs and behaviors were driven by deficit. She believed Mathilda didn't know enough, wasn't smart enough, and wasn't concerned enough. As you review the conversation, it becomes clear that Sandy's role is to TELL Mathilda what to do by explaining reasons. Sandy never acknowledges Mathilda's concerns as legitimate and does not demonstrate empathy. Indeed, the tone of the conversation is laden with negative judgment and dismissiveness, for example, when she says, "You can't keep Milo bubble wrapped forever." Importantly, it is highly unlikely that Sandy intends to be dismissive, argumentative, or appear as a know-it-all. Sandy is likely surprised and upset that an upper middle class, educated woman such as Mathilda actually believes vaccines are harmful and unnecessary, and her emotional response to this recognition may spill over into ineffective and unhelpful nonverbal and verbal communication.

Patients (and parents) like Mathilda pose important challenges to health care professionals: The fact that she is educated and upper middle class may mean she is less likely to automatically trust experts and professionals, and is confident and articulate enough to argue back. Further, she may have a consumer or customer mentality in which she expects her health care professionals to serve her and respond to her needs, rather than be experts whose advice is automatically followed.

Rather than focus on a deficit model for understanding Mathilda's beliefs and behaviors, Sandy would have been better off operating within a contextualizing model for understanding. The contextual model is one in which listening, rather than telling, dominates and in which judgment is suspended and practitioners and patients try to understand each other through respectful dialogue.

Consider how this situation could have evolved differently:

Mathilda: Well, of course I know you HAVE to say that and try to convince me to get Milo vaccinated, but you seem pretty intelligent so I'm sure you don't really believe it either, do you?

Sandy: Hmm. Tell me more about what you think about vaccines, Mathilda.

Mathilda: Well, it's not just about what I think, it's about the truth and what's best for Milo. I've been doing a lot of reading and discussion, you know. I just want what's best for my baby.

Sandy: Of course you do! You've been so conscientious throughout the pregnancy, and you've done everything to ensure he's had the best start in life.

Mathilda: Thank you! So I've been reading some work by this doctor. He's a medical doctor, I think, called Wakefield. His studies have shown that vaccines cause autism. And you know, my nephews, both of them, were diagnosed with autism right after they were vaccinated.

Sandy: I see. Of course, that would be something that would concern you or any mother. Go on.

Mathilda: Well, after I saw this Wakefield work, well, I found a group of new mothers online. There's a chat room and group, and well, we connected online at first, and now it turns out we live close by, so I've become friends with a lot of them.

Sandy: Okay. Do all of them agree that their babies should not be vaccinated?

Mathilda: No, I'd say it's about 50/50.

Sandy: The mothers who are going ahead and getting their babies vaccinated, tell me a bit about them.

Mathilda: Well, some of them are pretty aggressive about it, and as soon as they find a mother who doesn't get the vaccines for their child, they refuse to see them, have the kids play together, all of that.

Sandy: What do you think about that?

Mathilda: It's rude! And such an unnecessary overreaction. They make it seem like we are pariahs or something, when all we want is what's best for our baby.

Sandy: What do you mean it's an overreaction?

Mathilda: Nobody gets measles or mumps any more, and who even knows what this rubella thing is?

Sandy: We've actually been seeing a few cases here at the clinic in the past year, especially of measles. Did you see the story on the news about the school in the suburbs?

Mathilda: No. What happened?

Sandy: Let me see if I can find the link to the website to send to you.

As can be seen, the tone and direction of this conversation is completely different than the previous version. In this conversation, Sandy is asking many more questions, and giving Mathilda an opportunity to tell her story and explain how she has arrived at her views and beliefs. There is no judgmental language delivered by Sandy, and (one hopes) this is accompanied by nonjudgmental nonverbal cues. Rather than immediately move to correct each piece of misinformation uttered by Mathilda in real time, Sandy allows Mathilda the opportunity to continue to talk without interruption. This represents respect. Further, Sandy repeats on several occasions that Mathilda is a good mother who wants only the best for her baby Milo. This positive affirmation is also important because it demonstrates respect, and it is actually most likely true. Importantly, toward the end of this section of the conversation, Mathilda provides an opening for Sandy to do something important. In response to Mathilda's contention that "nobody gets measles or mumps any more," Sandy's response is to bring in real-world evidence from her own practice and from the local community. Rather than simply saying, "Yes, people do still get measles," which may appear theoretical, abstract, or suspiciously fake, Sandy is showing her real-world examples from Mathilda's local community.

An important component of the public understanding of science is the notion that immediate, first-hand sources of evidence are far more impactful on decision making than remote, expert-driven research in other places. Rather than trying to change Mathilda's mind by citing an abstract research study or large-scale statistical data, Sandy is using examples—anecdotes—close to home to illustrate her point. This can be a difficult technique for scientifically trained health professionals to use on a routine basis. Scientifically oriented individuals are taught that large-scale, statistically oriented data are more trustworthy and impactful than individual stories and anecdotes, and from a scientific credibility perspective, this is true. However, such data can be overwhelming and incomprehensible to some patients, who instead may be more likely to respond to individual stories and cases. This paradox highlights an important component of the theory of public understanding of science and how it can be applied to structuring effective communication in challenging situations.

It is perhaps naïve and unrealistic to believe that if Sandy continues to take this approach and use this type and tone of communication with Mathilda that she will change her mind today and get Milo his scheduled vaccines. In all likelihood, Mathilda and her husband are in a precontemplation stage where they are not even considering changing their minds and behaviors, especially because they have clearly invested much time and energy in developing their beliefs and articulating their stance already. Instead, they are now seeking out individuals who will only confirm, rather than challenge, what they know and believe to be true. Open confrontation and frank disagreement in such a situation will not work, and instead in all likelihood, will only irritate and alienate Mathilda and drive her to leave the practice and the conventional health care system entirely. Sandy's second, carefully calibrated conversation was focused on building rapport and a relationship by establishing common ground (i.e., acknowledging that Mathilda wants the best for her child), demonstrating respect through verbal and nonverbal cues, and assuming a listening, rather than telling, stance in the conversation. The best that Sandy can hope for in today's conversation is keeping connected with Mathilda, and allowing for another, further conversation at a later date. Of necessity, this will mean Milo will likely not get his scheduled vaccinations when he should, thereby exposing him (and his community) to some unnecessary and unfortunate risk. There is, however, no other real alternative at this point. It will take Mathilda and her husband time to move from precontemplation to contemplation regarding vaccinations, and it will take time for Sandy to establish trust and rapport to build a relationship strong enough to act as a counterweight to what Mathilda already believes. Optimistically, and with time and patience, it should be possible to continue this type of conversation, applying principles of the public understanding of science in order to help Mathilda make more informed decisions regarding the health of her son.

Interested in Learning More?

Aikenhead G. Science communication with the public. In: Stocklmayer S, Gore M, Bryant C, eds. *Science Communication in Theory and Practice.* Dordrecht, The Netherlands: Kluwer Academic Publishers; 2001.

Dubé E, Gagnon D, MacDonald N. Strategies intended to address vaccine hesitancy: review of published reviews. *Vaccine.* 2015;33(34):4191–203.

Helps C, Leask J, Barclay L, Carter S. Understanding non-vaccinating parents' views to inform and improve clinical encounters: a qualitative study in an Australian community. *BMJ Open.* 2019;9:e026299.

Miller J. Public understanding of, and attitudes toward, scientific research: what we know and what we need to know. *Public Underst Sci.* 2004;13:273–294.

Smith T. Vaccine rejection and hesitancy: a review and call to action. *Open Forum Infect Dis.* 2017;4(3):ofx146.

Receiving Mixed Messages:
Communicating Across Barriers

Interprofessional, person-centered care involves aligning both verbal and nonverbal communication in a manner that is responsive to patients and their caregivers. This alignment relies heavily on the ability of the professional to observe and accurately assess and identify the verbal and nonverbal messages being transmitted by the patient or caregivers, and in turn, respond appropriately, proportionately, and effectively to engage and sustain dialogue and to build rapport and trust.

At times, this can be a challenge, particularly if the health professional is not able to accurately or confidently decipher verbal and nonverbal messages being transmitted, or when mixed messages are being transmitted. Mixed messages involve situations where there is inconsistency, lack of alignment, or outright contradiction between WHAT is being said (i.e., verbal communication) and HOW it is being said (i.e., nonverbal communication).

Consider the following scenario:

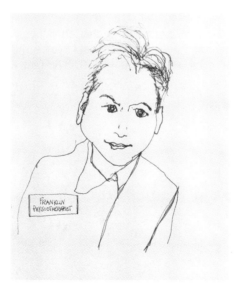

Franklin, Physiotherapist

Franklin is a physiotherapist working with a new patient, Benny Al-Soukra. Benny was driven to the clinic today by his wife Laverna, who is sitting in on the session, "Just so I can remind Benny of everything you've said that of course he's going to forget." Franklin is attempting to provide instruction to Benny on how to navigate steep stairs in their house safely and comfortably following his surgery. In the course of providing this education, Laverna constantly interrupts with statements like, "Oh, he'll never remember this" or "You see what I have to deal with every day. He's just hopeless, isn't he, doctor?" In response, Benny rarely says anything and doesn't even appear to display any kind of nonverbal reaction. On occasion, he will quietly "hrmph," but even that is relatively infrequent. The education session is frustratingly ineffective for Franklin; between Laverna's constant interruptions and belittling of Benny, and Benny's passivity and lack of interest in what's going on, Franklin feels like just standing up and saying, "What am I even doing here wasting my time with you people. When you two get your act together, call me, but until then, good luck to the two of you!" Of course, Franklin might feel like saying this, but he doesn't. Instead he smiles, soldiers on, and starts to wonder if he made a mistake becoming a health care professional.

This is a difficult and complex situation. On the one hand, Benny, the patient, is sending strangely mixed messages that are difficult for Franklin to understand. His passivity and lack of interest in his own health is strange, but perhaps an understandable response to Laverna's hectoring. Laverna's behavior toward her husband borders on rude; although it's clear she loves him and is concerned, she's also so dismissive of him and demeans him publicly, and these mixed messages are difficult for Franklin to interpret and respond to. Finally, Franklin recognizes he himself is sending mixed messages. He's trying to look and act professional by pretending to ignore all that's going on around him with a smile on his face, but he recognizes that in not calling out Laverna on her interfering behavior and Benny on his passivity, he is as much a part of the problem as the two of them are.

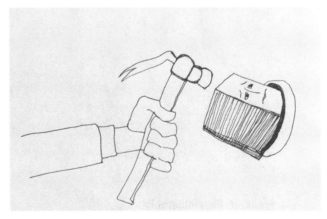

Conveying a mixed message is sometimes like hammering a square peg into a round hole—it doesn't make sense and it just doesn't work.

Situations such as this frequently arise because people—including health care professionals—are not confident or able to clearly and directly express their thoughts and feelings in a coherent manner. In many situations, strong emotions interfere with the formulation, articulation, and verbal expression of thoughts, and in the process, both the emotion and the thought are distorted as a thinking and feeling battle for supremacy. Because communication requires the ability to send, receive, and respond appropriately to nonverbal and verbal messages, how can this be addressed?

Psychologists suggest that the root cause of such mixed messages is frequently connected to our inability to appropriately express emotion. Distortions that emerge because of this inability not only affect nonverbal messages sent, but fundamentally skew attempts to communicate verbally due to the cognitive overload produced by this situation. Learning how to more effectively, appropriately, and clearly express our emotions can provide a pathway to preventing mixed messages and reducing the stress and cognitive overload that compromises communication.

Emotions are data, and emotions are important for communicating meaning and intent. For Laverna, it's clear through her behavior that she is irritated. Is she irritated because her husband is a burden and she is tired, or is she irritated because she is worried for Benny's health and well-being and is responding to his passivity and seeming lack of interest? These are two entirely different reasons to express irritation, and through her verbal and nonverbal communication, it's simply not clear which one she is experiencing. For Franklin, and for Benny, this lack of clarity makes it difficult in turn for them to respond appropriately and accordingly, and so the situation spirals even further toward a crisis.

It may be tempting to believe all that matters is that Laverna knows what kind of irritation she is experiencing and why it is happening. Most psychologists agree that knowing one's own motivations and reasoning is important, and this in itself will help to improve verbal and nonverbal communication, but only somewhat. Self-awareness, however, does not by itself solve the problem of mixed messages entirely. Beyond self-awareness must come the skill of knowing how to appropriately express emotion.

Both self-awareness and the skill of appropriately expressing emotion consume psychological energy and can be exhausting, contributing to cognitive load and further inhibiting capacity for relationship building. If self-awareness is not automatic or does not come naturally, this in itself will contribute to anger and irritation. The skill of emotional expression appears to be connected to emotional intelligence. For example, those who are more extroverted may have a tendency toward and greater capacity for verbalizing or talking out loud, rather than inside their own heads, which makes emotional expression somewhat easier and more natural. Those who are more agreeable will tend to be more emotionally expressive around positive emotions, which in turn draws people to them and makes them more comfortable. From this perspective, emotional intelligence may provide some people with built-in advantages with respect to emotional expression.

For those who, by nature, are more introverted or less agreeable, it will be necessary to invest time and psychological energy to learn to be either more verbal or more receptive of positive emotion as a way of enhancing expressiveness. Importantly, although this may not come easily or naturally, it can be learned, practiced, and rehearsed so it can be done with minimal expenditure of psychological energy. It requires a conscious choice and deliberate action, and a willingness to try to go beyond one's normal comfort zone. For natural introverts, it can be helpful to develop a series of patterned phrases that can be called on to express emotions with a minimal amount of thinking or energy required. Most often, such patterned phrases are successful when they are framed as "I" statements. For example, if Franklin were a strong introvert and getting frustrated with Laverna and Benny's behaviors, his natural tendency might be to say, "You two are driving me bananas!" This will, of course, be received defensively by the couple and may end up escalating the tension. Instead, Franklin should consider saying something like, "I'm feeling really drained right now; I'm not sure I have the energy to continue." The difference is important. By focusing on his experience and his response, not on what Laverna and Benny are doing, Franklin is able to send a clear signal and statement regarding his emotional state in a much less threatening way. It will now be up to Laverna and Benny to respond appropriately to this statement in order to continue to move the dialogue forward.

Similarly, if Franklin were less agreeable, his natural tendency may be to say, "Stop it, you two. Your bickering is driving me crazy!" A more agreeable way of framing his emotional state is to focus on the positive emotions that are at play, saying something like, "I can see how much you care about your husband, Laverna, and that's so important for his recovery. Let's take a step back for a moment to check in with Benny to see how he is feeling."

Learning to express emotion in this way can reduce cognitive load and minimize the risk of sending mixed messages that are misinterpreted—for example, Franklin pretending he doesn't hear what Laverna is saying, and just continuing to smile and go along teaching Benny.

A fundamental principle to remember is that people are more comfortable with and will be more responsive toward the expression of positive rather than negative emotions. All difficult, emotional situations are an amalgam of both positive and negative: For example, Laverna's behavior represents both her annoyance with Benny and also her love and concern for him. Training oneself to focus on the positive part of this amalgam and use that as the foundation for subsequent verbal communication can help enhance the quality of interactions.

Beyond emotional intelligence traits such as agreeableness and extroversion, another important influence is that of culture. For example, American culture demands that the answer to the question, "How are you?" be "Great!" or "Fantastic!" a tendency that is difficult to understand for people from many other cultures and countries. If a person were to answer that question with "Fine" or "Okay," it might be interpreted as "something is really wrong with me." In contrast, in a country like Germany, the same question of "How are you" (in German, "Wie gehts?") is interpreted as an invitation to truly sit down and converse deeply about modern life, philosophy, and personal struggles. To many Germans, the American cultural imperative that demands the answer "I'm awesome!" seems both superficial and silly, a desire to mask the expression of authentic feeling and emotion. To many Americans, the German response may come across as unrelentingly dour and depressing.

Understanding the culturally appropriate perimeter of emotional expression is part of learning how to express one's emotional self within a specific context. In increasingly multicultural communities, traditional national cultural norms may not be as important as local community norms. For example, for Laverna and Benny, at their age and with their cultural background, the kind of bickering that irritates and frightens Franklin may simply be the socially appropriate way for long-married couples to interact with one another. Franklin's well-intentioned attempt to calm them down may not only be unnecessary and unhelpful, it might actually backfire and cause both Laverna and Benny to resent his interference. Despite this, Franklin's emotional response to the bickering is still an issue he must manage, either by redirecting his clients' behaviors or by finding a way to come to terms with and accept it without experiencing a strong personal emotional response.

This bias toward positivity that is prevalent in American culture has led some psychologists to suggest that there is a cultural bias away from authenticity and genuine sharing between people, and in the longer term, this fundamentally limits the quality of relationships of all kinds. From this perspective, interpersonal relationships are based on shared experiences, which means the ability to freely share emotions and feelings with one another. In an environment or culture where one is always expected to be "great" or "awesome," and there is no cultural space for answering the question "How are you?" honestly, it may inhibit formation of meaningful interpersonal relationships.

One important strategy to help manage this cultural bias is to develop a vocabulary and a capacity to differentiate between levels of intensity around emotions. For example, if you were to ask Franklin (after the interaction with Laverna and Benny), "How are you?" and encouraged him to avoid the positivity bias and be honest, he may respond, "I can't stand them! All they do is argue. It makes me hate my job." When we first use words to articulate our emotional state, there is a tendency to upwardly amplify and distort the intensity of the emotion we are feeling. In Franklin's case, "hate" is an extremely strong word. Once spoken, however, the labeling of an emotion in such a strong way starts to take on the sense of self-fulfilling prophecy. When we say "I hate this" out loud, we actually talk ourselves into experiencing this high level of intense emotion. If Franklin trained himself to respond to the question "How are you" by more accurately and appropriately saying, "I'm exhausted. It was very draining for me emotionally listening to this couple argue all the time. It makes me question how effective I am in my professional role," the intensity of his emotion has been significantly recalibrated.

Accurate calibration of the intensity of emotion one is experiencing and finding the correct words and vocabulary to express this intensity is an incredibly valuable skill in helping to improve communication and prevent the delivery of mixed messages. It requires a measure of self-awareness and insight, and also the desire and willingness to be as authentic and transparent as possible with oneself and with others. Avoiding the natural, lazy response to immediately escalate to the highest intensity level of emotion and instead demonstrate flexibility in understanding the difference between being ticked, pissed off, irritated, angry, or furious is important. Equally important, many health care professionals are themselves multilingual and multicultural and, consequently, will have their own, calibrated understanding of how typical or usual cultural conventions regarding communication of emotion apply. Reflecting on your own background, beliefs, biases, and behaviors will help you to better understand how and why you interpret patients' responses, which can help you to better respond to patients in ways that help them feel more comfortable and open.

How might Franklin apply these lessons to help him manage his current difficult situation with Laverna and Benny? Franklin recognizes that his emotional state is turning negative due to the bickering he is being swept into. He does not know its cause or if this is normal for this couple, but he does recognize he needs to do something about it to prevent it escalating further or to prevent him from completely disconnecting from this pair and losing professional interest in them.

Franklin: Okay, Benny, let's take a look and see how you're doing with those exer-
                 cises we discussed last time.

Laverna: Yeah, Benny, go ahead and show him how little you've done. Honestly, I
                 tell you, if it wasn't for me, he wouldn't get out of bed in the morning!

Benny: Hrmph.

Franklin: Sure, okay, so Benny would you like to—

Laverna: I just don't know what to do. Benny, sit up straight!

Benny: I am, stop bugging me!

Laverna: I'm worried to death about him, you know? He just doesn't seem to take
                 any interest in doing anything to help himself.

At this point, Franklin can feel an emotional response; he is feeling irritated by Laverna's bossiness and Benny's passivity and rather than simply fake it or ignore it, he is going to address this.

Franklin: Laverna, Benny, I'm starting to feel a bit caught in the middle between you
                 two.

Laverna: Why? What are we doing?

Benny: I'm not doing anything.

Franklin: Laverna, it's so great you are so worried for Benny and looking out for
                 him, and Benny, you're so lucky to have a wife who cares for you so much.

Laverna: See, I told you so, Benny.

Benny: Hrmph.

Franklin: And Benny, it's so great that you have Laverna to help you and keep push-
                 ing you forward, and Laverna, it's so great that Benny knows that when
                 you're pushing him, it's only because you care.

Laverna: Hrmph.

Benny: Yeah.

Franklin: So, I want to do the best possible job for both of you, to help Benny get as
                 healthy as he can be. We're all going to need to work together, all three of
                 us, right?

Laverna: Of course, that's why we're here.

Franklin: Great, so let's start working together by helping me to keep up with
                 the two of you. Can we agree that only one person speaks at a time?

	I'm having a hard time following you both and that's making it difficult for me to do my job.
Laverna:	Silly boy, that's how we always are. That's how old married people are! Don't you know anything?
Franklin:	Well, I hope one day I'll get there, to the place the two of you are now.
Benny:	God forbid.
Laverna:	Shhh, Benny, let the boy talk.
Franklin:	But for now, I need to have a little bit more space to focus on Benny to see how he's been doing with the exercises we discussed. Benny?
Benny:	Well, I get tired. And it's not very interesting.
Franklin:	Okay, then, what do you do when you aren't motivated?
Laverna:	That's what I'm here for.
Franklin:	Benny, is that working for you? Having Laverna push you when you can't push yourself to do your exercises?
Benny:	Well, I don't like it, you know
Franklin:	Go on.
Benny:	I don't like it, but I guess I know it's good for me. I wouldn't do anything without her pushing me, I guess.
Laverna:	Hallelujah! A nice word from Benny after all these years!
Franklin:	Okay, kids, that's what I needed to hear, so let's settle down again and focus on these exercises.

In this conversation, Franklin used a variety of techniques. First, he focused on "I" statements rather than "you" statements to express his emotional state by discussing how he was feeling and how he was responding rather than what Laverna and Benny were doing. This reduced defensiveness on the part of his clients. Second, Franklin carefully calibrated his language to accurately and appropriately convey the intensity of his emotional response: He wasn't angry or furious, he was feeling overwhelmed. In using the correct word to describe this intensity of emotion, he was able to communicate his needs more effectively to Laverna and Benny. Third, in choosing to communicate his emotional needs, Franklin also opened up the possibility of Laverna and Benny discussing their emotional needs in a more appropriate and transparent way, using words rather than negative nonverbals such as "hrmph" or a hectoring tone of voice. Fourth, Franklin used gentle, self-deprecating humor, acknowledging his youth and inexperience with respect to married life. Finally, but perhaps most importantly, Franklin was able to leverage his agreeableness and use the positive emotions (Laverna's concern for Benny, and Benny's appreciation for Laverna pushing him) that were part of this complex situation rather than focus on the negative emotions (passivity and nagging).

In a text-based format such as this, it is difficult to convey the nonverbal communication Franklin may have used to reinforce his verbal statements and to ensure no mixed messages were being sent. Franklin should ensure everyone remained seated and that he demonstrated an open body posture while in his chair, feet squarely planted on the ground, facing forward, arms relaxed at his side with appropriate gesturing, and (most importantly) ensuring that he alternate eye contact, focus, and attention equally between Laverna and Benny to demonstrate he is not playing favorites with either of them. Franklin should speak in a natural and relaxed tone of voice, perhaps a bit more softly than normal in order to shift Laverna and Benny into a more respectful tone with one another. These nonverbal cues will be more effectively transmitted and received if they are aligned with the verbal statements Franklin is making. By not mixing his messages and ensuring consistency in what he says and how he says it, Franklin is better able to express his immediate current emotional needs in a way that will be understood by Laverna and Benny and will allow them to respond appropriately.

Expressing emotion can be difficult, especially for health care professionals who are trained to check their feelings at the door and always be professional in interactions with patients. Being professional does not mean ignoring, suppressing, or diminishing one's own emotional response to a difficult situation. Your emotional response to a difficult situation is an important source of data regarding what is really going on. Use this data wisely and let it help shape your interpretation and clinical judgment and decisions. Learning to ensure your emotional response is proportionate and that you communicate it in an effective and helpful manner may come more naturally to those who are by nature extroverts and agreeable. For others, it is a skill that can be learned using patterned responses such as "I" statements and expressing the correct intensity of emotion using the right words to allow others to respond more appropriately. All human beings experience emotional responses and, therefore, must learn how to express themselves emotionally in a socially and contextually appropriate way.

Interested in Learning More?

Kothari D, Krakower D, Sullivan A, Abdeen A, Stead W. Mixed messages: ambivalence among specialist providers regarding communication practices. *J Grad Med Educ.* 2013;5(3): 528–529.

Linder J, Friedberg M. Mixed diagnoses and mixed messages. *JAMA Intern Med.* 2016; 176(5):718–719.

Ray C, Floyd K, Tietsort C, et al. Mixed messages: I. The consequences of communicating negative statements within emotional support messages to cancer patients. *J Patient Exp.* 2019. doi:10/1177/2374373519873781.

Rosenthal M, Chen C, Hall K, Tsuyuki R. Mixed messages: the blueprint for pharmacy and a communication gap. *Can J Pharm.* 2014;147(2):118–123.

CASE

13 | Saying "No" in Person-Centered Care

Person-centered care is built on a foundation of mutual respect, understanding, empathy, and concern for the best interests of patients and clients and their caregivers, families, and communities. Helping people differentiate between what they want by way of health care and what they need can be challenging, and, at times, it is not only reasonable, but it is necessary and appropriate for health care professionals to say "no" to a request.

Consider the following scenario:

> Silvio Sylvester comes to the clinic today suffering from a sore throat, muscle aches, and general fatigue. He is convinced he has the flu and wants antibiotics to deal with it. Benji is Silvio's primary care provider and does the assessment and workup, concluding that Silvio is likely suffering from a mild viral infection that would not respond to or benefit from use of antibiotics. In the past, Silvio has always simply gotten whatever he's asked for, so he is surprised when Benji refuses to provide him with the antibiotic he was expecting to receive.

It is important to recognize that person-centered care does not mean or imply that patients get everything they want; health care professionals have multiple responsibilities, including ensuring appropriate use of medications such as antibiotics. As is well known, inappropriate prescribing of antibiotics creates significant issues with respect to unnecessary and preventable side effects for patients, as well as heightening the potential for emergence of dangerous antibiotic resistance and proliferation of so-called superbugs. Viral infections will not respond to antibiotic treatment; using antibiotics in Silvio's case is both unnecessary and irresponsible, and it is Benji's duty as a health care professional to support antibiotic stewardship and responsible use by not simply agreeing to Silvio's request.

Learning to respectfully and clearly say "no" to a patient is challenging, but it is an essential skill for any practitioner. Being clear yet empathetic, supportive yet nonjudgmental, and kind but firm requires sophisticated interpersonal communication skills. General principles to guide such conversations include the following.

Do not engage in arguments. In this case, Silvio is not feeling well and, in most cases, people visit health care professionals when they are at their worst. As a result, they may

315

have less capacity for patience, understanding, and effective listening. When people are feeling unwell, they simply want what they want then want to leave. In refusing to provide Silvio with the antibiotic he thinks he needs, it is likely that there may be an escalation of discussion toward an argument. Learning to redirect conversations and learning not to argue in such a situation are essential.

Be clear. Sometimes, in an effort to maintain good relationships or appear civil, there is a temptation to be vague and say something like, "Well, let's see about that" or "That's something to think about." If you are clear that your answer to a request is "no," it is important to not provide false hope or suggest otherwise. An attempt to be nice and conciliatory may actually backfire and produce resentment and accusations regarding your intentions. Lack of clarity will simply increase the likelihood of an argument and prolong a painful discussion unnecessarily.

Be consistent. If Benji had recently provided Silvio (or someone Silvio knows) with an antibiotic for a similar situation, it will be challenging to refuse to provide one now. Unfortunately, it can be difficult at times for patients to accurately assess and appraise what a "similar situation" actually is; in this case, the signs and symptoms of a viral infection (which would not respond to antibiotics) and a bacterial infection (for which antibiotics may be appropriate) may look and feel similar to a patient even though they are, in reality, very different things. Health care professionals need to recognize that patients talk to one another and look for patterns in the way practitioners do their jobs. If they sense inconsistency in treatment, that may be viewed as unfairness, prejudice, or discrimination. Being consistent in your practice is an essential component of having the authority to fairly and appropriately say "no" to patients with unreasonable requests.

Ensure you understand and acknowledge why the patient is asking in the first place. Silvio, like most patients, is in discomfort and is likely concerned about his health, and of course wants to advocate as best as he can for his own well-being. He is neither selfish nor stupid in asking for antibiotics, but he is incorrect in believing they will help him in this situation. Recognizing that, in the vast majority of cases, patients with unreasonable requests actually have reasonable intentions and good reasons for asking is essential, and acknowledging this to the patient as part of your conversation, is an important way of building rapport and trust and improving the likelihood of a successful interaction. When you understand the underlying reason for an unreasonable request, you can tailor your communication and the education you provide in a more targeted and focused way, and avoid appearing to dismiss the patient or diminish their intelligence and motivations. Most importantly, it ensures you explain your decision rather than simply saying "no" and leaving it at that, which will produce more questions and anger from the patient.

Explain your decision. Simply saying "no" without providing the patient with an explanation and education regarding your decision making is likely to result in the patient feeling dismissed and insulted. When explaining and educating, it is important to use terms and language that are well-understood by the patient, at his or her level. Do not talk down to patients, but, equally, do not use overly complex medical terminology or jargon. Importantly, avoid using vaguely insulting turns of phrase such as "in lay language, this means. . ." or "for a patient like you, it may be easier to explain it like this. . . ."

Use policies as a tool for best practice and for communication with patients. Many organizations rely heavily on policies as a tool to guide day-to-day practice. Policies are objective, impersonal, legalistic documents that can be one way of deflecting blame and criticism in difficult conversations. By indicating that there is a clinic policy preventing use of antibiotics in viral infections, a different, more collegial tone will be established rather than saying, "No, I am not going to give you antibiotics." It is important to be careful in the way policy is invoked or used as a reason for saying no. If it is overused, patients will become irritated by the bureaucratic paralysis you are supporting, and this may worsen your relationship with them. Judicious use of policies can, however, provide a starting point for discussing alternatives.

Always provide alternatives. Rather than simply saying "no," it is helpful to say "no, and . . .," indicating what other options the patient may have to manage the situation. Ideally, providing multiple options for the patient to choose from can provide patients with a greater sense of control and autonomy, despite the initial denial of the request.

Be kind, calm, and patient. Effective use of nonverbal communication, empathetic and effective listening, and attention to tone of voice, body language, and posture are essential. The word "no" is inherently negative, but it can be softened considerably with nonverbals that indicate you are nonjudgmental and supportive. Using empathetic statements such as "I know this isn't want you wanted" or "I can see this is upsetting to you" acknowledges the patient's feelings and validates them. Alternatively, using a phrase such as "I wish antibiotics could be used in viral infections—it would really help so many people—but sadly, they just don't work that way" can also highlight your commitment to engage with the patient.

How might Benji go about having this challenging conversation with Silvio? Consider the following approach to applying these principles in this case.

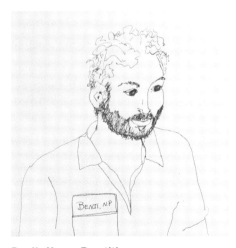

Benji, Nurse Practitioner

Benji: Okay, Silvio, I've completed the assessments, and the good news is that it looks like you've got just a mild viral infection.

Silvio: Phew! Great, I was worried it was going to be something worse than that, considering how terrible I've been feeling. So some antibiotics should fix me up fast?

Benji:	These viral infections can throw you for a loop, for sure. But the other good news is that you won't be needing any antibiotics either. These kinds of infections will usually clear up in a few days or a week, and you'll be back to normal.
Silvio:	Oh. But, well, it's really busy for me at work right now and I really need to get over this fast. Last year when I had this exact same thing you gave me some great antibiotics and they really worked well.
Benji:	I remember that. Yes, last year you had a bacterial infection. Antibiotics don't work against viruses or viral infections, what you have now. They only work against bacterial infections, what you had last year.
Silvio:	But, it's the same thing! I mean I had exactly the same symptoms: the cough, the aches, all of that.
Benji:	You might remember that last year you had a really spiky fever too? During the assessment, you specifically said you didn't have a fever this time.
Silvio:	Yeah, that's right, no fever.
Benji:	And as well when you sneeze or bring up phlegm: You mentioned it was clear and didn't have a particular color to it?
Silvio:	Yeah, but it still feels the same as last year.
Benji:	For sure. Viral and bacterial infections often feel the same to patients, but it's those small things—the fever, the phlegm—that help us to tell them apart. Antibiotics just don't work against viruses.
Silvio:	Well, couldn't I try them? I mean what's the harm? It worked so well last year.
Benji:	Sure, antibiotics do work well against bacteria. But do you remember last year, when you were taking the antibiotics, there's always a risk of some side effects, things like nausea or stomach upset, or even diarrhea.
Silvio:	That's right. I remember that now, but it got better after a few days, and still, my flu got so much better so much quicker!
Benji:	I really wish antibiotics worked for viral infections, but they just don't. What's worse is if you take an antibiotic right now, during a time where you really don't need to, there's a risk you'll develop resistance.
Silvio:	Resistance?
Benji:	If you're taking an antibiotic unnecessarily, the bacteria that are already in your body learn to trick it, learn to fight back against it, and those bacteria go on and multiply and you end up having a whole bunch of new bacteria that will also be resistant to that antibiotic and potentially a lot of other antibiotics as well. So that means in the future, if there's a time where you actually really need an antibiotic, there might not be one that will be able to work for you any longer.

Silvio:	Really? That's sounds scary.
Benji:	Have you heard or read anything about superbugs? These are bacteria that have evolve defenses against all the antibiotics we have, and it's a huge problem because superbugs are really difficult or impossible to treat. These superbugs probably evolved because too many people were taking too many antibiotics for viral conditions, like yours, and that was the breeding ground for resistance to develop. Not just in individuals, but across societies and countries.
Silvio:	Wow!
Benji:	I hope that makes sense now. An antibiotic just won't work for you, and the risks, in terms of side effects and resistance, are just too great. But don't worry, there's a few other things that will help you that won't have the same problems.
Silvio:	Okay.
Benji:	First, it's important to get the small things right. Get plenty of sleep, try to eat well—lots of fruits and vegetables—and drink lots of water. That will make sure you are as strong as possible to allow your body to fight this infection as effectively as possible.
Silvio:	Sounds good.
Benji:	And make sure you wash your hands frequently. Viral infections spread from person to person because of hand contact when you shake hands or touch doorknobs. Washing your hands regularly, using water and soap, or using hand sanitizer, can really cut down on that spread. Equally important, people can reinfect themselves. Just when you are getting better, it's possible, for example, you'll rub your nose then scratch your eye and bingo! You might transmit an infection—a stronger version of the same virus—right back into your system. Keep washing your hands and be careful about touching your face, nose, mouth, and eyes.
Silvio:	Wow!
Benji:	Finally, after a couple of days, throw away your toothbrush.
Silvio:	What?
Benji:	Yup, your toothbrush. It's another way people reinfect themselves. Viruses love the warm, moist environment of a bathroom where you keep your toothbrush. Get a new toothbrush in a few days. And make sure you don't share towels with other people, and change your towels regularly over the next week. Same thing with your pillowcases. Basically, anything that can be a way of reinfecting yourself just as you're getting better is something you want to deal with.
Silvio:	That's a lot of work. Wouldn't it just be easier for you to give me an antibiotic?

Benji: As I said, I wish I could but it wouldn't work and it would actually be more risky to you in the long run. That's why the clinic has specific policies that prevent us from giving medications in a case like yours. So even if I wanted to, I am not allowed to. I know it seems so easy, take a pill a few times a day, but in your case, an antibiotic just isn't going to work. Try these other strategies, though, and I think you'll be surprised by how fast you'll get over these symptoms.

Silvio: Okay, thanks.

Of course, not all patients will be as pleasant, open, and cooperative as Silvio. His need for antibiotics was clearly driven by a misunderstanding and lack of awareness regarding their use in viral infections, and this was something Benji was able to address effectively through the education he provided. Benji used many of the strategies previously discussed, including being clear about his intention to not provide antibiotics, providing reasons and a clear rationale for his decision, providing a menu of alternative courses of action for Silvio to consider, expressing empathy and support while at the same time saying "no," and invoking policy to highlight that he had no other options in this case.

In some cases, the conversation may not be as smooth: For example, increasingly, primary care providers are experiencing significant pressure from patients to inappropriately prescribe, dispense, or provide narcotics and painkillers, or to complete insurance or workplace compensation forms regarding mobility limitations or sick leave requests. In Silvio's case, his desire for antibiotics was based on a genuine and real lack of knowledge and awareness regarding the differences between viral and bacterial infections and the consequences of inappropriate antibiotic use. Regrettably, in some cases, patients may have other reasons for their requests.

Still, even in difficult situations involving, for example, opioids and painkillers, it is essential to remember the same principles and approaches will apply. Do not assume that those seeking potent narcotic medications are selfish or dangerous and to be dismissed quickly without empathy or the benefit of a conversation. Every patient has their own story and reason for the requests they are making, and taking the time to get this story and these reasons will help you to determine the best path forward in explaining why you must say "no." In some cases, you will need to be prepared for anger and disappointment—a strong emotional response to your refusal to go along with the request. Recalling lessons from previous chapters and case studies in this book, it is important to react and respond empathetically and appropriately to the emotional and nonverbal cues that are being transmitted to you, rather than fixate on providing education and your explanation at a time when the patient has little cognitive capacity to process facts because they are managing complex negative emotions. Use of empathizing statements, reflecting and acknowledging the patient's emotional response and state, and taking the time to listen to the patient's concerns are all important strategies to help manage such situations. Specific communication strategies to consider for such difficult situations include the following.

Use the nonverbal communication techniques you want your patient to use. Don't ask or tell a patient to calm down. Model calmness yourself by, for example, speaking in a slow, even, low tone of voice; minimizing excessive hand gestures; and avoiding dismissive nonverbal cues such as eye-rolling. Consider shifting your position or moving so the patient follows you, and encourage the patient to take a seat, but give them the control over where.

Where excessively or alarmingly emotional statements are made or questions asked, and the patient expects a response, avoid using words and instead use empathetic fillers such as "uh-huh" while maintaining positive eye contact and body language. This can help you find common ground and keep the patient connected to you.

Take a step back and try to find specific reasons for the amplified emotion displayed by the patient. A comment such as "This is clearly very important to you. Can you help me understand the specific reasons why?" can help shift from an emotional to a more cognitive tone and processing style.

Be mindful of HOW you say no, including the nonverbals that accompany it along with tone of voice, gestures, body language, etc. Saying "no" while maintaining an open body posture, a smile, and empathetic eye contact may not come naturally, but it can go a long way to defusing tension.

Ask—rather than tell—the patient if they are ready to work with you to brainstorm alternatives to what they initially requested. If they are not yet ready, do not push them further. An invitation to further discussion can be helpful, such as, "We can talk about other options later, once you've had a chance to think this over," or "If anything changes with your condition, let's look at other options."

Avoid the temptation to leapfrog directly to reassurance and empathy without first explicitly acknowledging the patient's experience of the conversation. The patient needs to hear that you actually get it, that you understand where they are coming from, even if you don't agree with it.

What if, in the case involving Silvio, he had been much less open to Benji's educational approach and instead became angered when he said no to his request for an antibiotic? How might the conversation have evolved differently?

Benji: Unfortunately, antibiotics don't work for viral infections, so they wouldn't do you any good.

Silvio: What? That's nuts! Of course they work, that's what helped me the last time. Look, are you going to give me what I need to get better?

Benji: It's not about me giving you what—

Silvio: So you're not? That's pathetic. What kind of a health care professional are you anyway?

Benji: Silvio, please, let's try to—

Silvio: Don't tell me what to do. I mean, if you're not going to even bother to help me when I'm sick. . . .

Benji: (not taking the bait, and using silence effectively)

Silvio: I don't understand, it's not fair, you are supposed to be trying to help me to get better.

Benji: Absolutely, that's exactly what I'm trying to do. Help you.

Silvio:	Then why won't you give me the drugs I need?
Benji:	Help me to understand why you think the antibiotics are so important for you right now.
Silvio:	Because I'm really, really sick and I need to get better.
Benji:	When I said that you have a viral infection and antibiotics don't work for viral infections, what were you thinking?
Silvio:	I don't know. Like you didn't want to help me or something.
Benji:	Ummm.
Silvio:	I mean, I really feel crappy. I need something to get better. I can't afford to miss work, I might lose my job, then what'll happen to me and the kids?
Benji:	You're dealing with a lot right now. Even if your health was 100%, which I know right now it's not, you've got a lot on your plate.
Silvio:	Thanks, yes, it's hard. I just need to feel better.
Benji:	I really wish an antibiotic would do that for you. Or some other magic pill. I really wish there was something like that. But there isn't. Do you feel like discussing other options, things you might be able to do that will help you get better as fast as possible?
Silvio:	You're really sure an antibiotic won't work for me this time?
Benji:	Yes, I'm really sure. But that doesn't mean there aren't other things we can try to help you.

Unfortunately, in some cases, your professional responsibility to say "no" to a patient's request may result in a negative short-term outcome: Patients may become angry, withdraw, and threaten to leave your practice (or report you to a supervisor or a regulatory body). This, in turn, may trigger a strong immediate defensive and emotional response from you, which may make implementation of the suggestions in this case challenging. Managing your own emotional responses and state should be the priority; you will not be able to provide education, demonstrate empathy, and describe your reasons effectively if you are consumed with your own emotions during the conversation. In such situations, it may be best to find a way to call a time out, providing both you and the patient with much-needed time and space away from one another to allow you to gather your thoughts, manage your emotions, and identify a pathway forward to effective communication.

Few of us feel good when we must say "no" to our friends, our family, our children. Most human beings, including health care professionals, want to be liked and want to appear to be positive and collaborative. In general, the way human beings do this is by saying "yes" and graciously agreeing to requests made by others. Health care professionals have unique responsibilities to patients, the health care system, and society as a whole. Stewardship of resources (such as antibiotics), enforcing guidelines, and ensuring patient safety are all reasons why, at times, every health care professional will need to say "no" to a patient's request. Learning to say "no" in a respectful way that empowers and enlightens the patient by providing them with education, alternatives, and choices to make can help you to sustain or even improve your relationships while still fulfilling your responsibilities for safe and effective patient care.

Interested in Learning More?

Carlsen B, Norheim O. "Saying no is no easy matter": a qualitative study of competing concerns in rationing decisions in general practice. *BMC Health Serv Res.* 2005;70.

Epstien D. When evidence says no, but doctors say yes. *The Atlantic.* February 22, 2017. Available at: https://www.theatlantic.com/health/archive/2017/02/when-evidence-says-no-but-doctors -say-yes/517368/. Accessed April 2, 2020.

Hardavella G, Aamli-Gaagnat A, Frille A, Saad N, Niculescu A, Powell P. Top tips to deal with challenging situations; doctor-patient interactions. *Breathe.* 2017;13(2):129–135.

Kee J, Khoo H, Lim I, Koh M. Communication skills in patient-doctor interactions: learning from patient complaints. *Health Prof Educ.* 2018;4(2):97–106.

Paterniti D, Fancher TL, Cipri CS, Timmermans S, Heritage J, Kravitz RL. Getting to "no": strategies primary care physicians use to deny patient requests. *Arch Intern Med.* 2010;170(4):381–388.

Pomey M, Ghadiri D, Karazivan P, Fernandez N, Clavel N. Patients as partners: a qualitative study of patients' engagement in their healthcare. *PLoS One.* 2015;10(4):e0122499.

14 | When Pronouns Trigger Conflict

Although there has been increasing recognition and social acceptance of fluidity in gender and sexual identity, there is by no means universal agreement as to how individuals (e.g., loved ones, coworkers, employers, health care professionals) can best support and interact in difficult situations. Recently, one of the most contentious and well-publicized of such situations involves the use of pronouns, and those individuals who feel their biological and psychosocial identities may not align. Some transgendered people (individuals with a gender identity or gender expression that differs from the sexual identity assigned at birth), transsexual people (those who desire medical intervention to transition from one assigned sexual identity to the other), and nonbinary individuals have expressed discomfort with the use of binary pronouns such as *he* or *she* in everyday conversation. In some cases, this discomfort has resulted in formal requests—sometimes demands—that other individuals address them using a nongendered neutral pronoun such as *they*. In turn, this request or demand can, in some cases, trigger disagreement or conflict because others in the community may reject or refuse to support use of the pronoun *they*. These individuals may have misgivings, frank disregard for, or even open hostility toward the notion of nonbinary identity or transgenderism, and as a result, refuse to accede to such a request. In other cases, some individuals may be overwhelmed or confused by the request to use what has historically been a plural pronoun (i.e., *they*) in the context of a single individual. Other requests (e.g., use of the bespoke term *zhe* rather than he or she) may similarly cause distress, argument, or outright animosity.

For most health professionals, the existence of nonbinary gender identities, fluidity in sexual identity, and the reality of transgenderism will most likely result in accepting a patient's request to use a specific pronoun. Although not universal, most health professionals try to provide person-centered care and, if politely asked, will respond and use the pronoun suggested by their patient. In some cases, the health professional will be fully supportive and endorse this request. In other cases, individual health professionals may have personal qualms or disagreements regarding this request, but ultimately decide that it is their professional obligation and/or ethical duty to accede to the request even if they personally are in disagreement.

In some situations, however, a well-intentioned health care professional may find that their professional choices and behaviors can actually contribute to or escalate conflict within a family unit, and as a result, the professional may need to demonstrate extraordinarily sophisticated communication and interpersonal skills to maintain civility among all participants in a meeting.

Consider the following situation:

Joey is a 9-year-old who has experienced considerable bullying, psychological distress, and diagnosed depression for the last 5 years. Through extensive counseling and assessment, it has emerged that Joey has experienced significant gender dysphoria. Although assigned to the male sex at birth, Joey has always felt like a girl and has always been more interested in activities more traditionally and stereotypically associated with girls. Through one-on-one counseling with an expert in child and adolescent psychiatry, this realization has been transformative for Joey because Joey finally has words to describe the feelings experienced all these years. The impact on Joey's family has been significant. Joey's mother Caroline is distraught and mourning what she calls "the death of my son" but is slowly coming to understand the complexity of the situation and wants to support Joey in whatever comes next. Joey's father, Gerry, is adamantly negative and has increasingly isolated himself from his family as this story has unfolded. Gerry believes this is a phase, cannot understand this notion of "boys who think they're girls," and is resentful toward Caroline, Joey, and the health care professionals involved. In such a complex situation, both specialists and the primary care team are involved to support the family moving forward. Today, there is a meeting with Joey's primary care provider, Peter, the clinical nurse practitioner.

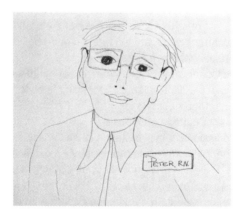

Peter, Clinical Nurse Practitioner

Peter: Hello, everyone, thanks for coming in today. We have some information from the university teaching hospital now about Joey's assessment and I just wanted to go over what they've said about him and where—

Joey: "Them." Could you, I mean, if it's all right with you, could you not use words like "him" or "he" if you're talking about me and I'm, like, right here?

Peter: Sorry?

Joey:	It's just, well those words like "he" and "she" don't . . . they're not right, you know? They don't really apply to me.
Peter:	Oh, okay. Joey, can you tell me what you'd prefer?
Caroline:	(trying to be helpful) Well, at home we use pronouns like "they" or "them," something that isn't clearly, well, you know.
Gerry:	(dismissively) Oh great, here we go again!
Caroline:	Gerry, please.
Peter:	(sensing the conflict brewing between the parents and trying to prevent it) Oh, of course, Joey, if that's what will make you comfortable, I'm happy—
Gerry:	(sounds defeated) Because everybody has to do what little Joey wants. He's 9 years old! What does a 9-year-old know about what he wants?
Caroline:	Gerry, not here. This isn't the place.
Gerry:	(getting more resistant) It's never the place. This is crap, I tell you, absolutely garbage.
Joey:	(dismissively) Dad, please.
Gerry:	Yeah, if you get to tell people what to call you, well, don't call me that word "Dad" then, either, okay?
Caroline:	Gerry, how can you—
Gerry:	(turning to Peter, with hostility) And you, you're going along with this? You're the reason this is all happening anyway! What the hell kind of medical people are you? He—yeah, HE—is 9 years old! Let him be 9 years old! Treat him like a 9-year-old!
Peter:	Gerry, we're all just trying to hear what Joey has been going through to help hi—I mean them. (stumbling on what pronoun to use)
Gerry:	(belligerently) Do you hear yourself? How ridiculous you sound? This is total garbage. You're total garbage. I mean, look at you, you're a guy— well, you're supposed to be one at least—and you're a NURSE, so of course you'd want to do this to Joey.
Caroline:	(increasingly angry) You're out of control, Gerry, stop it now. Look, Joey's crying, and you're making a fool of yourself!
Gerry:	(standing up) I'm not staying another second if this *nurse* insists on call- ing my son "them." It's Peter and people like him that are putting all these ideas in Joey's head anyway. So, what's it going to be, Peter?

This is clearly an extremely difficult situation for all four individuals involved. In this case, the health care professional is being put into the middle of a highly emotional family situation, and on top of it, is being verbally abused and demeaned simply by trying to do his job. Still, Peter recognizes that he is there to support his patient, Joey. This family meeting has careened wildly out of control, and there may even be a risk of the family fracturing apart completely.

What can or should Peter do? In response to Gerry's inappropriate and unacceptable provocation, and the heightened emotions everyone is experiencing at this moment, the next sentence Peter says will fundamentally shift both the balance of power in the marital and family relationship and may cast in stone the way this family moves through this difficult situation. Of course, when a situation such as this occurs in the real world, and it does, Peter would have only a moment to gather his thoughts, manage his emotions, and determine what to say or do in response to Gerry's statement: "So, what's it going to be, Peter?"

What might be going through Peter's mind at a time like this? First, he is likely experiencing a strong immediate emotional response to the emotions being demonstrated, recognizing that he is the only other adult male in the room and, therefore, perhaps, considered a fair target for abuse by Gerry. Second, Peter may also be experiencing an emotional counterresponse of his own based on how Gerry has challenged his masculinity and professional choices. Third, the sight of a vulnerable child crying and afraid and the fear expressed by Caroline will also add further emotional fuel to this already combustible situation. Even before considering any of the words spoken, the emotional tone of the conversation has been overwhelming.

Gerry is, in a seemingly threatening way, trying to force Peter to make a choice. Say "him" or "them," pick my side or the other side, and suffer the consequences of your choice. Peter has already demonstrated his desire to provide person-centered care to Joey, and has already acceded to Joey's request for use of nonbinary pronouns in everyday conversation. Whether this accession is grudging or wholehearted is not known, but at the very least Peter has shown he wants to be an ally to Caroline and Joey.

Highly emotional situations such as this, in which multiple professional, personal, and medical issues are simultaneously colliding, often result in individuals believing that there must be a single, stark, binary choice or answer: "So, what's it going to be, Peter?" Although Peter may be experiencing an intensely personal and emotional response to all that is swirling around him in the room, it is essential that—in his response to Gerry's provocation—he does not take the bait and believe he must actually respond directly to what Gerry is asking him to do. At this point, if Peter were to say or demonstrate "I'm with Joey and Caroline," the affront to Gerry could have devastating, potentially violent, consequences. Gerry's emotional escalation suggests he has invested a tremendous amount personally in the direction of this conversation. To be this distraught means Gerry is particularly vulnerable to losing face if Peter disagrees with him, and this could be just the escalation required to turn this into a truly violent situation. Conversely, if in the emotional heat of this moment, Peter succumbs to his own fears and anxiety and says or demonstrates agreement with Gerry, it will have absolutely devastating consequences for Joey and Caroline. It will prove to them that this bad behavior will ultimately win and it will likely demoralize them in ways Peter cannot predict.

Peter faces a dilemma. In general, one should avoid making assumptions about others' behaviors and simply ask them what they are thinking and feeling in an attempt to better understand and more appropriately and proportionately respond. However, in cases where intense emotion and potential conflict is escalating, it may simply not be possible or reasonable to ask a question such as "Tell me how you're feeling?" In a situation like this, where Peter himself has become part of the situation and is no longer a dispassionate observer or outside mediator, he will need to think on his feet and quickly decide how best to proceed. To do so may require Peter to use his powers of observation and focus on what Gerry has, and has not, said and Gerry's body language, affect, and posture. These can provide important clues as to what may be going on inside Gerry and can provide a first approximation of what might be a helpful next step in this situation. In essence, Peter needs to be able to buy a few moments to gather his thoughts, de-escalate the current situation, and select his next verbal and nonverbal communications carefully to avoid escalation and begin the process of de-escalation.

The concept of losing face may be helpful to understand Gerry and this situation without making assumptions about what Gerry is thinking and feeling. The term *losing face* is an idiom that captures a complex amalgam of cognitive and emotional elements associated with losing the respect of others or feeling that you have been humiliated and experienced public disgrace. Face is sometimes described as an image one has of oneself or a way of comparing ourselves to generally approved-of social attributes—it is part of the arena in the Johari Window. Face contributes to our sense of self-worth and our ability to know our status within a hierarchy. As a result, most human beings invest a considerable amount of time, energy, emotion, and thought in maintaining face and presenting the best possible version of themselves to others in order to enjoy the benefits that come from this. Losing face is equated with public humiliation and diminishment and can have enormous psychological and practical consequences.

What might be motivating Gerry's hostility toward the seemingly innocuous request to replace one pronoun with another? For many people, children and families are an important part of self and an important component of the face they present to the world. In this case, much of Gerry's emotion may stem from the concern about losing face with his friends and social community. There may be gender role and cultural amplifiers at work here. For example, men and fathers may experience strong and negative emotional responses to Joey's situation, given entrenched and socially reinforced beliefs regarding appropriate roles for males and females in society. Within East Asian cultures, face may be disproportionately important and drive behaviors. Of course, Gerry's ego needs and desires to preserve face within his friendship communities should not excuse his behavior or negate Joey's needs and wants; however, this may help explain the forcefulness of his reaction to the question of pronoun choice.

We hope that Peter has the presence of mind in the heat of this moment to recognize that Gerry alone does not get to dictate whether a binary answer (i.e., "he" versus "they") is all that exists in this case. This is a complex situation, and each person will be on their own trajectory in terms of acceptance, understanding, and empathy. No matter what happens next, Gerry is and always will be Joey's father. He is also Caroline's husband. Although it may be understandably easy to vilify and diminish Gerry as a brute, this further escalates the emotion of the situation, paradoxically may reinforce an inappropriately hypermasculine face, and makes it ever more challenging to find the common ground everyone, especially Joey, so desperately needs at this moment.

There is no simple or perfect response in this case, but one approach that may be helpful for Peter is to remember the fundamental equation of conflict: Conflict = Intellectual Disagreement + Emotional Involvement. When the emotional involvement part of this equation becomes overwhelming, it is not possible to focus on the actual intellectual disagreement at hand or to look for a resolution. Peter's first priority, therefore, needs to be finding a way of defusing the incredibly high level of emotion in the room. Let's return to where the conversation left off to see what Peter might be able to do at this point.

Gerry:	(getting more resistant) It's never the place. This is crap, I tell you, absolutely garbage.
Joey:	(dismissively) Dad, please.
Gerry:	Yeah, if you get to tell people what to call you, well, don't call me that word "Dad" then, either, okay?
Caroline:	Gerry, how can you—
Gerry:	(turning to Peter, with hostility) And you, you're going along with this? You're the reason this is all happening anyway! What the hell kind of medical people are you? He—yeah, HE—is 9 years old! Let him be 9 years old! Treat him like a 9-year-old!
Peter:	Gerry, we're all just trying to hear what Joey has been going through to help hi—I mean them. (stumbling on what pronoun to use)
Gerry:	(belligerently) Do you hear yourself? How ridiculous you sound? This is total garbage. You're total garbage. I mean, look at you, you're a guy— well, you're supposed to be one at least—and you're a NURSE, so of course you'd want to do this to Joey.
Caroline:	(increasingly angry) You're out of control, Gerry, stop it now. Look, Joey's crying, and you're making a fool of yourself!
Gerry:	(standing up) I'm not staying another second if this *nurse* insists on calling my son "them." It's Peter and people like him that are putting all these ideas in Joey's head anyway. So, what's it going to be, Peter?
Peter:	(Remains seated and calm and maintains eye contact with Gerry but not in an aggressive or penetrating way. Maintains a small, nonthreatening body language and tries to communicate with his eyes and the way he holds his mouth that he is not judging Gerry, but that he understands how painful this is for him, and giving Gerry the time he needs to de-escalate the conflict himself, to save face.)
Gerry:	(still advancing) Well?? Mr. Nurse-Man? What do you say? What do you have to say for yourself?
Peter:	(as before)
Caroline:	(moving to stand up) Gerry, Gerry!
Peter:	(Looking calmly at Caroline, signaling nonverbally and with his eyes that she too should remain seated, remain calm, and not get involved. He signals the same thing nonverbally to Joey.)
Gerry:	It's . . . I . . . oh forget it. (sits back down, looking defeated)

Peter: Thank you, Gerry. I can see how difficult this is for you, and for Caroline, and for Joey.

Gerry: (grunting) Hrmph.

Peter: We have several families here at the clinic with experiences similar to yours.

Gerry: (looking surprised) You do? We're not the only freak show?

Caroline: (exasperated) Gerry!

Peter: (calmly) We have families that are at different points in the process, some a little farther ahead, some just starting. Every family manages this differently. But we try to work with each family to keep them working, talking, living, and moving forward together. Together as a family. You don't need me to tell you how hard this is, but maybe it would help if you were able to meet with other families just like yours to share your experiences?

Gerry: (abruptly) No. Well, maybe. I don't know, maybe not yet.

Peter: (smiling) It's just one idea. Let's talk about some other ideas you might all want to consider. . . .

The sequence of events and Peter's communication in this case are difficult to describe in words because he elected to manage this situation using nonverbal cues and gestures. When anger emerges due to losing face, words are frequently unhelpful and can, in some cases, actually trigger further problems. By remaining seated, and therefore lower in space than Gerry, Peter sent a strong nonverbal cue that he was no threat to Gerry and that he had no quarrel with him. By maintaining eye contact without being aggressive or penetrating with it, Peter sent another strong nonverbal cue that he was going to stand his ground and not be intimidated, but that he was also open to communication of any sort with Gerry, when Gerry was ready. By projecting a face to Gerry that communicated openness and no judgment, Peter was able to say without words, "I can see (and feel?) this is so, so difficult for you Gerry. And we aren't going to leave you behind, but we all need help to know what all of us need right now to move forward." However, had Peter actually SAID these words in the emotional heat of this situation, it could not have succeeded.

A case such as this demonstrates the importance of nonverbal communication, especially where there are strong emotions. Verbal communication is of course powerful, but there will be situations where words or a specific word will actually trigger or escalate conflict. In this case, there was no way for Peter to proceed to find common ground and to return civility to the conversation without first de-escalating the emotion in the room. With Gerry's emotions running so high, there was no cognitive space available for Gerry to actually process words and their meanings. The only viable communication in such a situation would have to be built around nonverbal cues and nonverbal gestures. An important lesson from a case such as this is that, in some situations, words and verbal communication are both unhelpful and counterproductive in managing a difficult interpersonal situation. This is not to say that silence is the answer. Although Peter did not say anything out loud, through his eye contact, body language, posture, and position, he conveyed and communicated an immense amount of empathy and understanding, and this was what was needed to move through what easily could have become a crisis.

And what of Joey and Joey's needs? Once the immediate emotional situation has been somewhat defused, what does Peter say or do next in order to demonstrate support for the entire family: Gerry, Joey, and Caroline? Clearly, given what has preceded this point in the conversation, it is not appropriate or safe for Peter or anyone to hector or try to force Gerry to accede to Joey's request regarding the pronouns. At best, we can surmise that Gerry is still in precontemplation (if not outright denial) of the reality of Joey's situation. Gerry will need time and space to figure out his own emotions and his own thoughts. This cannot be rushed, and it will not be well served by ostracizing him, diminishing or insulting him, or attempting to force him into something he has such strong and violent feelings about. Importantly, part of this shift will also involve Gerry figuring out for himself or with the help of a professional counselor how he can manage his own concerns regarding losing face.

Once some measure of civility has returned to the room, Peter will have many options to consider. He could ask Joey and Caroline to leave for a few moments to speak with Gerry alone to simply allow Gerry an opportunity to speak candidly and share his own struggles. This is rarely helpful, however; in dividing the family physically in this way, it perpetuates the notion of secrets being kept from one another and will make it more difficult to find common ground. He could suggest another health care professional be involved to work with Gerry in processing his emotions. In situations such as this, peer support groups and peer mentors can be an invaluable support. Other parents who have experienced a similar journey with their children could provide Gerry with insights that no health care professional really could. Similarly, Joey could benefit from peer mentors and peer support; others who have had similar experiences may help Joey in many different ways. It would likely be highly unproductive to ask Gerry to apologize or reflect on his behavior right now. Emotions will still be high and feelings will still be raw, and this action might be construed by Gerry as insulting or diminishing. Equally, however, Peter should also demonstrate his solidarity with Caroline and Joey; without being preaching or obvious, Peter should continue to use Joey's preferred pronouns in their conversation, but do so in a way that is neither crowing nor triumphant, but instead in a quiet, matter-of-fact kind of way. This will send a strong message to both Caroline and Joey that Peter believes in person-centered care and communication, and that Peter's most important priority is Joey. Peter can reasonably expect that, in the context of what has just happened, the first time the pronoun "them" is used to refer to Joey, Gerry will become upset. The key will be the tone of voice Peter uses. If Peter is quiet, calm, measured, nonprovocative, and above all confident in his tone of voice using the pronoun "them," it will send a message to the entire family of what Peter thinks and how he intends to behave. It will also send the message that he is not judging Gerry for his choices and behaviors, and wants to be open to the entire family as they move through this difficult time.

It is essential to recognize that societal norms and expectations are continuously evolving. What is suitable and appropriate at the time you are reading this (and the time that this case was written) may or may not be applicable in a different time. Similarly, even within this time, different communities have different perspectives that must also be reconciled as best as possible. For example, in some communities, it is becoming increasingly common to send a signal of solidarity and support through written communication by including an email signature statement indicating one's preferred pronoun choices. At the end of each email, where one would normally see a person's name, degrees, address, and contact information, there may be an additional statement such as "Preferred pronouns: she/her" or "Preferred pronouns: they" to alert readers of the email to the individual's wishes. Although other individuals may object to this as a form of compelled speech, others suggest that this approach provides greater clarity and the opportunity for civil discourse. Society's and individual's perspectives on issues such as this will change and evolve, and health care professionals must consider their role in fostering and encouraging greater understanding and acceptance.

The focus of this chapter has been on the question of pronoun choices, but beneath this issue, there are clearly many other important psychological and social issues that need to be understood. In such complex situations, communication becomes even more important than ever. Recognizing the power of nonverbal and verbal communication to help manage challenging situations such as this will help both Joey and the family to move forward as best as possible.

Interested in Learning More?

Agana M, Greydanus D, Indyk J, et al. Caring for the transgender adolescent and young adult: current concepts of an evolving process in the 21st century. *Dis Mon.* 2019;65(9):303–356.

Imborek K, Nisly N, Hesseltine M, et al. Preferred names, preferred pronouns and gender identity in the electronic medi5-53.cal record and laboratory information system. *J Pathol Inform.* 2017;8:42.

Klein D, Paradise S, Goodwin E. Caring for transgender and gender-diverse persons: what clinicians should know. *Am Fam Physician.* 2018;98(11):645–653.

Rosendale N, Golman S, Ortiz G, Haber L. Acute clinical care for transgender patients: a review. *JAMA Intern Med.* 2018;178(11):1535–1543.

Sallans R. Lessons from a transgender patient for health care professionals. *AMA J Ethics.* 2016;18(11):1138–1146.

Steuer K, Davis K. Respecting gender identity in healthcare: regulatory requirements and recommendations for treating transgender patients. *GPSolo eReport.* March 1, 2017. Available at: https://www.americanbar.org/groups/gpsolo/publications/gpsolo_ereport/2017/march_2017 /respecting_gender_identity_healthcare_regulatory_requirements_recommendations_treating _transgender_patients/. Accessed April 2, 2020.